Chesneys' Radiographic Imag

Chesneys' Radiographic Imaging

John Ball TDCR
Formerly Principal
South West Wales
School of Radiography
Morriston Hospital NHS Trust
Swansea

Tony Price HDCR
Radiology Services Manager
Glan-y-Môr NHS Trust
Neath General Hospital
Neath
West Glamorgan

Sixth Edition

**Blackwell
Science**

© 1965, 1969, 1971, 1981, 1989, 1995 by
Blackwell Science Ltd
Editorial Offices:
Osney Mead, Oxford OX2 0EL
25 John Street, London WC1N 2BL
23 Ainslie Place, Edinburgh EH3 6AJ
238 Main Street, Cambridge
  Massachusetts 02142, USA
54 University Street, Carlton
  Victoria 3053, Australia

Other Editorial Offices:
  Arnette Blackwell SA
  1, rue de Lille, 75007 Paris
  France

  Blackwell Wissenschafts-Verlag GmbH
  Kurfurstendamm 57
  10707 Berlin, Germany

  Feldgasse 13, A-1238 Wien
  Austria

First published under the title
Radiographic Photography 1965
Second edition 1969
Third edition 1971
Reprinted 1975, 1976
Fourth edition (under the title *Radiographic Imaging*)
1981
Reprinted 1984, 1987, 1988
Fifth edition 1989
Reprinted 1990, 1992 (twice)
Sixth edition 1995

Set by DP Photosetting, Aylesbury, Bucks
Printed and bound in Great Britain
at the University Press, Cambridge

DISTRIBUTORS
Marston Book Services Ltd
PO Box 87
Oxford OX2 0DT
(*Orders:* Tel: 01865 791155
      Fax: 01865 791927
      Telex: 837515)

North America
  Blackwell Science, Inc.
  238 Main Street
  Cambridge, MA 02142
  (*Orders:* Tel: 800 215-1000
           617 876-7000
         Fax: 617 492-5263

Australia
  Blackwell Science Pty Ltd
  54 University Street
  Carlton, Victoria 3053
  (*Orders:* Tel: 03 347-5552)

A catalogue record for this book is available from the
British Library

ISBN 0–632–03901–9

Library of Congress
Cataloging-in-Publication Data
Radiographc imaging.—6th ed./revised and edited by
  John Ball, Tony Price.
      p.   cm.
    Rev. ed. of: Chesneys' radiographic imaging. 5th
  ed./revised and edited by John Ball, Tony Price, 1989.
    Includes bibliographical references and index.
    ISBN 0–632–03901–9
    1. Radiography, Medical.   I. Ball, John,
  TDCR.   II. Price, Tony, HDCR.   III. Chesneys'
  radiographic imaging.
    [DNLM: 1. Radiography.   WN 200 R1285 1995]
  RC78.R2356   1995
  616.07'572—dc20
  DNLM/DLC
  for Library of Congress   95-5293
                                                  CIP

Contents

Preface to the sixth edition

Only six years have elapsed since we handed over to our publishers the manuscript for the 5th edition of *Chesneys' Radiographic Imaging*. But during that brief period a veritable revolution has been taking place in diagnostic imaging.

In the clinical field, the impact of digital technology is ever more apparent, and while radiologists become increasingly involved in interventional procedures, radiographers are expanding their roles into new areas, including those formerly the province of their radiologist colleagues.

In education, the last remaining pre-registration diploma students are completing their DCR courses, and undergraduate radiography students already seem part of the established scene. Meanwhile, traditional post-diplomate studies such as the HDCR, DMU and DRI are being abandoned in favour of post-graduate diplomas and higher degrees, with more and more radiographers tackling masters degrees and doctorates.

We have attempted, in this latest revision, to reflect developments in the clinical field by incorporating new material, pruning away some of the old, and where appropriate, by changing the emphasis of what remains. Digital technology has been given a higher profile, with new sections introduced on digital picture archiving and communication systems (PACS) in Chapter 15, and computed radiography (CR) in Chapter 28. However, for this edition, we have delayed discussing these topics in full detail until it becomes clearer exactly which system (if any) will become the universally accepted standard. A description of dry silver imaging has been introduced into Chapter 23, while Chapter 29 includes a new section on receiver operating characteristics (ROC). In Chapter 16, the section on the distorted image has been rewritten and more fully illustrated, while in Chapter 12 we have expanded the discussion of health and safety in processing areas.

As new technologies and techniques gain in importance, others fall by the wayside. Hence, for example, we have relegated xeroradiography from its former full chapter status, to a subsection of Chapter 28. The continued decline in the importance of darkrooms is reflected in our revision of Chapter 12.

The changes in radiography education suggested to us that both undergraduates and postgraduate students may well use our book in a more questioning spirit than hitherto. It has therefore been revised with this in mind. Early on in the revision process, in what can only be described as a moment of madness, we optimistically committed ourselves to referencing source material as an aid to our readers. There have been moments when we regretted taking that decision! We soon discovered, not unexpectedly, that many aspects of radiographic practice are empirically based, and while there is no shortage of anecdotal evidence to support these practices, there is a paucity of up-to-date, high-quality published research, particularly from radiographers. We sincerely hope that the recent changes in radiography education will encourage radiographers not only to undertake much needed original research, but also to *publish* the fruits of their work in the scholarly journals. We look forward to referencing the results of such activity in our next edition.

The time we spent on restructuring the logical framework of *Chesneys' Radiographic Imaging* for its fifth edition has proved a sound investment: we have been able to revise the present edition without further restructuring. However, in response to a suggestion by our publishers, we have introduced decimal numbering of paragraphs and have revised all cross-references accordingly.

Once again we are pleased to acknowledge the help we have received from many individuals and organizations during the revision period. From the organizations we would particularly like to thank Agfa-Gevaert, Wardray Products, Chris Bull of 3M for providing us with up-to-date information on dry silver imaging, Ges Shilvock of Dupont, Gary Walford of Fuji, Ken Hinds and Jane Furnival of Kodak, David Blake of Laser Line for his help with the section on PACS, and Eddy Klarich of Photosol.

We also thank the numerous individuals who were kind enough to send us their comments as users of the fifth edition: we have listened to, and for the most part acted upon their advice. As always, we have been sustained in our efforts by the tremendous help, support and encouragement offered by our friends and colleagues in South Wales and elsewhere. Any credit which may be received for this sixth edition is their as much as ours. In particular, we are indebted to the following individuals with whom we debated many ideas and proposals: Tracy Adams and Mark Arnold, whose constructive criticisms prompted us to rethink the section on image distortion in Chapter 16; Karen Eckloff, whose practical experience of QA testing has been incorporated into Chapter 18; Val Bradshaw, Malcolm Ebdon, Adrian Moore, Adrian Rolls and Martin West. We would like to make special mention of Brian Murphy, former principal of West Mercia School of Radiography, who died suddenly in December 1994 after a short illness. His advice, support and friendship over more than 30 years have had a major influence on the revision of this book. We will miss him greatly.

We thank Lisa Field of Blackwell Science for reminding us (but not *too* frequently) that we had a deadline to meet. And lastly, we thank our families – Chris and Gareth, Liz and Dave – for tolerating our moods and our absences (in spirit as well as in body) particularly on being reminded of the approaching deadline! We *will* keep the lawns trimmed – next year.

John Ball and Tony Price
January 1995
Swansea

Preface to the first edition

This book is not about photography; it is about a number of subjects which are grouped together under the title Radiographic Photography in the syllabus of training for the Membership Diploma of the Society of Radiographers. The word camera appears in this book comparatively seldom and those who would seek in its pages for light on their studio lighting must remain perpetually unillumined.

In the first and last analyses, we should recognize that good radiography, though it may depend upon a knowledge of theoretical concepts, in fact is a practical skill. The subjects in their syllabus of training, summarized in the term radiographic photography, are important to radiographers because they are realistic subjects: knowledge and appreciation of them significantly affect the quality of the end-product – the radiograph. It seems strange that no textbook has yet been written for radiographers about radiographic photography and that their teachers must build courses of instruction on manufacturers' pamphlets and photographic manuals in a wider category. The authors hope that this book may fill what appears to be a gap among the aids to those who must learn and the tools of those who must teach.

In attempting to meet the needs of student radiographers, as we believe that they are not scientists and may have only irregular knowledge of chemistry, we have kept to a minimum the appearance of mathematical expressions and have avoided chemical formulae. Of great convenience to those in the know, such shorthand can be only profoundly baffling to those who are not. We hope that we have made to radiographic photography the practical approach which its character deserves.

The syllabus of training for the M.S.R. Diploma has directed the selection of material for this book. While it has been written for the education of student radiographers, we know that in some places greater detail is given than may be required for the M.S.R. course. It seems a proper principle to include in a textbook something more than the minimum demanded by a particular course of study; perhaps especially so in a field of knowledge which is fertile of development. This aspect of the book may attract at least some postgraduate readers who wish to prepare for the Higher Examination of the Society of Radiographers.

From inclusions to an omission. This book has given no space to the reproduction of photographic faults in radiographs. Possibly this may appear a serious defect to its critics. However, it must be evident to radiographers of experience that if the catalogue of such errors is to be usefully extensive, apart from any attempt to make it complete, a large number of illustrations is necessarily required: even then it is certain that someone at some time would be confronted in the viewing room with a bizarre radiographic appearance for which no reference here would enable the radiographer to account. Reproduction on paper of certain classic faults is much less satisfactory than their visualization on original films. We would suggest that for student radiographers a more useful exercise than looking at such copies is always the handling and examination of the real material. Why should they not be permitted some limited experiment from which to form their own library of malpractices in handling radiographs?

No man is an island and, perhaps more than many others, authors of textbooks are dependent on links with certain mainlands of learning and material. We are aware that the substance of this book has been strengthened because a number of people each have given to us generous measures of their knowledge, ability and not least of their time. We are glad of an opportunity to offer to them an expression of our thanks, though the small gesture is incommensurate with the gift received.

We are grateful to Dr D.M. Alexander, consultant radiologist at the Coventry and Warwickshire Hospital, for reading Chapter 14 and discussing it with us; and to Miss A. L. Hebden, medical photographer at the same hospital, who took photographs, with most welcome expedition, of a step-wedge and of parts of the Odelca and Hansen equipment. Dr J. F. K. Hutton, consultant radiologist at the General Hospital, Birmingham, receives our thanks for kindly reading Chapters 12 and 13 and giving his comments. Mr W. Hurt, medical photographer at the Birmingham Children's Hospital, came to our aid at very short notice and provided illustrations to show the appearance of a granular pattern at different degrees of photographic enlargement.

From Mr K. W. Goddard we have had the stimulus of early interest in the project and we appreciate his help in reading the manuscript of Chapters 11, 6 and 7 and in mobilizing for us some of the resources of Kodak Ltd who have loaned many illustrations and supplied other material. With Kodak we must associate Mr Sydney Marshall who has been most helpful as informant, reader and commentator.

We would like to thank Mr John Bennett and Mr R. Greenway, each of whom supplied a personal communication of immeasurable value on automatic processing and respectively read Chapters 6, 7 and 8, and 9. We are grateful also to Mr R. J. Hercock for his kindness in giving close attention to nearly a third of the manuscript and to us so much of his time.

It has been necessary in some parts of this book to provide working descriptions of certain equipment. In the absence of practical contact with the apparatus concerned such accounts may be troublesome to follow, but they are no less than impossible to write. With this problem we have appreciated energetic help from Mr C. W. Mead who has made available opportunities to examine certain fluorographic equipment, supplied technical data and given useful commentary on the resultant chapters of the manuscript. We are grateful too to Mr P. Spencer for having so willingly put us on similar good terms with a Ken-X processor and for freely loaning relevant material. Finally we owe to the knowledge and helpfulness of Dr George Parker, who read Chapters 15 and 16, the reassurance that our own pristine ignorance of some photographic optics has been successfully eliminated.

This book would have been poorly illustrated had it depended solely on the artistic ability of either of its authors. Nearly all the diagrams and photographs have been given to us through the courtesy of certain manufacturers, learned journals and publishers, and to these collectively we are most grateful for such practical assistance, in some cases on a very generous scale. We give sincere appreciation to the following: Cuthbert Andrews; The Fountain Press; Ilford Ltd, particularly Mr J. James of X-ray Sales and Mr D. H. O. John of the Techno-Commercial Dept (X-ray Division); the *Journal of Photographic Science*; Kodak Ltd, particularly Mr K. W. Goddard of the Medical Sales Division; N.V. Optische Industrie, De Oude Delft, The Netherlands; Pako Corporation, Minneapolis, USA; D. Pennellier and Co. Ltd; Philips Electrical Ltd; Philips Technical Library; *Radiography*, the

Journal of the Society of Radiographers; Theratronics Ltd; Watson and Sons (Electro-Medical) Ltd, particularly Mr G. R. Woodall, Publicity Manager; X-ray Sales Division, Eastman Kodak Co., Rochester, New York.

D. Noreen Chesney
Muriel O. Chesney

Part 1
Introduction

Chapter 1
Introduction

Medical diagnosis is essentially the extraction of anatomical and physiological information from a subject (the patient) and the interpretation of this information in such a way that corrective treatment may be prescribed. Diagnostic radiography provides one method by which the information can be obtained. The radiographic image presents the information in a *visual* form which is relatively easy for a trained observer to understand.

It is useful to examine more closely the flow of information from the patient to the observer. It may be considered in three distinct stages.

Stage 1: The formation of an invisible or 'aerial' X-ray image
This is the ordered pattern in the X-ray beam which has been transmitted through the patient.

During the radiographic examination of a patient, an X-ray beam of uniform intensity passes from the X-ray tube into the patient. At this stage the beam carries no information about the patient. As the beam penetrates through the body tissues it becomes modified, or is **modulated**, each part of the beam being attenuated to a degree which depends on the particular tissue structure through which it has passed. When the beam finally emerges from the patient it is no longer uniform. It displays a pattern of intensities which carries information about the structures the beam has penetrated. We shall refer to this pattern of intensities as the **invisible X-ray image**. Figure 1.1 illustrates the formation of a simple X-ray image.

Chapter 3 provides a detailed account of the formation of the invisible X-ray image.

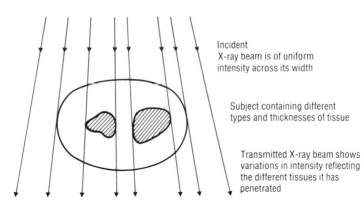

Incident X-ray beam is of uniform intensity across its width

Subject containing different types and thicknesses of tissue

Transmitted X-ray beam shows variations in intensity reflecting the different tissues it has penetrated

Fig. 1.1 X-ray beam is modified as it penetrates through tissue structures.

Stage 2: The conversion of the invisible X-ray image into a visible light image
This can be achieved in a number of ways:

(1) By employing the **photographic effect** of X-rays on a sheet of sensitive film. When a photographic film is exposed to X-radiation and is then chemically processed, it becomes permanently darkened to a degree which depends on the level of exposure it has received. Photographic material used for this purpose is known as **direct-exposure X-ray film**.

(2) By employing the **xeroradiographic process**. An electrically charged imaging plate is exposed in a similar way to an X-ray film. It reacts to exposure by leaking the charge from exposed areas, while retaining the charge on unexposed areas. During processing, fine **toner** powder, which is blown across the surface of the plate, adheres to the charged areas forming an image which is transferred permanently onto a paper-based receptor. Chapter 28 discusses the characteristics of xeroradiographic images.

(3) By employing the **fluorescent effect** of X-rays on a sensitive screen. When a fluorescent screen is exposed to X-radiation, it emits visible light whose brightness depends on the level of exposure it receives. The visible pattern of light produced by the fluorescent screen may be recorded permanently on a sheet of photographic film placed in intimate contact with the screen. A fluorescent screen used in this way is known as an **intensifying screen**, while the film which records its image is referred to as a **screen-type X-ray film**. The image it records is similar in appearance to that displayed on direct-exposure X-ray film. An X-ray film (either direct exposure or screen type) which carries this visible pattern of light and dark is known as a **radiograph**. Chapters 4–17 provide a detailed account of the production of a radiograph. Alternatively, the visible light image emitted by a fluorescent screen (the **fluoroscopic** image) may be amplified by a device known as an **image intensifier**, resulting in a smaller but much brighter image which may itself be recorded on miniature photographic film (known as **fluorographic film**) or viewed by a television camera and displayed on the screen of a television monitor. Chapters 19–23 provide a full account of the production and recording of the fluoroscopic image.

(4) By employing the process of **photon stimulated luminescence**. A phosphor-coated **imaging plate** is exposed in a similar fashion to an X-ray film. The energy absorbed is stored in the phosphor layer until stimulated by photons from a laser which systematically scans the imaging plate. When stimulated in this way, the phosphor emits light whose brightness is related to the original X-ray exposure. The light output is detected and converted to a digital signal from which a computer reconstructs an image displayed on a TV monitor and recorded (for example) with a laser imager. Such a system is known as **computed radiography** (CR). Chapter 28 provides further details of computed radiography.

Stage 3: The viewing, perception and interpretation of the visible image
The diagnostic image, whether it be on photographic film or on a television screen, must be viewed and understood before a diagnosis can be made.

The diagnostic information carried by such images can only be communicated effectively to an observer under optimum viewing conditions. Viewing of the radiograph is discussed in Chapter 14, while viewing of television images is considered in Chapter 22. Additionally, the physiology and psychology of the observer have an important influence. Chapter 29 is devoted to a study of this aspect of radiographic imaging.

Other imaging technologies
Chapters 24–28 describe some of the diagnostic imaging techniques currently available which supplement, and in some cases have replaced, conventional radiography. Chapter 29 includes reference to the perception and interpretation of these images.

Chapter 2
Image Characteristics

On several occasions in Chapter 1 we employed the term *image* to describe a recognizable pattern carrying useful information. In this chapter we examine the meaning of the term image and we study the general features possessed by images.

2.1 What *is* an image?

The dictionary (Sykes, 1987) tells us that an image is:

- An optical appearance;
- A form or semblance;
- A mental representation;
- An idea or conception.

Thus, the term image may be applied to a picture such as a photograph, a painting or a sketch which has a real physical existence. But it may also be applied to an idea or concept which has a mental rather than physical existence.

If asked to imagine an object such as an apple, a *mental* image of an apple comes to mind. The existence of this visual image helps us to grasp the concept of an apple. Being shown a photograph of an apple has a similar effect.

Of course, a photograph of an apple represents only one aspect of an apple: its visual appearance. It provides no representation of the taste, smell or feel of the apple. It is left to our mental processes to imagine these other non-visual characteristics of an apple which we remember from past experiences.

Thus, we may surmise that visual images are of two types:

(1) *Real images:* those having a real, physical existence such as photographic or radiographic images which are accessible to scientific measurement and objective study.
(2) *Mental images:* those generated as mental pictures within our own minds and which are accessible only to subjective study.

It is our task in the remainder of this chapter to explore those important characteristics of real images which can be studied objectively, and which are an inherent feature of images such as those recorded on a radiograph or displayed on a television screen.

Real images consist of patterns of light intensity and possibly variations in colour. The patterns of light are created in one of three ways.

*(1) Viewing by **reflected** light from a surface*
The surface contains pigments which reflect varying amounts (and/or colours) of the light incident upon them (see Fig. 2.1). The text and the illustrations in this book are all viewed by reflected light and the absorbent pigment used is ink. In radiography, xeroradiographs (see section 28.7) are viewed by reflected light. Photographic images intended to be viewed in this way are known as **prints**.

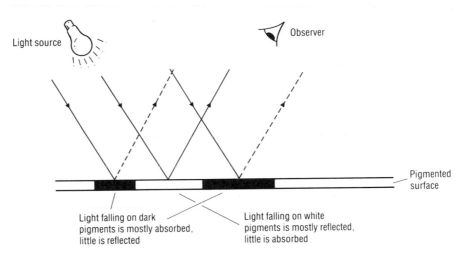

Fig. 2.1 Viewing an image by reflected light.

*(2) Viewing by light **transmitted** through a semitransparent layer*
The layer contains pigments which transmit varying amounts (and/or colours) of the light incident upon them (see Fig. 2.2). The image on a conventional radiograph is viewed by transmitted light. In this case the light-absorbing pigment is metallic

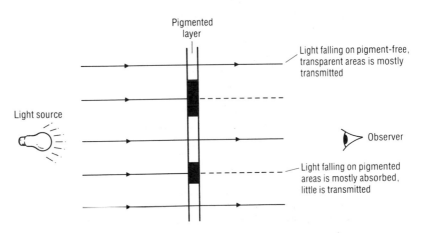

Fig. 2.2 Viewing an image by transmitted light.

silver. A photographic image intended to be viewed by transmitted light is known as a **transparency**.

(3) Viewing by light emitted from a fluorescent layer
Exposure to X-rays or to an electron beam stimulates the fluorescent material to emit varying amounts of light (see Fig. 2.3). The fluoroscopic screen image and the image on the television screen are produced in this way.

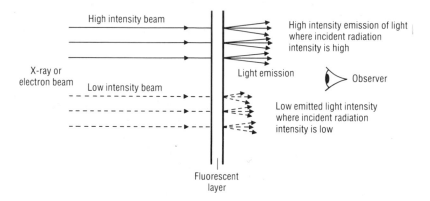

Fig. 2.3 Viewing an image by fluorescence.

Notice that viewing an image by reflected or transmitted light requires an external light source, e.g. a 'reading' lamp or an X-ray illuminator ('viewing box') respectively. Viewing a fluorescent image does not require such light sources.

2.1.1   *Image characteristics*

Real images display four essential characteristics:

(1) Noise;
(2) Contrast;
(3) Sharpness;
(4) Resolution.

2.1.1.1   Noise
Real images consist of two components:

(1) A meaningful pattern or **signal** carrying information about the subject, and
(2) A spurious, chaotic pattern or **noise**, carrying no information about the subject.

These two components are superimposed in the image. The presence of noise limits the amount of information which can be extracted from the image. In particular, the finer details of structure may be lost by being swamped by the effect of noise (HPA, 1977).

Origin of the term noise
Noise may seem an unlikely term to apply to a visual image which is silent. The use of the term probably originates from radio engineering, where the quality of

reception of radio signals is often impaired by background noise (e.g. hisses and whistles), particularly when the original signal is rather weak and the radio receiver is being used with maximum amplification. The effect of such noise on the information communicated via a radio link is very similar to the effect of noise on the information carried by an image.

Signal-to-noise ratio

Under optimum conditions the magnitude of the signal is very much greater than the magnitude of the noise. The **signal-to-noise ratio** is said to be high. Under adverse conditions the signal-to-noise ratio is low, and much information is lost.

Appearance of noise

It is not uncommon for a radiographic image to be fogged, perhaps due to an accidental exposure to scattered radiation in the X-ray room, or to poor conditions of storage. When such a radiograph is examined its image appears as viewed through a mist or fog. The information content of the image is reduced. Some information is lost entirely, whilst that which remains is more difficult to see. The fogging contains no information about the subject of the radiograph. Such fogging is an example of one form of image noise.

Another type of noise may be seen on a television image. In this case, the image appears as if viewed through a snowstorm. The screen displays a very large number of small white specks which appear superimposed on the image. Again, the effect is to reduce the information content of the image. Such an appearance may be due to inferior design of the electronic circuitry employed, causing **electronic noise**. However, in many cases the basic cause is that the signal being displayed is too weak, and the specks represent the *absence* of information, rather like the spaces left by missing pieces in a jigsaw puzzle. It is possible for a similar effect to occur in the image on a radiograph, except that in this case the image appears to have a large number of very small black specks superimposed on it, giving it a grainy or mottled appearance commonly known as **quantum mottle** or **quantum noise**. Quantum noise on radiographs is discussed more fully in section 7.11 and on the television image in sections 19.2.2.2 and 22.3.2.

2.1.1.2   Contrast

To be able to identify a feature on an image, it must appear different from its surroundings. On a radiograph, a structure must be of a different optical density (shade of grey) from adjacent structures. On a television image, the structure must be of a different luminance (brightness). The term **contrast** is used to describe these differences in density or luminance. If the differences are great, the structure will stand out well from its surroundings and we say the contrast is **high** (or **good**). If the differences are small, it is difficult to identify the structure against its background. The contrast is said to be **low** (or **poor**) (Pizzutiello & Cullinan, 1993).

Demonstrating contrast

It is helpful to investigate the effect of different levels of contrast by adjusting the contrast control on a monochrome television set (or on a colour TV with the colour control adjusted to give a monochrome image).

High contrast With a high level of contrast the image produced appears harsh, with lots of dense blacks and brilliant whites. Details may be lost in the highlighted areas and in the deep shadows, but the boundaries between the dark and light areas appear sharply defined.

Low contrast With the contrast level at a minimum the image appears dull, lacking in any true blacks and whites. However, inspection of the highlighted areas and the shadows reveals detail that was absent in the high-contrast image.

It is often the case that while a high-contrast image is more pleasing to the eye, it is the *lower*-contrast image which reveals more information.

Optimum contrast

We have seen that it is a simple matter to control the contrast of a television image. The optimum level of contrast is usually about midway between the extremes available, although the exact setting selected tends to be a matter of personal preference and depends also on the nature of the subject.

The contrast of the image on a radiograph is more difficult to control. Adjustment of the X-ray tube kilovoltage and control of scattered radiation are just two methods available to the radiographer by which the radiographic image contrast may be influenced. Again, the optimum contrast level tends to be neither very high nor very low, and is different for different subjects. It is also true that different individuals have different concepts of what constitutes optimum contrast: a radiograph judged by one radiographer or radiologist to be correctly exposed may well be criticized by another. A further complication is that in a single radiographic image the optimum contrast for one structure may be different from the optimum contrast for another. For example, in a postero-anterior chest radiograph the image contrast is usually chosen to give maximum information about the lung fields. However, the contrast within the region of the mediastinum is very poor. To achieve optimum contrast in this region, it is necessary to produce a more penetrated radiograph. Unfortunately, the penetrated image of the chest offers very little contrast in the lung fields. The eventual contrast of the image on a radiograph is determined essentially at the moment of the X-ray exposure; there is very little scope for adjustment afterwards. A major advantage of **digital** imaging systems (see section 22.4) is that they enable image contrast to be manipulated freely and repeatedly *after* exposure.

There are a number of factors which determine the contrast of an image. In section 3.1.1 we shall examine the way that contrast is generated in the transmitted X-ray beam, while later on we investigate the influence of the recording medium on image contrast. Section 16.3 provides an analysis of contrast as seen on a radiograph, while section 22.3.4 examines contrast in the television image.

2.1.1.3 Sharpness

Contrast was described as the *difference* in blackening (optical density) or *difference* in luminance between two adjacent areas of an image. Sharpness is concerned with *how suddenly* blackening changes at the boundary between adjacent parts (Pizzutiello & Cullinan, 1993). Consider Fig. 2.4, which shows two areas A and B of different optical densities (D_A and D_B).

The boundary between the two areas appears very sharp because there is a sudden change in the value of density at the boundary. If we were to scan across the boundary, taking readings with a **microdensitometer** (a device which can measure optical density), we would expect a trace of density against distance to appear, as shown in Fig. 2.5, with a vertical rise between A and B.

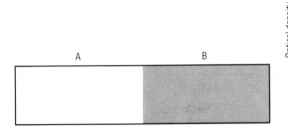

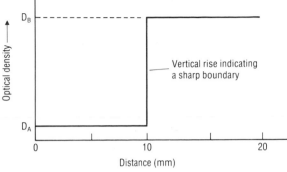

Fig. 2.4 Two areas A and B of different optical densities separated by a sharp boundary.

Fig. 2.5 Microdensitometer trace of density across the boundary between A and B in Fig. 2.4.

Suppose, however, we examined the boundary with a microscope so that we could identify the individual specks of pigment forming the image. The boundary would no longer appear so sharp (Fig. 2.6).

Redrawing the microdensitometer trace with an enlarged scale of distance (Fig. 2.7) shows that there is not a vertical rise in density at the boundary but a more gradual change, shown as a slope. It is this which characterizes the appearance of sharpness (or unsharpness) at the boundary. The steeper the slope, the more sharp the image appears: the shallower the slope, the more blurred the image. In fact, no image is perfectly sharp; thus, we tend to discuss the *un*sharpness of images rather than their sharpness (Kodak, 1982).

We are revealing here a subtle difference between the concepts of **unsharpness** and **lack of sharpness**. Unsharpness is an objective concept which, as we shall see in the next section, can be measured. On the other hand, sharpness is our *subjective*

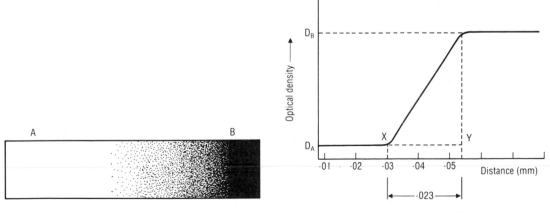

Fig. 2.6 Enlarged view of the boundary in Fig. 2.4 showing the unsharp nature of the change in density.

Fig. 2.7 Microdensitometer trace of density changes across the boundary in Fig. 2.6 with an expanded scale of distance. The distance XY over which density is changing is a measure of unsharpness.

perception of unsharpness, and depends on contrast as well as unsharpness. We judge one image boundary to be sharper than another, even though they are both equally unsharp, if the contrast of the first image is greater.

Specifying unsharpness
Image unsharpness may be expressed in several ways; for example, by means of **transfer functions** such as:

(1) Edge spread function;
(2) Point spread function;
(3) Line spread function;

or as a simple numerical quantity (Rossman, 1969; Workman & Cowen, 1994).

(1) *Edge spread function (ESF)* The microdensitometer trace that we have described above, showing the variation in image density across a boundary, is an example of an **edge spread function**, but it is usual to express the density values across the boundary in relative terms, giving a range of 0 to 1. The object whose image we have analysed must possess a perfectly sharp edge. It is doubtful whether we shall ever image such an object in clinical radiography but ESF is, nevertheless, a useful concept. It is one way in which unsharpness may be specified. From it, we can express unsharpness numerically by stating the distance over which the density is changing; e.g. $XY = 0.023\,\text{mm}$ in Fig. 2.7. (Contrast can be expressed as the *change* in density; $D_B - D_A$.)

(2) *Point spread function (PSF)* The tissues and organs which we image in our everyday work as radiographers consist of a number of minute **points** of anatomical detail. It would seem more sensible to base our measure of unsharpness on the images of points rather than edges. A point structure in an object (e.g. a minute hole in a sheet of lead) should produce a sharp image. In practice, the image of a point will be unsharp and will appear as a small blurred disc. A microdensitometer trace across the centre of the disc will show a *gradual* rise in density towards the centre. Again, relative values of density are employed. The measurement of density at the centre is plotted as unity, while the measurements of background density, well away from the centre, are plotted as zero.

Such a trace is known as a **point spread function** (Fig. 2.8), but there are technical problems in producing it. For example, it is difficult to be certain that the microdensitometer has scanned across the exact centre of the image. Also, the trace should be repeated in different directions to build up a complete picture of the symmetry, or otherwise, of the image. For these reasons, the PSF is unfortunately of limited practical use.

(3) *Line spread function (LSF)* The problems in obtaining a trace of the PSF can be overcome by replacing the point structure by a **line** structure (e.g. a narrow slit in a sheet of lead) which produces a line image. The microdensitometer can scan across the line image, at right angles to it, and produce a trace of the variations in density it experiences. Relative values are used, as with ESF and PSF. There are now no problems in alignment of the scanning sensor. The trace is known as the **line spread function**. The LSF is a most useful method of defining the unsharpness of an image (Fig. 2.9).

From the LSF we can extract a single numerical value, which may be quoted as a

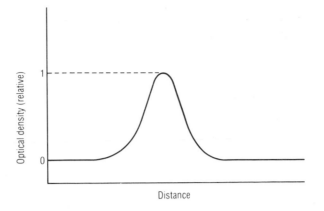

Fig. 2.8 Point spread function. The microdensitometer trace across the image produced by radiographing a minute hole in a lead sheet.

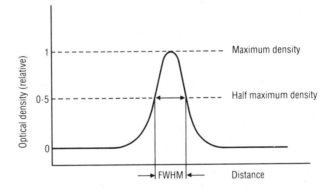

Fig. 2.9 Line spread function. The microdensitometer trace across the image produced by radiographing a narrow slit in a lead sheet. From the LSF the full width at half maximum (FWHM) measurement can be obtained which provides a simple measure of unsharpness.

simple measure of unsharpness. It is shown on Fig. 2.9 as the FWHM measurement (full width at half maximum) (Cowen and Coleman, 1986).

A statement sometimes quoted in radiography is that an image whose unsharpness is < 0.1 mm will appear to be sharp under 'normal viewing conditions' (Kodak, 1968). However, as we have seen, our perception of unsharpness seems to be determined more by the **density gradient** than by the simple measure of unsharpness referred to above. Density gradient depends both on unsharpness and on density difference (contrast). Thus, an image of high contrast may appear sharper than one of low contrast, even though both images possess the same measured unsharpness. Figure 2.10 illustrates this point.

Note that we have described unsharpness in terms of density changes as seen on a radiograph. We must remember that on a fluorescent image, unsharpness is described in terms of changes in screen luminance rather than density, but in other respects the concept of image unsharpness is similar.

It is the task of the radiographer to ensure that image unsharpness is kept to the

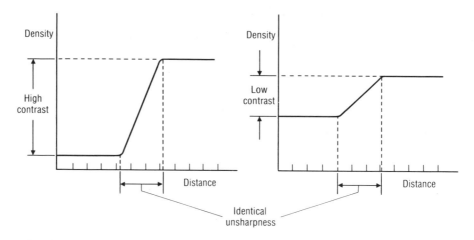

Fig. 2.10 Microdensitometer traces of two density edges of equal unsharpness but different density gradients. The high contrast image with a steep density gradient *appears* sharper than the low contrast image.

minimum. Only by understanding the factors which contribute to unsharpness can this be achieved. As we work through this book we shall be investigating the many causes of image unsharpness; e.g. section 16.1 provides a concise analysis of their relative importance in the image on a radiograph, while section 22.3.1 looks at unsharpness in television images.

2.1.1.4   Resolution

The resolution of a system is its ability to demonstrate closely spaced structures in the subject as separate entities in the image. For example, the trabeculae of cancellous (spongy) bone form a network of very fine threads. It is a supreme test of an imaging system to be able to demonstrate this trabecular pattern in all its detail. Any significant unsharpness causes the images of the individual trabeculae to merge together, and much of the detail is lost. A system which is able to meet this challenge is said to demonstrate **high resolution**, while a system which cannot reproduce such detail offers **lower (or poorer) resolution**.

Measurement of resolution

The resolution of a system may be assessed subjectively by imaging a suitable test object. The object should contain a mesh or grid of closely spaced lines, alternately radiopaque and radiolucent, whose spacing is accurately known (Fig. 2.11). Each line and its corresponding space is known as a **line pair**. The spacing of the line pairs is expressed as a **spatial frequency**, usually quoted in line pairs per millimetre (lp/mm). From the image, the closest spacing (highest spatial frequency) which can be detected is noted and this value may be used to specify the resolution of the imaging system. Some of the film–screen systems used in radiography permit image resolutions around 20 lp/mm (Cowen *et al.*, 1990), whereas an image on an image intensifier–television system may achieve a resolution barely approaching 2 lp/mm (MDD, 1994).

Modulation transfer function

The resolution of different imaging systems may be compared objectively by

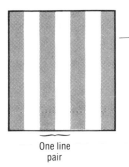

Resolution test object consisting of
alternate radiopaque and radiolucent lines

One line
pair

Fig. 2.11 The concept of line pairs. If one line pair occupies 0.1 mm the spatial frequency is 10 line pairs per millimetre (lp/mm). This is sometimes written as '10 cycles mm^{-1}' or just '10 mm^{-1}'.

reference to the **modulation transfer function** (MTF) of each system. The MTF is a method of assessing the success with which modulations of structure (detail) in an object are transferred into modulations of density or luminance in the image. The magnitude of the modulations in image and object are compared. An MTF of unity means that the image reproduces exactly the variations in the object. It is a characteristic of imaging systems that, as the detail in the object becomes finer, the ability of the system to record that detail becomes progressively reduced. In other words, as spatial frequency increases, modulation transfer function decreases. This relationship is therefore generally displayed as a graph of MTF plotted against spatial frequency. Figure 2.12 shows the typical appearance of an MTF curve for an X-ray film–screen system.

Commercially manufactured resolution test objects are available for the purpose

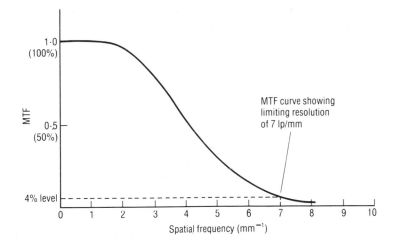

Fig. 2.12 Appearance of a typical modulation transfer function curve. As spatial frequency increases MTF reduces. It is often stated (e.g. Jenkins, 1980) that the spatial frequency at which MTF = 0.04 (4%) represents a threshold resolution below which detail is no longer visible. Resolution is thus sometimes quoted in terms of this threshold value or **resolution limit** (RL) in line pairs per millimetre (Cowen *et al.*, 1990).

of determining the resolution of radiographic imaging systems (Workman & Cowen, 1994).

Factors limiting resolution
The resolution of a radiographic image is influenced at almost every stage in the process of image production. If we consider each step in this process as links in a chain, then the quality of the final image can be no better than that of the weakest link. As radiographers, we must identify the weakest links and try to improve them. But we must realize that in improving one aspect we may weaken another. There is a complex interrelationship between many of the factors concerned, including all of the image characteristics discussed in this chapter. Only when we have studied all the ramifications of image production will we be able to understand fully how resolution may be optimized.

2.2 Conclusion

We have now completed the introductory part of the book. In the next chapter we examine in detail the process of production of the invisible X-ray image.

Part 2
The Invisible X-ray Image

Chapter 3
Production of the Invisible X-ray Image

Characteristics of the invisible X-ray image
    Subject contrast
    Sharpness
    Noise
    Resolution

In Chapter 1 we described diagnostic imaging as a method of information transfer from a subject (the patient) to an observer. We analysed the transfer into three distinct stages:

(1) The formation of an invisible X-ray image;
(2) The conversion of the invisible X-ray image into a visible light image;
(3) The viewing, perception and interpretation of the visible image.

In this chapter, we shall consider the first stage in detail and examine the origin and characteristics of the invisible image in the X-ray beam emerging from the patient.

Figure 3.1 shows the beam from an X-ray tube entering a patient. Careful examination shows that there will be slight differences in intensity between the

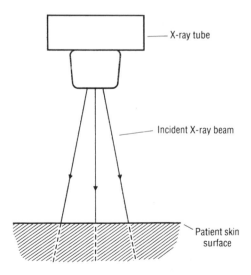

Fig. 3.1 X-ray beam entering a patient. Peripheral rays have further to travel than the central ray and are therefore of slightly lower intensity. In practice such differences in intensity are minimal for small field sizes or large focus–skin distances.

central ray of the beam and the peripheral rays, because of the different distances they have had to travel. These differences are entirely predictable and certainly do not constitute information about the patient. For our present purposes, we shall assume that the beam entering the patient is of *uniform* intensity.

As the beam penetrates through the patient's tissues, it is attenuated such that the beam which eventually emerges from the patient is reduced in intensity compared with the incident beam. Moreover, the amount by which its intensity is reduced varies at different points across the beam, because beam attenuation depends on the type and thickness of tissue through which it has passed. Thus, the X-ray beam now carries a pattern of varying intensities which reflects the anatomy of the tissues that it has penetrated. We can think of this pattern of intensities as an invisible or **aerial image** (Pizzutiello & Cullinan, 1993). It is this image which must be made visible to form the radiographic image with which we are all familiar.

3.1   Characteristics of the invisible X-ray image

Although the pattern of X-ray intensities is invisible at this stage, we can examine it in terms of the four essential image characteristics discussed in Chapter 2: contrast, sharpness, noise and resolution.

3.1.1   *Subject contrast*

The term **subject contrast** is often used to describe the differences in X-ray intensity that we are discussing, to distinguish it from the differences in optical density or luminance to which the term contrast is normally applied. It is a shortened form of **radiation contrast in the subject** (Chesney & Chesney, 1981) and it must not be confused with the term **subjective contrast**, which has a quite different meaning, to which we shall refer in section 29.2.6.

Without differences in intensity, i.e. without subject contrast, we cannot achieve any visible contrast in the eventual radiographic image. It is therefore vital that subject contrast is present.

3.1.1.1   **What are the causes of subject contrast?**

(1) Differential attenuation
Subject contrast is a consequence of the **differential attenuation** of the X-ray beam in passing through the patient. You will recall from your study of radiation physics that diagnostic X-ray beams are attenuated in two ways as they pass through matter: by **photoelectric absorption** and by **Compton scattering** (Ball & Moore, 1986).

Differential attenuation, and hence the subject contrast created, depends on:

(1) The differences in **thickness** of the anatomical structures in the patient.
(2) The differences in the physical nature of the body tissues, such as the **effective atomic number** and **physical density** of the tissues. In the case of body tissues, density does not vary greatly between different tissues unless air or gas is present, but there may well be sufficient differences in effective atomic number to create reasonable subject contrast.
(3) The presence of a radiological **contrast agent**. If there are insufficient *natural* differences in atomic number or density of the tissues, a contrast agent may be

introduced to produce an artificial change. A **positive** agent containing iodine or barium sulphate produces an increase in atomic number, whilst a **negative** contrast agent such as air produces a reduction in density. Sometimes both types of contrast agent are used simultaneously, as in the **double contrast** technique for investigation of the stomach or large bowel.

(4) The **X-ray tube kilovoltage** employed. Since the attenuation due to photoelectric absorption is heavily dependent on the atomic number of the tissues, we try to ensure that most of the attenuation which occurs is due to this process rather than to Compton scattering. Photoelectric absorption predominates at low energies, so we tilt the balance in its favour by keeping the X-ray tube kilovoltage low. As the kV is raised and the amount of photoelectric absorption reduces, so we find that subject contrast (and the eventual radiographic image contrast) begins to decrease. Hence, the well known (but not so well understood!) rule:

> To increase contrast, reduce kV; to reduce contrast, increase kV.

Bone tissue has about *twice* the atomic number of the softer tissues of the body, and this is sufficient to create good subject contrast between bone and soft tissue over a wide range of kilovoltages. In other cases, e.g. the breast, the tissue differences are much smaller, and subject contrast may be inadequate unless very low kilovoltages are used. At very high kilovoltages, e.g. approaching 150 kVp, the Compton effect is the dominant attenuating process. It is not always appreciated that under these conditions, the production of adequate subject contrast depends almost entirely on the ability of the Compton effect to discriminate between different structures (Hay, 1982). Because high kV techniques are comparatively uncommon, it is perhaps understandable that radiographers are far more familiar with the *negative* aspects of the Compton effect (namely scatter) than with its *positive* contribution to image contrast.

(5) The X-ray **beam filtration** used. Increasing the filtration of the X-ray beam has the effect of raising its effective photon energy by removing its low energy component. This influences the predominance of the photoelectric absorption process in a similar way to the raising of tube kilovoltage, and causes a reduction in subject contrast. In situations such as mammography (soft tissue radiography of the breast), where subject contrast is very low, it is common practice to use the **minimum** permitted beam filtration (currently 0.5 mm aluminium equivalent: NRPB, 1988). In conjunction with the selection of low kilovoltages, this ensures that differential attenuation is maximized.

(2) Scattered radiation

When the primary beam from the X-ray tube interacts with matter, **scattered radiation** is produced. Scattered radiation travels along different paths from the primary beam and may well seriously degrade the quality of the invisible X-ray image by reducing subject contrast.

Figure 3.2 shows the production of scattered radiation within the patient. Some of the scatter will itself be absorbed inside the patient, but some will escape in all directions. A proportion of the scattered radiation will travel forward in the general direction of the transmitted primary beam. Any image receptor (e.g. film–screen system or image intensifier) positioned to detect the transmitted primary beam will also be exposed to scattered radiation. The effect will be to increase overall the intensity of radiation received and to reduce the relative variations in intensity

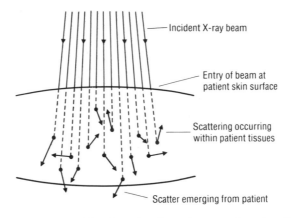

Fig. 3.2 Scattering of X-ray beam within the patient. Scattering occurs in random directions but forward scatter emerging from the patient may affect the image receptor, causing fogging of the image. Note that the diagram does not show transmission of primary rays.

which the image detector is attempting to record. Subject contrast and the signal-to-noise ratio will be reduced.

The presence of scatter *always* has a negative effect on subject contrast but, with care, its effects on image quality can be minimized.

3.1.1.2   How may the effects of scatter on subject contrast be minimized?
There are two basic approaches:

(1) Reduce the amount of scatter produced *at source* by:
   (a) **Collimating** the primary beam ('coning down') so that as small a volume of the patient as possible is irradiated. This also has the advantage of reducing the radiation hazard to the patient.
   (b) Reducing the proportion of **forward scatter** from the patient. It is scatter directed from the patient to the image receptor which constitutes the greatest problem. This can be controlled to some extent by virtue of the fact that the proportion of forward scatter decreases as the energy of the beam is reduced. If high kilovoltages can be avoided, then the problem of forward scatter is eased. However, there may be pressing reasons why it is essential to use high kilovoltages. In such cases, extra care will need to be taken to prevent forward scatter from reaching the film.
   (c) Reducing tissue thickness by application of a 'compression band' where appropriate. In suitable cases, e.g. radiography of the abdomen, this has the effect of displacing some of the patient's tissues away from the primary beam, thus reducing the actual volume of tissue irradiated (Fig. 3.3). It has the added advantages that exposure factors can be reduced and the patient is more effectively immobilized. (Note that although the term compression is commonly employed to describe this practice, little if any tissue compression occurs. **Tissue displacement** is a more accurate description of the technique.)
   (d) Taking care to remove or to protect from radiation any objects placed near to the patient or image receptor which might act as sources of scatter. For example, when radiographing the A-P projection of a patient's knee, the unaffected limb can act as a source of scatter unless it is adequately shielded

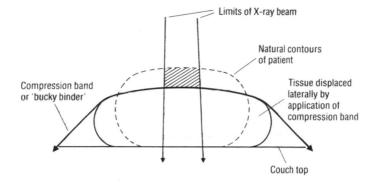

Fig. 3.3 Effect of tissue displacement. Hatched region indicates increased tissue volume the beam must penetrate if a compression band is not used. Application of compression modifies patient contours from the original (broken line) to a flatter contour (solid line) by displacing tissue laterally.

by judicious collimation of the primary beam. This phenomenon calls into question the well known practice of producing an A-P projection of both knees side-by-side on the same film, *with a single exposure*, when a bilateral examination is requested. Although this practice may save time, the scatter generated by each knee will reduce the subject contrast of the image of its fellow, particularly if the knees in question are larger than average. The image quality, and therefore diagnostic value of the examination may be compromised. The cassette housing the intensifying screens and X-ray film, and the tray holding the cassette are also potential sources of scattered radiation. The use of a lead backing layer in the cassette helps to prevent loss of subject contrast due to **back scatter**.

(2) Protect the image receptor from scatter by:

(a) The use of a **secondary radiation grid** (Aichinger, *et al.*, 1992). The purpose of such a grid is to transmit the primary beam onto the image receptor with as little attenuation as possible, but at the same time to obstruct the passage of scattered radiation from the patient (see Fig. 3.4). The grid is constructed from a series of radiopaque slats and radiolucent interspaces. The alignment of the slats and interspaces is carefully arranged so that the primary X-rays, arising from the X-ray tube focus and therefore travelling in predetermined directions, are able to pass through the interspaces comparatively unhindered. The scattered rays, whose directions differ from those of the primary rays, are absorbed when they collide with the radiopaque slats which form the walls of the interspaces.

Unfortunately, grids are unable to discriminate fully between primary and scattered radiation. They do not transmit *all* of the primary rays. Some are absorbed by the slats, producing the appearance of 'grid lines' on the image. Others are slightly attenuated as they penetrate the supposedly radiolucent interspaces and the front and back protective covering of the grid.

Additionally, grids do not absorb *all* of the scattered rays: some rays may be travelling in directions which enable them to pass through an interspace; others may be of high enough energy to penetrate through the radiopaque slats. This is particularly so when a high kilovoltage technique is employed because the forward scatter produced is then more penetrating.

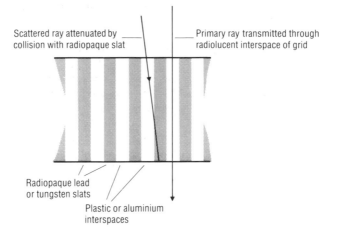

Scattered ray attenuated by
collision with radiopaque slat

Primary ray transmitted through
radiolucent interspace of grid

Radiopaque lead
or tungsten slats

Plastic or aluminium
interspaces

Fig. 3.4 The secondary radiation grid (magnified cross-section) which selectively attenuates scattered radiation while transmitting much of the primary radiation with little attenuation.

(b) Employing an **air gap** (e.g. 30 cm) between the patient and the image receptor. The intensity of the scattered radiation arising from the patient reduces markedly with distance over the first few tens of centimetres of its travel because its divergence is so great (Fig. 3.5). The intensity of the primary beam over the same path is reduced very little because by this stage it is nearly parallel. Thus, by the time the radiation reaches the image receptor, the intensity of the scattered radiation has been reduced to an acceptable level, whilst the intensity of the primary beam is only slightly reduced.

It is a common misconception to believe that the air gap technique works

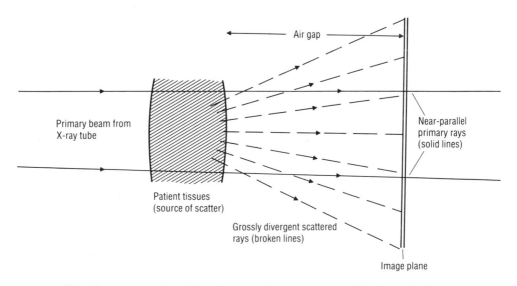

Air gap

Primary beam from
X-ray tube

Near-parallel
primary rays
(solid lines)

Patient tissues
(source of scatter)

Grossly divergent scattered
rays (broken lines)

Image plane

Fig. 3.5 Air gap technique. The percentage reduction in intensity of the scattered radiation in crossing the air gap is far greater than that experienced by the primary beam. Thus at the image plane the intensity of scatter is small relative to that of the primary rays and a satisfactory image can be formed.

because the scattered rays are *absorbed* by the air present in the air gap. This is not so.

The analogy illustrated in Fig. 3.6 may help with our understanding of this problem. Consider how the illumination from a reading lamp changes as one moves further away. The illumination may be perfectly acceptable at a distance of, say, one metre. But at a distance of three or four metres, the illumination from the lamp is totally inadequate for reading. Compare this with the illumination of sunlight. Moving a few metres closer to or further from the sun makes not the slightest difference to the level of illumination that it provides. The reason is that in the case of the reading lamp (and of scattered X-radiation) the *percentage change* in distance from the source is large, but in the case of sunlight (and of primary X-radiation) the percentage change in distance is very small.

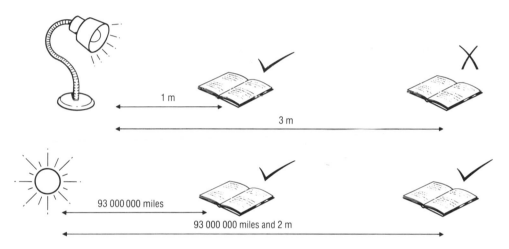

Fig. 3.6 The reading lamp analogy. Moving the book 2 m further from the lamp makes a great difference to the level of illumination. Moving the book 2 m further from the sun makes no noticeable difference.

3.1.1.3   When should we use a grid or air gap?

Before leaving the topic of scattered radiation we should point out that when examining parts of the adult patient, such as the distal extremities (e.g. hands, wrists, feet, ankles, etc.), and in neonatal radiography, the volume of tissue irradiated may be small enough for us to dispense with the use of a grid or air gap. The more proximal extremities (shoulders, knees, etc.) are regions where the use of a grid is certainly worthy of consideration, particularly with larger patients. Grids become very necessary for radiography of the adult skull, spine and trunk, with the exception of the chest (for lung fields), where in most cases the use of a grid is optional.

The use of the air gap is more limited. It is commonly used in conjunction with high kilovoltage techniques (> 120 kVp) for the chest (Jackson, 1964; Evans, 1991). An air gap is unavoidable during radiography of the neck in the lateral projection, and it is an essential feature of the magnification technique of **macroradiography** (see Chapter 26), but in neither of these examples is the air gap introduced primarily in order to control scatter.

It is *not* necessary to use both grid and air gap simultaneously.

3.1.2   *Sharpness*

In order to explain the sharpness of the invisible X-ray image, we need to consider the geometry of image formation.

3.1.2.1   **Image geometry**

(1) Point focus

Figure 3.7 shows the ideal situation in which the source of X-rays is a **point focus**; i.e. it has zero area. The beam is shown passing through the patient's tissues, which are assumed to be uniform except for a single small structure (A) which we could imagine to be perhaps a small calcified lesion or opacity. The transmitted beam is of uniform intensity, except where it has had to penetrate through A. The distribution of the transmitted intensity across the image plane XY is shown in Fig. 3.8, which demonstrates that there is an abrupt change in intensity as we pass under the 'shadow' of the structure A. The X-ray image is perfectly sharp. (Compare this with the **point spread function** (PSF) described in section 2.1.1.3. (Note that because of the divergence of the X-ray beam, the width (W) of the image of A is greater than the width of A itself; i.e. the image is magnified.

(2) Finite focus

Now let us consider a more realistic X-ray source: one which has a finite area (Fig. 3.9). From the extreme edges of the source we have traced the paths of four rays, each of which passes through the tissues without penetrating the opacity A. We use these rays to define the regions L, M and N on the image plane XY.

Consider the distribution of transmitted intensity across XY. In region L, intensity is at its maximum since none of the X-rays arriving at L have passed

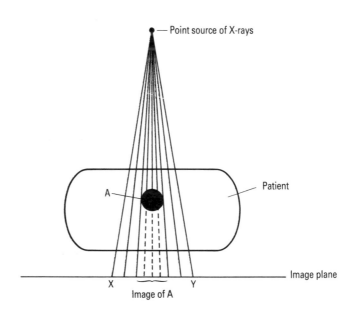

Fig. 3.7 X-ray image production from a point source. The image of A is sharp, but magnified.

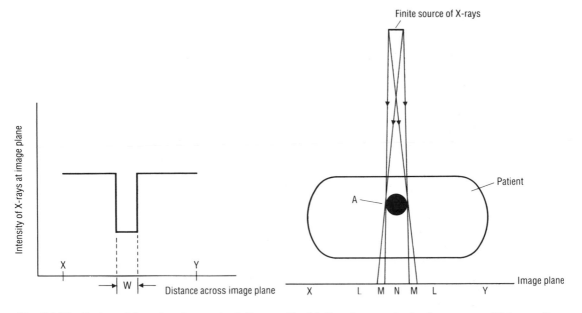

Fig. 3.8 Distribution of intensity of transmitted X-rays across the image plane XY in Fig. 3.7.

Fig. 3.9 X-ray image production from a source of finite area. Rays traced from the edges of the source divide the image plane into regions labelled L, M and N (see text for explanation). M is penumbra.

through the opacity. In region N, the intensity is at a minimum because all of the X-rays arriving at N have had to penetrate the opacity. In region M, the intensity lies between the extreme values because while some rays arriving at M have had to pass through the opacity, others have not. Figure 3.10 shows a plot of the intensity distribution across XY. It demonstrates that there is no longer an abrupt fall in

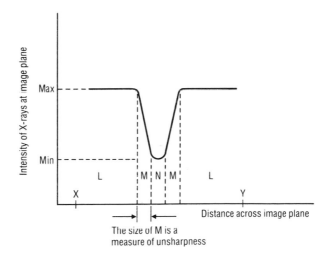

Fig. 3.10 Distribution of intensity of transmitted X-rays across the image plane XY in Fig. 3.9.

intensity as we move into the shadow of the opacity. There is a region (M) of partial shadow or **penumbra** in which intensity changes gradually from its maximum to its minimum value. The image is no longer perfectly sharp and the size of the penumbra is a measure of the unsharpness present.

3.1.2.2   Geometric unsharpness

The formation of unsharpness due to a penumbra is a direct consequence of the finite size of the X-ray source. The image unsharpness which results is known as **geometric unsharpness**, often abbreviated U_G. It is a matter of simple geometry to establish the factors which determine the magnitude of geometric unsharpness present. Consider Fig. 3.11, which shows a finite source of X-rays (S), a point (P) in an object, and the image plane (I) which would normally be occupied by the film–screen cassette or image intensifier input phosphor. At the image plane, the image of P is represented by CD. The image of P *should* be a point, but because of the finite size of the X-ray source it is imaged as a disc whose diameter is CD.

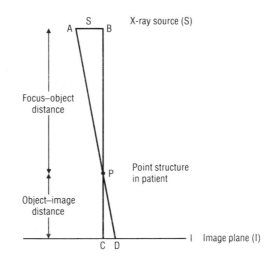

Fig. 3.11 Geometry of image formation and geometric unsharpness. Triangles ABP and CDP are geometrically similar. AB is the focal spot size; CD is the penumbra size (geometric unsharpness) therefore

$$\text{Geometric unsharpness} = \frac{\text{Focal spot size} \times \text{object}-\text{image distance}}{\text{focus}-\text{object distance}}$$

Triangles ABP and CDP are geometrically similar (their corresponding angles are equal). It is a property of similar triangles that the ratio of their bases (AB/CD) is equal to the ratio of their heights (BP/CP), i.e.

$$\frac{AB}{CD} = \frac{BP}{CP}$$

Rearranging this gives:

$$CD = \frac{AB \times CP}{BP}$$

or

$$\text{Geometric unsharpness} = \frac{\text{focal spot size} \times \text{object}-\text{image distance}}{\text{focus}-\text{object distance}}$$

Thus, we can see that geometric unsharpness depends on three major factors:

(1) *Focal spot size:* reducing focal spot size reduces geometric unsharpness. Note that it is the **apparent** or **effective** focal spot size which determines geometric unsharpness, *not* the **real** size of the focus. We could add, therefore, that for a given real focal spot size, geometric unsharpness depends on the X-ray tube **target angle**. Furthermore the apparent size of a focus alters at different points in the beam. Figure 3.12 shows that at the anode end of the beam (B), the apparent focus is smaller than at the cathode end (C) because of foreshortening. In practice, variations in geometric unsharpness due to this effect are usually masked by other forms of unsharpness.

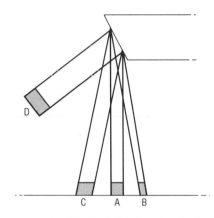

Fig. 3.12 Variation in the apparent size of the focal spot along the axis of an X-ray beam. A, B and C are three apparent focal areas. D is the actual focal area.

(2) *Object–image distance:* reducing object–image distance reduces geometric unsharpness. This is the origin of the radiographers' rule that the patient should be placed as close as possible to the cassette (or image intensifier). In cases where we are unable to fulfil this condition, the other factors determining geometric unsharpness must be modified if satisfactory image quality is to be maintained. The air gap techniques discussed earlier (section 3.1.1.3) require consideration along these lines.

Note that object–image distance is often referred to as **object–film distance**, and the abbreviation OFD is employed.

(3) *Focus–object distance:* increasing focus–object distance reduces geometric unsharpness. Focus–object distance is a concept not normally considered in diagnostic radiography, except from the viewpoint of radiation dose to the patient. But we often refer to **focus–film distance** (FFD) or source–image distance (SID). However, focus–object distance (FOD) is merely the difference between FFD and OFD:

FOD = FFD − OFD

It is therefore correct to say that increasing FFD reduces geometric unsharpness; hence, we can justify the use of long FFD values for chest radiography and for the lateral projection of the neck.

3.1.2.3   How can we minimize geometric unsharpness?

We have seen that there are three major parameters upon which geometric unsharpness depends. Changing any of them will affect the magnitude of this form of unsharpness. Let us now consider each modification in turn.

(1) Reduction of focal spot size

We can do this by selecting the smallest focal spot available on the X-ray tube. A reduction in geometric unsharpness will occur *as long as the other factors remain constant.* However, the rating (maximum output) of the X-ray tube falls when focal spot size is reduced (Carter, 1994), and we may find that the disadvantages introduced because of the fall in X-ray output outweigh the improvement in geometric unsharpness.

(2) Reduction of object–image distance

In general, we should arrange that the object–image distance is at a minimum. With radiography of the extremities this is rarely a problem, but in other cases thought may need to be given in deciding how to achieve minimum object–image distance. Even the use of a bucky table increases the distance between patient and cassette. The patient's own tissues may add to the problem; for example, in radiography of the lateral projection of the adult lumbar spine it is inevitable that the object–image distance will be large (25–35 cm). In many cases, the choice of whether to do an antero-posterior or postero-anterior projection depends on our assessment as to which gives the smaller geometric unsharpness.

(3) Extension of focus–object (or focus–film) distance

Diagnostic radiography is not usually undertaken with an FFD of less than about 90 cm because to do so would increase geometric unsharpness unduly and would also increase the radiation hazard to the patient unnecessarily.

Extending the FFD much beyond 100 cm introduces other problems. The intensity of the transmitted beam reduces with increasing distance, and to achieve an adequately exposed radiograph requires the selection of higher exposure factors. This may lead to the abandonment of the use of the fine focal spot in favour of the higher output offered by the broad focus. This in turn negates any improvement gained in geometric unsharpness. Only in selected cases does an overall improvement result.

There is thus no single solution to the problem of minimizing geometric unsharpness. Each case must be treated on its merits. The particular procedure adopted as standard for each radiographic examination has been determined over the years partly as a result of considerations such as we have described, and partly by trial and error. It is tempting to undertake radiographic examinations using the standard procedures without stopping to consider whether optimum image quality will result. But as professional radiographers and students of radiographic imaging, it is important that we gain an insight into the arguments for and against each procedure, perhaps bringing fresh ideas to the subject and making modifications if necessary.

3.1.2.4   Edge penetration

The finite size of the X-ray source is not the only cause of unsharpness in the invisible X-ray image. The nature of the structures that we are imaging may itself lead to unsharpness. Figure 3.13 illustrates an enlarged view of a small round opacity in the tissues of a patient. Examine the passage of several rays through the opacity. Ray 1 must penetrate the full thickness of the opacity and is heavily attenuated. Ray 2 traverses a smaller thickness and is attenuated to a lesser extent. Ray 3 passes almost tangentially to the opacity and is attenuated even less.

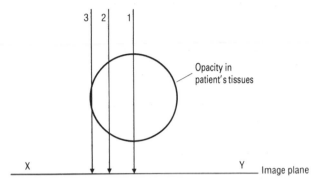

Fig. 3.13 Edge penetration. Three rays penetrating through a small, rounded opacity. Ray 1 suffers maximum attenuation, ray 3 minimum.

A trace of the distribution of transmitted intensity across the image plane XY is shown in Fig. 3.14. The gradual change in intensity demonstrated, confirms that the X-ray image is unsharp (Wilks, 1987). The cause of the unsharpness is the manner in which the X-ray beam penetrates the edges of the opacity. This form of unsharpness, due to **edge penetration**, is an inherent feature of X-ray imaging and would be present even if there were no geometric unsharpness.

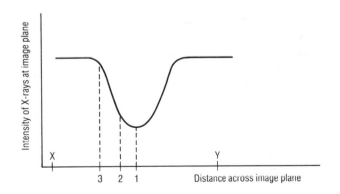

Fig. 3.14 Distribution of intensity of transmitted X-rays across the image plane XY in Fig. 3.13. The *gradual* change in intensity confirms that the image is unsharp due to edge penetration.

3.1.2.5 Movement (kinetic) unsharpness
The patients that we investigate are dynamic subjects: many of the tissues and organs are in motion, e.g. peristaltic movements of the gut, and cardiac and respiratory movements. In some cases, the patient as a whole may be in motion during the investigation, e.g. if restless or uncooperative or inadequately immo-

bilized. The effect of movement of the subject is to cause corresponding changes in the pattern of intensities forming the invisible X-ray image.

Such changes may lead to unsharpness in the final image if they occur during the time required for the image receptor to record the invisible X-ray image. Movement unsharpness, often abbreviated U_M, is dependent on the speed of response of the image receptor and we shall discuss its importance later (Chapters 16 and 17).

3.1.3   *Noise*

In Chapter 2 we described noise as that component of an image which carries no information about the subject. The presence of noise, and in particular the existence of a low **signal-to-noise ratio**, reduces the quality of the image.

We referred to three kinds of image noise:

(1) Fog – perhaps due to the presence of scattered radiation;
(2) Quantum noise – due to the quantum nature of the X-ray beam;
(3) Electronic noise – due to limitations in the electronic processing of the image.

In the present chapter we are confining our discussion to the characteristics of the invisible X-ray image in the beam transmitted through the patient, before any electronic processing takes place. Thus, electronic noise does not concern us at this stage. However, both image fog and quantum effects are relevant.

(1) Image fog
During our discussion of subject contrast earlier in this chapter (section 3.1.1), we described the damaging effects of scattered radiation on image quality. We showed that it reduces subject contrast. It results in a lowering of the signal-to-noise ratio by producing an overall fogging effect on the image. We have seen how the effects of scatter may be minimized.

Note that there are several other ways in which fog may be produced in the *final* radiographic image (e.g. safelight fog), but they occur later in the image-forming process and will be discussed under different headings.

(2) Quantum noise
The X-ray beam which produces the invisible X-ray image is not continuous. It can be thought of as a stream of particles (quanta or photons) of radiation energy. Each quantum, by its presence in the transmitted beam, carries information about the tissues of the patient. The greater the photon flux or the higher the density (concentration) of photons present in the transmitted beam, the greater is its information content. If the photons are spread too thinly, the gaps between them may become significant and lead to a 'grainy' appearance in the image.

3.1.3.1   **How can the effects of quantum noise be minimized?**
There are two basic ways to achieve this:

(1) Ensure that there is a sufficiently high density of photons in the incident beam. This is achieved by the selection of adequate exposure factors, producing a high enough X-ray intensity in the beam transmitted through the patient.
(2) Ensure that the image receptor is able to detect and process a high proportion of the quanta to which it is exposed, i.e. that it has a high **quantum detection efficiency** (see Chapter 5).

Note that only the first of these methods affects the quantum noise in the invisible

X-ray image, but if such noise is present at this early stage, there is little that can be done to correct the problem later. It may be possible to eliminate the grainy appearance of the final image by reducing image contrast and/or by increasing unsharpness, but the missing information, which is characterized by quantum noise, is lost forever.

3.1.4 Resolution

As we saw in Chapter 2, the resolution of an image depends on contrast, unsharpness and noise. In the context of the invisible X-ray image we must try to achieve the optimum resolution at this stage, so that during the later stages of the production of the visible radiographic image the inevitable losses which occur do not result in degradation of image quality to the extent that resolution of detail becomes unacceptably poor.

The consistent achievement of high-resolution final images depends on a sound knowledge of each step in the sequence of processes which lead to that final image. Moreover, we must also be aware of the relationships between the individual processes: the effects of each on the others. A study of the modulation transfer function (MTF) introduced in Chapter 2 will help us to quantify the relationships between the different contributory factors, which are discussed in Chapter 16.

3.2 Conclusion

We have described in some detail the process of formation of the invisible X-ray image and the characteristics possessed by this image. Such emphasis is justified for two reasons:

(1) If the invisible X-ray image is of poor quality, it is extremely difficult to produce an adequate standard of final visible image. The use of computer enhancement of image quality is well known in modern radiography (e.g. in computerized tomography, in digital subtraction techniques and more recently in computed radiography) and is most successful in the manipulation of contrast. But an image which suffers badly from geometric unsharpness is beyond help. It is therefore essential that the greatest attention is paid to the production of the highest quality X-ray image at this early stage.

(2) It is during the production of the invisible X-ray image that the radiographer has probably the greatest scope for control of image quality, particularly in conventional radiography. Care taken at this stage pays dividends in terms of the quality of the final image. Control of scattered radiation, selection of exposure factors, immobilization of the patient and minimization of geometric unsharpness are aspects which should always be given serious consideration *before* making an exposure.

In the next series of chapters (4–18) we consider the use of X-ray film and film–screen systems as image receptors in the production of a conventional radiograph.

Part 3
The Radiograph

Chapter 4
Photographic Principles

Having studied the method by which the invisible X-ray image is produced, we can now move on to examine how such an image is recorded and converted into a visible form. The traditional way in which X-ray images are recorded is by using the photographic effect of X-radiation on sensitive emulsion, and we shall concentrate on this method in the next few chapters.

4.1 The photographic effect

Some chemical compounds undergo subtle structural changes when they are exposed to electromagnetic radiations such as visible light, ultraviolet radiation or X-rays. The changes in most cases are not immediately visible, but they are associated with an alteration in the chemical behaviour of the substance such that in certain chemical reactions the exposed material responds differently from similar materials which have *not* been exposed to radiation and whose structure has therefore not been affected. By careful chemical processing, it is possible to differentiate between exposed and unexposed materials, producing visible differences between them and thus creating a visible image (Horder, 1958).

The effect on the chemical nature of the material is known as the **photographic effect** of radiation and the chemical processing necessary to make the invisible changes visible is known as **photographic development**. In this chapter we shall discuss the changes which occur in photosensitive materials and also some aspects of their manufacture and performance. The chemical processing of the photosensitive materials used in radiography is discussed more fully in Chapter 9.

4.2   Photosensitive materials

Radiography is a specialized application of the photographic process, but the light-sensitive agents employed in radiography are the same as or similar to those used in photography generally and are known as **silver halides** (Fuji, 1983).

4.2.1   *Silver halides*

The silver halides are a group of chemical compounds consisting of atoms of the element silver combined with atoms of the halogen elements: bromine, iodine and chlorine. The compounds thus formed are silver bromide, silver iodide and silver chloride. These compounds are used because they are particularly sensitive to light (and X-rays). When they are exposed to these radiations, they undergo changes which enable them to form a photographic (or radiographic) image. In radiography, silver bromide is the most commonly used photosensitive agent. Silver iodide is used in smaller amounts, but silver chloride is only used in special applications.

4.2.1.1   **Physical properties of silver halides**
Silver halides are white or pale-yellow crystalline salts similar in appearance to common salt. The links between the silver and halogen atoms are described as **ionic bonds**. Ionic bonds occur when positive and negative **ions** (atoms which are electrically charged) are locked together by the electric forces of attraction between them. In silver halides, the silver ions are positively charged and the halide ions are negatively charged. The electric forces fix the positions of the silver and halide ions in a regular three-dimensional crystal structure or **lattice** (Fig. 4.1).

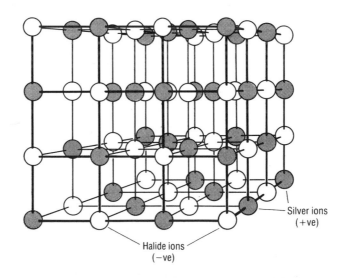

Silver ions
(+ve)

Halide ions
(−ve)

Fig. 4.1 The crystal lattice structure of silver halides. The perspective view shows a 4 × 4 × 4 matrix of silver and halide ions forming a cubic crystal. The connecting lines represent the electric forces holding the ions in place

4.2.1.2 Chemical properties of silver halides

Pure silver halide crystals are relatively stable and do not readily suffer chemical breakdown. Under certain conditions, however, it is possible to neutralize all the positively charged silver ions in a silver halide and convert them to **atoms** of metallic silver. This conversion is achieved by donating negatively charged electrons to the silver ions. A chemical which provides a supply of electrons for this purpose is known as a **reducing agent** and is said to **reduce** the silver halide to silver.

The chemical reduction to silver of a silver halide sample which has been exposed to radiation takes place much more rapidly than the reduction of an unexposed sample. This difference in rate of reduction is a key feature of photographic processing, and photographic development is primarily a process of chemical reduction (Pizzutiello & Cullinan, 1993).

4.2.1.3 Effects of exposure on silver halides

What happens when a silver halide is irradiated?

We have said that invisible structural changes occur in silver halide crystals when they are exposed to light or X-radiation. Let us now examine the nature of these changes (Hay, 1982; Fuji, 1983).

Figure 4.2 shows the regular arrangement of silver and bromine ions in a crystal of pure silver bromide. Note that only a single lattice plane is illustrated since it is difficult to show clearly in two dimensions the true three-dimensional nature of the lattice. Figure 4.3 shows the passage through the crystal of a photon of light (or X-radiation). Frequently, particularly with X-rays, a photon penetrates right through the crystal and emerges unscathed. In such cases, the crystal suffers no change in its structure: its exposure to radiation remains undetected. In other cases, however, a photon is absorbed in the crystal (Fig. 4.4). It interacts with a bromine ion, causing it to release an electron. The electron is then free to move about inside the crystal, but within a very short time (of the order of 10^{-11} s) it becomes lodged in a low-energy electron trap near the surface of the crystal, known as a **sensitivity speck**.

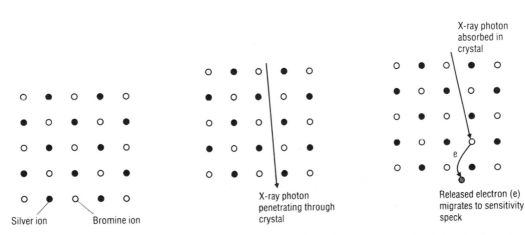

Fig. 4.2 The arrangement of silver and bromine ions in a silver bromide crystal.

Fig. 4.3 The passage of an X-ray photon through a crystal of silver bromide.

Fig. 4.4 The interaction between an X-ray photon and a bromine ion. The electron released migrates to a low energy electron trap or 'sensitivity speck'.

Sensitivity specks are produced by the deliberate introduction of traces of 'impurities' into the silver halide during its manufacture.

As it collects more and more electrons, each sensitivity speck acquires a negative electric charge. The charge becomes strong enough to draw towards the sensitivity speck those positively charged silver ions in the crystal which are not firmly held in the lattice. As the silver ions arrive, they each gain an electron which neutralizes their charge and transforms them from silver ions into atoms of metallic silver.

4.2.1.4   Significance of the formation of metallic silver

In normal circumstances, the number of silver atoms created in the way we have described amounts to only a few hundred per crystal – certainly too few to make a noticeable difference to the appearance of the crystal. However, this tiny collection of silver atoms has a critical effect on the chemical behaviour of the silver halide crystal. In particular, it renders the crystal much more vulnerable than unexposed crystals to attack by the reducing agent in photographic developer. The sensitivity speck now acts as a **development centre** in exposed crystals, enabling them to be reduced completely to silver during the development process. We shall examine development more fully in Chapter 9.

4.2.1.5   The latent image

The existence on a film of numbers of silver halide crystals possessing development centres is said to constitute a **latent image**. A latent image is defined as an **invisible** image formed as a result of exposure to radiation, and which may later be made visible by photographic development. The explanation we have provided for the formation of the latent image is based on the **Gurney–Mott theory**. Although this theory is still widely accepted in radiography, its status has been challenged by the **Mitchell theory** which arose from research into solid state physics. There are close similarities between the two theories, but they differ in the way they explain the early stages in the formation of silver atoms at the sensitivity speck of an exposed silver halide crystal (Gunn, 1994).

4.2.1.6   Differences between silver halides and metallic silver

The conversion from silver halide to metallic silver of exposed parts of a radiographic image is important because the two substances have different properties:

(1) Silver halides can be converted into soluble compounds by the action of chemicals known as **fixing agents**. Metallic silver is unaffected by fixing agents and remains insoluble. This provides a means of separating silver halide from metallic silver.

(2) Metallic silver is opaque to light and its presence can easily be seen as a darkened area against a light background. The blackened parts of a radiographic image are formed from metallic silver.

(3) Silver halides are sensitive to light, while metallic silver is not. An image which contains traces of silver halide can be expected to undergo changes if exposed to light. Such an image will not be permanent. However, an image formed entirely by the presence of metallic silver will not be affected by light and is essentially permanent.

To make use of silver halides in image-recording materials, they must be available in a convenient form commonly known as **photographic emulsion**.

4.3   Photographic emulsion

Photographic emulsion is the photosensitive layer on an X-ray film. It is a suspension of microscopic crystals of silver halide in gelatin. The emulsion of X-ray films is coated onto a supporting layer of transparent plastic film known as the base. Let us examine the two essential ingredients of a photographic emulsion: gelatin and silver halide.

4.3.1   *Gelatin*

An essential property of gelatin is that it can exist either as a liquid or as a solid 'jelly' and it can easily be transformed from one state to the other, e.g. liquid gelatin **sets** into a solid gel when it is cooled. Pure gelatin is used as the suspending medium and **binding agent** for the silver halide particles.

4.3.1.1   Functions of the gelatin emulsion binder

(1) It is the medium in which silver halide crystals form and grow during the chemical production of the silver halides (see below).

(2) It maintains the silver halide crystals uniformly distributed in the liquid emulsion prior to coating onto the film base so that they do not settle out or form local concentrations. Uneven distribution would cause unacceptable 'patchy' variations in blackening in the final radiographic image.

(3) Gelatin does not react chemically with the silver halides that it holds in suspension. Indeed, it may *increase* the ability of the silver halides to store the latent image resulting from exposure until processing takes place.

(4) It allows the film base to be coated evenly with warm liquid emulsion, which is then chilled and allowed to set. It is later dried and chemically hardened but retains enough flexibility to resist the normal mechanical stresses to which X-ray films are subjected during their lifetime.

(5) In its solid state, it can be wetted and then allows penetration by the chemical agents used during photographic processing. Gelatin is permeable, and when an X-ray film is immersed in a processing solution the gelatin absorbs water and softens, allowing the active agents in the solution to diffuse through the emulsion and react with the silver halide crystals held in suspension.

(6) It holds firmly in position the metallic silver particles which form during development, preventing them from clumping together. The result of such clumping would be unwanted graininess in the final image.

(7) Gelatin is a **transparent** medium, enabling the silver image it will carry to be viewed without difficulty.

4.3.2   *Silver halides*

As we have seen, crystals of a silver halide such as silver bromide undergo subtle structural changes when exposed to light or to X-rays. It is vital that the halides used in the emulsion of X-ray film have no previous history of exposure to radiation when they are incorporated into photosensitive emulsion. To ensure that this is so, the silver halides are actually synthesized in the liquid gelatin which will later form the emulsion.

Silver halides are a product of the chemical reaction between silver nitrate and an alkali halide such as potassium bromide. They are formed as part of the production of photographic emulsion during the manufacture of X-ray film. The production of emulsion and manufacture of X-ray film are highly complex processes and we shall only outline the broad principles involved. The entire procedure is carried out in conditions of absolute cleanliness, with temperature and humidity closely controlled. All light is excluded and the atmosphere is dust-free. Rigorous quality control is maintained throughout.

4.3.3   Production of photographic emulsion

(1) Solutions of silver nitrate and potassium bromide (and other alkali halides) are added at controlled rates and in measured quantities to liquid gelatin. Rather more bromide is used than the chemical reaction requires (see section 9.2.1.1 for the reason why).

(2) On mixing, the silver nitrate and potassium bromide react to form potassium nitrate (in solution) and a precipitate of tiny insoluble crystals or **grains** of silver bromide dispersed uniformly through the gelatin. If the mixing process is carried out rapidly, all the grains produced will be of roughly equal size. There is said to be a *narrow* **grain size distribution** (GSD). Such an emulsion has high-contrast characteristics. If the mixing process is more prolonged, those grains produced early in the process are able to grow to a significantly larger size than those produced towards the end of the mixing process, and a *wide* GSD results. An emulsion produced in this way will exhibit lower-contrast characteristics (Kodak, 1980). Note, however, that there are many other factors which influence the contrast of a radiographic image.

(3) The unwanted potassium nitrate is removed from the gelatin by allowing it to set, shredding it, and then washing it in water. The potassium nitrate diffuses from the gel into the water, while the insoluble silver halides remain.

(4) The gel is re-liquefied and undergoes repeated cycles of heating and cooling (processes known as **ripening** and **digestion**) to encourage the halide grains to grow in size and to allow sensitivity specks to form. The **average grain size** affects the sensitivity (speed) of an emulsion to exposure. An emulsion with relatively large grains will respond to lower levels of radiation (light or X-rays) than an emulsion with smaller grains. Thus, it is during these stages that the basic speed characteristics of an emulsion are largely determined.

(5) Finally, prior to coating onto the film base, other agents are added to the suspension, e.g.:

(a) **Sensitizers** to increase the response of the emulsion to radiation and to control its sensitivity to different colours of light (spectral sensitivity);

(b) **Antifrothing agents** to prevent the formation of air bubbles during coating which would otherwise produce imperfections in the emulsion layers on the film;

(c) **Plasticizers, hardeners, wetting agents, antifoggants, bactericides** and **fungicides**. These agents are included to enable the emulsion to survive the rigours of photographic processing later in its life (see Chapter 9).

4.3.4   The coating process

The liquid photographic emulsion is coated onto a suitable base, such as the transparent polyester plastic film referred to earlier.

To aid adhesion, the base is precoated with a thin **subbing layer** or **substratum,** which helps bind the emulsion to the base.

During coating it is essential that a constant thickness of emulsion is applied over the entire area of film base. Any local differences in thickness would result in optical density variations in the final image, because the sensitivity of an emulsion depends partly on its coating thickness. Once the liquid emulsion has been applied, it is allowed to set firmly onto the base. Finally, a thin protective **supercoat** of pure gelatin is applied.

It is common practice for X-ray films to have emulsion applied to *both* sides of the base material in order to increase sensitivity. Such films are said to be **duplitized** or double coated. Figure 4.5 shows a magnified cross-section through duplitized X-ray film. Single-coated X-ray films have a gelatin layer applied to their reverse (non-emulsion) side.

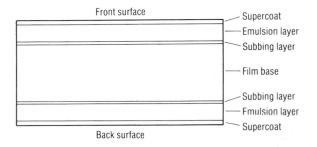

Fig. 4.5 Cross-section through duplitized X-ray film. Emulsion layers are coated on *both* sides of the base material to improve sensitivity to exposure.

Coating of the flexible X-ray film base is a continuous process and the completed product is wound onto large rolls. Later, the film is cut into the shapes and sizes (18 × 24 cm, 24 × 30 cm, 35 × 35 cm, etc.) with which we are all familiar, before being packed for shipment to X-ray departments. Although extremely high standards of manufacture are maintained, occasionally a faulty batch of film is released to the customer. In such cases, identification of the **batch number** on the film box may help the manufacturer to trace the exact cause of the fault.

4.4　Light-sensitive and X-ray-sensitive emulsions

There are two fundamentally different conditions of exposure for the films used in X-ray departments:

(1) They may be exposed to the visible light emitted by fluorescent intensifying screens, cathode ray tubes or image intensifiers;
(2) They may be exposed solely to X-radiation.

It is not possible to design one all-purpose photographic emulsion which will perform well under both conditions, so the manufacturers of film supply two basically different types of film, possessing quite different emulsion characteristics. Let us examine these film types in more detail.

4.4.1　*Light-sensitive film*

Of course, *all* film is light sensitive, but the film to which we refer has its image produced as a result of exposure to light rather than to X-rays (e.g. X-ray screen-type film). The photographic emulsion used in these films *must* respond well to visible light exposure. Fundamentally, this means that the emulsion layer (or layers) on the film must absorb the energy of the visible light photons incident upon it. As many as possible of the photons must be absorbed in the emulsion, because any photons which are transmitted *through* the emulsion layers cannot release their energy to the emulsion and cannot trigger the photographic effect.

As we have seen (section 4.3.1.1), the gelatin emulsion binder is transparent, and it is the silver halide grains which must absorb the light photons. Silver halides *do* absorb visible light, particularly light from the blue–violet part of the electromagnetic spectrum, but a photon can only be absorbed if there is a silver halide grain in its path. To ensure efficient absorption, therefore, the emulsion must contain a high concentration of silver halide. This may be achieved by:

(1) Close packing of the silver halide grains;
(2) Increasing the size of the halide grains;
(3) Increasing the thickness of the emulsion layer;
(4) Modifying the shape of the halide grains.

In practice, maximum grain size is limited to avoid noticeable 'graininess' in the final image. Graininess may reduce the resolution of the image.

Emulsion thickness is limited for several reasons:

(1) Image resolution tends to reduce as emulsion thickness increases;
(2) Thick emulsion layers require longer processing times, because processing solutions take longer to penetrate through the emulsion;
(3) Most absorption of light occurs in the upper layers of the emulsion. There is therefore little to be gained by increasing emulsion thickness beyond an optimum depth. Figure 4.6 shows the penetration of light photons into a layer of photographic emulsion.

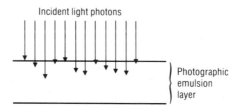

Fig. 4.6 Penetration of light photons into the emulsion layer. The majority of light photons are absorbed in the upper layers of the emulsion.

4.4.1.1 Duplitized film

The duplitizing of film is a method of gaining the benefits of increased emulsion thickness with few of the drawbacks. Duplitized film is designed for use with *two* intensifying screens and is still the most commonly used type of X-ray film in the X-ray department. Each emulsion coat on the film is exposed directly to the light emitted by the screen with which it is in contact. After processing there are in fact two images, one on each side of the film base, but because the base is so thin and the two images are essentially identical, when the radiograph is viewed the two images are superimposed and observed as one. Only on very close examination is it possible to detect the true dual nature of the image due to the **parallax** effect (section 5.1.1.2).

Advantages of duplitized film

The main advantages claimed for duplitized film used in conjunction with twin intensifying screens are:

(1) Increased sensitivity, i.e. adequate image density can be achieved from a smaller radiation exposure. This has two important consequences:
   (a) Radiation doses to patients and staff are reduced;
   (b) Wear on the X-ray tubes is reduced, thus extending their working life.
(2) Increased image contrast: the contribution made by film emulsion to the eventual contrast of the image is greater because of the greater effective emulsion thickness. This may enable higher tube kilovoltages to be employed without significant loss of contrast.

Disadvantages of duplitized film

(1) Loss of image quality: the use of a duplitized film and twin-screen system may introduce a *loss* of image quality compared with other image recording systems. For example, the **crossover** of light from each intensifying screen to the emulsion on the 'wrong' side of the film leads to a loss of sharpness in the image. This will be discussed further in Chapter 7. In some circumstances, such a loss of image quality is so serious that other systems which require higher radiation exposures must be used. Parallax effect produces *no* significant losses.
(2) Economic reasons: duplitized films use a higher coating weight of silver than single-coated films, and silver is an expensive and diminishing world resource.

It may be argued that considerations such as these could eventually lead to the demise of the duplitized film and twin-screen systems in favour of single-coated film used with a single intensifying screen.

4.4.1.2 Single-coated (single-sided) film

Many systems are now available which use a single-coated, screen-type X-ray film inside a cassette housing just one intensifying screen. Such a system is capable of a higher-quality image since it overcomes some of the problems inherent in twin-screen systems. The single-coated films employed possess a type of emulsion similar to that used with duplitized film, but the emulsion coat is applied only to one side of its base. Care must be taken when using such films because they must only be loaded into a cassette with their emulsion side in contact with the intensifying screen. To help identify the emulsion side of single-coated film in the darkroom, the manufacturer cuts a small notch into one edge of each film. If a film is held vertically, with the notch at the right-hand end of the upper edge, the emulsion side is nearest; see Fig. 4.7.

4.4.1.3 Spectral sensitivity

We have observed that for maximum effect the emulsion of screen-type X-ray films must absorb the light photons being received from the intensifying screen(s). It must be remembered that light can be of many different colours, representing different wavelengths of electromagnetic radiation. The spectrum is a display of the different colours arranged in order of wavelength (Fig. 4.8). Red light has a wavelength of about 700 nanometres (a nanometre (nm) is one millionth of a millimetre). Violet

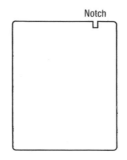

Notch

Fig. 4.7 Identifying the emulsion side of single-coated film. The emulsion side is facing if the film is held with the notch in the top right-hand corner as shown. Note that the size of the notch has been exaggerated for the sake of clarity.

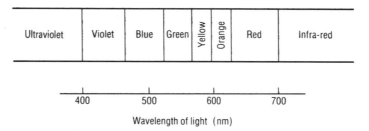

Wavelength of light (nm)

Fig. 4.8 The visible light spectrum. Note that there is no clear boundary between the different colours of the spectrum. Rather each colour merges gradually into the next. Many sources (e.g. Gunn, 1994) identify a seventh distinct colour between violet and blue (indigo).

light has a wavelength of about 400 nm. Ultraviolet and infra-red rays, with wavelengths outside these limits, are not visible to the human eye, but photographic emulsions can be made to respond to some of these invisible radiations.

It is found that light of different colours is absorbed differently in the emulsion, e.g. blue light is absorbed better than red light. The behaviour of emulsion in this respect is known as its **spectral response** and it is a critical feature of emulsion characteristics. During manufacture, colour sensitizers are incorporated into the emulsion to control its spectral response.

Without the use of sensitizers, a silver bromide emulsion is far more sensitive to blue, violet and ultraviolet light than to the rest of the spectrum, and is known as a **monochromatic** emulsion. Indeed, it may require prolonged or intense exposure to red light before any photographic effect is produced. This property of limited spectral response forms the basis for the safelighting employed in photographic darkrooms (see Chapter 12).

If sensitizers are incorporated, the spectral response can be extended into the green (up to 570 nm), known as **orthochromatic** emulsion, or even as far as the red (up to 700 nm) in a **panchromatic** emulsion (Fuji, 1983).

Ideally, a film emulsion should respond well to the particular wavelengths of light emitted by the fluorescent intensifying screen. If this is so, then the spectral response of the emulsion is said to be **matched** to the spectral emission of the screen phosphors. The use of film which is poorly matched to its intensifying screens leads to a loss of sensitivity and an increase in the required X-ray exposure.

We shall discuss the spectral response of film emulsion again, later in this chapter (section 4.5.6).

4.4.1.4 Effect of X-rays on screen-type film

We have discussed the effect of light from the intensifying screens on both double- and single-coated screen-type film, but these emulsion layers also receive a **direct** exposure to X-radiation. However, the effect of this is minimal, as can be seen if a simple experiment is carried out.

4.4.1.5 Testing the direct effect of X-rays on screen-type film

The effect can be demonstrated if the light from the intensifying screens in a cassette is prevented from reaching the film:

(1) Under safelight conditions in the darkroom, fold a sheet of opaque black paper around the film before it is loaded into its cassette, making sure that only part of the film is covered (Fig. 4.9);
(2) In the X-ray room, radiograph a suitable phantom onto the specially loaded cassette, using exposure factors appropriate to the film–screen combination employed;
(3) Process the film normally.

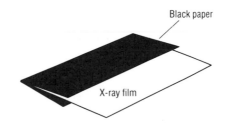

Black paper

X-ray film

Fig. 4.9 Protecting part of an X-ray screen film from light by enclosing it in opaque black paper before loading it into a cassette.

Warning

(1) Do not attempt to load or unload the cassette automatically in a 'daylight-handling' system: the paper would almost certainly cause a jam!
(2) Remember to dispose of the black paper before reloading the cassette when you have finished!

Examination of the processed film will reveal only a faint trace of an image on the area protected from light, while the unprotected area appears correctly exposed. Less than 5% of the image density is attributable to the direct effect of X-ray exposure in a film–screen system, the exact percentage depending on the speed of the system used. This does not mean, however, that such film need not be protected from accidental exposure to X-rays, e.g. due to careless storage of loaded cassettes in an X-ray room.

4.4.1.6 Other types of light-sensitive film

Modern imaging departments are using increasing quantities of light-sensitive film other than the traditional 'X-ray films'. Fluorographic film is popular for recording the images from an image intensifier. A range of films is available for recording the images from a laser imager or from cathode-ray-tube (CRT) screens during computerized tomography (CT), **radionuclide imaging** (RNI) and **diagnostic ultrasound**. Fluorographic, laser imager and CRT films have a single emulsion coat. The spectral response of these films is matched to the light source from which they receive their exposure. We shall examine films with such specialized applications in Chapters 21 and 23.

4.4.2 X-ray-sensitive ('direct-exposure') film

We will now consider those X-ray films whose images are produced entirely by the effect of direct exposure to X-radiation. Such films are no longer widely used in X-ray departments, but there remain a number of specialized applications, such as intra-oral dental radiography and foreign body detection, where the use of **direct-exposure**, (**envelope-wrapped** or **non-screen**) film is still justified.

The emulsion of direct-exposure film is designed to absorb as much as possible of the X-ray beam to which it is exposed. Despite using a specially formulated emulsion, the sensitivity of such films is poor compared with even the slowest film–screen system (Pizzutiello & Cullinan, 1993). The particular design features of direct-exposure film include:

(1) **Duplitization**: such film is invariably duplitized to gain the benefit of maximum emulsion thickness. Unlike light-sensitive film, there is no fall-off in photographic response as the emulsion thickness increases. The limiting factors here are:
  (a) The loss of image sharpness which occurs with increasing emulsion thickness;
  (b) The processing time: as emulsion thickness increases, so does the time taken for the processing chemicals to penetrate deeply into the emulsion and for the absorbed water to be evaporated from the emulsion during the drying stage. For best results, direct-exposure film needs significantly longer processing cycle times than other films;
  (c) Adhesion of the emulsion layer: there is a limit to the thickness of emulsion which can be securely coated onto the base.
(2) **Sensitizers**: the inclusion in the emulsion of additional sensitizing agents enables sensitivity to direct X-ray exposure to be increased. By this means the emulsion thickness need not be excessive, allowing the film to be more rapidly processed.

With the advances made recently in intensifying screen technology, it is increasingly difficult to justify the continued use of direct-exposure film solely on the grounds of superior image quality.

4.5 Describing photographic performance

It is often necessary in radiography to be able to evaluate and compare the performance of one film or one film–screen system against another. To facilitate these comparisons, we need to define the various aspects of the images being examined (e.g. density, contrast, etc.) and we require a convenient method for describing the performance of such image recording systems. The most widely used method available is known as the **characteristic curve**. It is an essential tool in **sensitometry**, the scientific study of the response to exposure of photosensitive materials. It illustrates graphically and concisely many of the critical features of the way a system responds to exposure (Workman & Cowen, 1994).

The performance of an image recording system is tested by subjecting it to a range of different exposures and then examining the photographic densities which result. But how are density and exposure defined? Let us examine these two concepts more closely.

4.5.1 *Density*

The result of exposing a film is that after processing a blackening effect is produced, the degree of blackening being dependent on the level of exposure received. How is blackening quantified? There are two approaches to the problem:

(1) **Transparency:** we can express the transparency of the image; i.e. we can measure the intensity (I_t) of light transmitted through the film and express it as a fraction or percentage of the intensity (I_0) of light incident on the film (see Fig. 4.10). **Fractional transmission** or **transmission ratio** is the ratio of transmitted light to incident light:

$$\text{Transmission ratio} = I_t/I_0$$
$$\text{Percentage transmission} = 100 \times I_t/I_0$$

A perfectly opaque area of an image has zero transmission ratio and zero percentage transmission. A perfectly transparent area has a transmission ratio of 1, and 100% transmission. As film blackening increases the transmission values reduce.

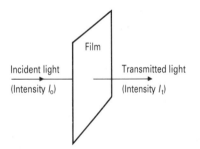

Fig. 4.10 Transmission of light through a film. The intensity of light incident upon the film is I_0; the intensity of light transmitted through the film is I_t. Transmission ratio is then I_t/I_0.

(2) **Opacity:** we can express the opacity of the image by inverting the transmission ratio. This gives us a quantity which increases as blackening increases (and as exposure increases):

$$\text{Opacity} = I_0/I_t$$

A perfectly transparent area of an image has an opacity of 1. A perfectly opaque area has an infinite opacity! The blackest part of a radiographic image has an opacity approaching 10 000. Thus, there is a vast range of values of opacity to contend with.

Because the action of radiation exposure is to *blacken* rather than lighten a film, it seems logical to select an approach based on the expression of opacity rather than transparency. However, the extreme range of values associated with this quantity requires further thought.

4.5.1.1 Optical density

One method by which the range may be reduced to more manageable proportions is to convert the opacity to its logarithmic value. For example, using logarithms to the base 10, an opacity of 1000 converts to 3 (because $1000 = 10^3$); an opacity of 10 000 becomes 4 ($10\,000 = 10^4$), and an opacity of 1 (perfectly transparent) becomes 0 (because $1 = 10^0$). Thus, the simple mathematical 'trick' of expressing opacity in logarithmic terms produces a much more useful quantity, which is termed **optical density** (or **photographic density**):

$$\text{Optical density} = \log_{10} \text{opacity}$$
$$= \log_{10} (I_0/I_t)$$

On a typical radiographic image, optical density values vary from about 0.2 in the most transparent parts, to 3.5 or 4 in the blackest parts of the image. The mid-grey tones which form what are often the most useful parts of the image have densities close to 1.

As well as giving a more convenient range of numerical values, there are other benefits to be gained by using this logarithmic concept of density:

(1) Density increases with exposure.
(2) Density of a photographic image is approximately proportional to the amount of silver present in the emulsion: a density of 2 has roughly twice the silver present compared with a density of 1.
(3) Combining densities is simple: the total density produced by superimposing a number of separate images is equal to the sum of their separate densities.
(4) The human eye seems to respond to differing tones in a way which is approximately logarithmic. A density of 2 *looks* twice as dark as a density of 1 (Fuji, 1983).

For the purpose of this discussion we have assumed the images being considered are transparencies, viewed by transmitted light. Were we to consider *print* images, which are viewed by reflected light, a different concept of density known as **reflection density** would be required, based on the reflection properties of the image rather than its transmission properties (Horder, 1958).

Note that for convenience, it is common to refer to optical density as just 'density' and in radiographic imaging it seems quite acceptable to do so. We shall generally use the abbreviated form in this book. Sometimes, however, to avoid confusion with the term density used in physics (meaning mass/volume), it is safer to employ the full title.

4.5.2 *X-ray exposure*

In conventional radiography, the image recording system is exposed to X-radiation. A film–screen system has its intensifying screens exposed to X-rays and a non-screen system has its film directly exposed to X-rays. It appears, therefore, that we need to measure the X-ray exposure involved. Note that the term 'X-ray exposure' is *not* synonymous with 'exposure factors'. It refers to a physical measure of exposure in units such as coulombs per kilogram (SI units) or roentgens (traditional units). To obtain such absolute measurements with consistency and accuracy is no easy matter. It is, however, quite possible to produce **relative** values of exposure.

4.5.2.1 Relative exposure

If a sheet of screen-type X-ray film is divided into (say) ten small areas and each area is exposed in a cassette using the same tube kilovoltage (kVp) and tube current (mA) but different exposure times, it is a simple matter to relate the X-ray exposure received by each area. For example, if an exposure time of 0.01 s is used for area A and 0.02 s for area B, it is reasonable to suppose that area B has received twice the X-ray exposure of area A; i.e. the **relative exposure** is 2 at B compared with 1 at A.

The area of film which has been given the smallest exposure is used as the baseline and is allocated a relative exposure of unity, and the other areas, subjected to higher exposures, then have relative exposure values greater than one. For example, areas A–I receive exposures of 1–256, as shown in Table 4.1. It is convenient to arrange that the values of relative exposure rise in geometric progression, i.e. each value is a constant multiple of the previous value, the multiple being 2 in the example quoted above. The reason for this is explained below.

Table 4.1 The relative exposures received by different areas of the film.

Area	A	B	C	D	E	F	G	H	I
Relative exposure	1	2	4	8	16	32	64	128	256

4.5.2.2 Log relative exposure

For a typical radiographic image, the range of exposure reaching different areas of the film–screen system is very great. The intensity of radiation producing the blackest parts of the image may be thousands of times greater than that producing the lowest densities. Thus, the values of relative exposure may vary from unity to several thousand. This causes problems of scaling if relative exposure is to be plotted on a graph.

As with density measurements, the answer lies in quoting the **logarithmic** value of relative exposure. A range of 1–1000 then becomes a range of 0–3. A series of relative exposure values which increase in geometric progression (e.g. 1, 2, 4, 8, 16, 32, ...) will produce a series of logarithmic values which increase in arithmetic progression (0, 0.3, 0.6, 0.9, 1.2, 1.5, ...) and will be evenly spaced if plotted on a graph. **NB** A log relative exposure value of zero does *not* represent zero exposure. Rather it represents the 'baseline' exposure value with which all other exposures have been compared. In fact it is not possible to express zero exposure as a logarithmic value.

It has been found that the log relative exposure method of quantifying the exposure received by X-ray films and film–screen systems is both convenient and reliable. Its applications extend beyond X-ray films to film materials such as those which record cathode-ray-tube images in which exposure to **light** alone is involved.

Having defined suitable methods for expressing the exposure received by a film or film–screen system and the image blackening which results, we can move on to consider how these two quantities are related. The relationship is conveniently described by means of a graph known as a characteristic curve.

4.5.3 The characteristic curve

The characteristic curve is a graph which illustrates the way in which a film or film–screen system responds to different levels of exposure. Different film emulsions, different intensifying screens and different film–screen combinations respond to exposure in different ways, and their characteristic curves reflect these differences. The characteristic curve is therefore a valuable tool for describing the sensitometric behaviour of a photographic recording system. Since the blackening produced on a film is intimately linked with the processing it has received, the shape of a characteristic curve is also dependent on processing.

The characteristic curve is a plot of optical density (D) against log relative exposure (log E). For this reason, the curve is sometimes known as a D log E curve. Alternatively, the graph may be called a **Hurter and Driffield** or H and D curve, after two pioneers in sensitometry (Kodak, 1981).

4.5.4 How is a characteristic curve produced?

We shall discuss the value of characteristic curves in the implementation of image quality assurance programmes in Chapter 18. However, it is necessary to look at the principles involved in order to understand more fully the meaning of characteristic curves. There are three basic stages involved:

(1) Exposing and processing the film.
(2) Measuring the densities produced.
(3) Plotting the curve.

We shall now examine each stage in turn.

4.5.4.1 Exposing and processing the film

To generate a characteristic curve we need to irradiate the film or film–screen system with a series of exposures which progress in known steps so that the relative exposure received by each step can be recorded. The relationship between one exposure and the next is known as the **wedge factor**. Its value should preferably be constant throughout the exposure range, in order to obtain evenly spaced points for plotting. To enable a well defined curve to be drawn, it is usual to provide 21 exposure steps related by a wedge factor of (say) $\sqrt{2}$ (i.e. 1.414). The smallest exposure must be such that no measurable effect can be seen on the film. The heaviest exposure should be greater than that sufficient to activate every silver halide grain in the emulsion, so that the maximum possible density is produced.

The exposure series can be achieved in one of two ways (Kodak, 1981):

(1) **Time-scale sensitometry** – with this method each area on the film is exposed to the same intensity of radiation, but the *duration* of the exposure is varied to provide the required range of relative exposures. If, as is often the case, an X-ray unit is used as the radiation source, then the exposure timer is the means by which exposure duration is adjusted.
(2) **Intensity-scale sensitometry** – in this case, each area on the film is exposed for the same length of time (usually all areas are exposed simultaneously) but the *intensity* of radiation on each area is varied. The exposure may be made either by using X-radiation or by using light.

X-ray exposure
With an X-ray exposure, the intensity variations are normally generated by passing

the X-ray beam through a stepped wedge made from a material such as aluminium (Fig. 4.11). The differential attenuation caused by the **step-wedge** creates the required range of intensities. The difficulty with this method is in finding the relationship between the intensities transmitted through the different step thicknesses. A process of **calibration** of the step-wedge must first be carried out to discover the wedge factor, which relates the intensities transmitted through successive steps, and therefore the relative exposures received by the film (section 4.5.5.5). However, the calibration obtained is only valid for one specific quality of radiation. If tube kV, type of high-tension generator or beam filtration are altered, a recalibration must be carried out. An additional complication is that the wedge factor is not the same for all steps on the step-wedge, because X-ray beam quality becomes modified by an amount dependent on step thickness during its passage through the step-wedge.

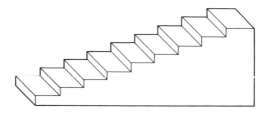

Fig. 4.11 An aluminium step-wedge. When radiographed, this test object transmits a range of different X-ray intensities to the image receptor beneath.

Visible light exposure
If the film is to be exposed to light rather than to X-rays, a commercially available device known as a **sensitometer** can be used. An internal light source produces a beam of uniform intensity. Before it exposes the film test strip, the light beam is passed through a light attenuator known as a **grey scale**. The grey scale transmits a series of stepped intensities whose relative values are known. Thus, the relative exposures received by the test film are easily obtained.

Once the film test strip has been exposed, by one of the methods indicated above, it is processed in the film processor in the X-ray department.

4.5.4.2   Measuring the densities produced
The optical density of each exposed step on the film test strip must be measured using a densitometer. Depending on its degree of sophistication, the densitometer may have an integral light source or it may need to be used on a normal X-ray illuminator; the density read-out may be from a digital display or from an analogue display using a pointer and calibrated scale. In either case, a value of density for each exposed area may be read off. These values should be tabulated alongside the corresponding values of relative exposure. The values of log relative exposure must be obtained (e.g. from an electronic calculator) and included in the table, as shown in Table 4.2.

4.5.4.3   Plotting the curve
The axes of the graph are scaled as shown in Fig. 4.12. The same scale should be adopted for both axes, e.g. if 2 cm represents a density change of 1 on the vertical axis it should also represent a change of 1 in log relative exposure on the horizontal

Table 4.2 Tabulation of results obtained prior to plotting a characteristic curve.

Area	A	B	C	D	E	F	G	H	I
Density	0.25	0.3	0.4	0.9	1.45	2.1	2.5	2.7	2.9
Relative exposure	1	2	4	8	16	32	64	128	256
Log relative exposure	0	0.3	0.6	0.9	1.2	1.5	1.8	2.1	2.4

axis. The vertical density axis extends from zero to a value beyond the maximum density achieved on the test strip. Typically, this will be about 3.5 for screen-type X-ray film but higher, perhaps up to 6.0, for direct-exposure film. The horizontal log relative exposure axis extends from zero to a value beyond the maximum log relative exposure given. Typically, this will be at least 3.0. The values of log relative exposure and corresponding density are then plotted and the points joined to form a smooth curve, as shown in Fig. 4.13. A more convenient method is to enter the data into a personal computer (PC). Most spreadsheet and database packages offer a range of charting and graphing options from which high quality characteristic curves can be produced without difficulty.

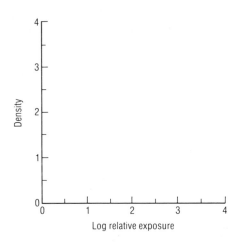

Fig. 4.12 Characteristic curve. The same scale is adopted for both axes. The density axis would need to be extended further for direct exposure film.

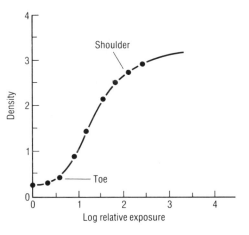

Fig. 4.13 Characteristic curve. After plotting the points from the tabulated values of density and log relative exposure, a smooth curve is drawn through the points. The **toe** and **shoulder** are indicated (see text).

4.5.5   *Features of the characteristic curve*

Reference to Fig. 4.13 shows that the graph possesses two sharply curved sections known as the **toe** and the **shoulder**. Thus, the curve is divided into three regions:

(1) The region to the left of the toe. Its features include: base density; fog; threshold.
(2) The region between the toe and shoulder. Its features include: contrast; gradient; film latitude; exposure latitude; speed and sensitivity.

(3) The region to the right of the shoulder. Its features include: maximum density; reversal.

Let us now examine the important features of each region.

4.5.5.1 The region to the left of the toe
This is sometimes referred to as the region of underexposure. Examination of this section of the characteristic curve shows that an increase in log relative exposure from 0 to 0.6 is accompanied by hardly any change in density. None of the exposures received by the film in this region is sufficient to produce any photographic effect. The density in this region arises from two sources:

(1) Base density – due to the absorption of light as it is transmitted through the polyester film base. This will be greater if the base has been tinted during manufacture (see section 5.1.1.2).
(2) Fog – i.e. the density produced by the development of silver halide grains which have received no intentional exposure. It has several causes:
    (a) **Age veil** – due to the unavoidable exposure of the film to natural background radiation.
    (b) **Storage fog** – due to poor storage conditions (see section 6.1).
    (Note that both of these forms of fogging increase with the age of the film and set limits on its shelf-life.)
    (c) **Chemical fog** – caused by the failure of the developing agents during processing to differentiate properly between exposed and unexposed silver halide grains.
    (d) **Safelight fog** – due to exposure to darkroom safelight illumination. For example, this may occur if film-handling time in the darkroom is excessive (see section 12.5.2.6).

Note that the total density of base plus fog is often referred to as **basic fog** or **gross fog**. Its value should not be greater than about 0.2.

Net density
Frequently, when plotting characteristic curves, gross fog is subtracted from each value of density measured. This produces a plot of **net** density against log relative exposure where:

Net density = Gross density – Gross fog

Figure 4.14 shows a characteristic curve of this type. Ideally, there should be an indication on the graph that net density has been plotted. Even without this information, the fact that the curve passes through the origin immediately identifies this type of characteristic curve.

Threshold
As exposure increases and we approach the toe of the curve, the film emulsion begins to respond to exposure and its density begins to rise above gross fog. This part of the curve is known as its **threshold**. On a correctly exposed chest radiograph, the subphrenic region usually receives an exposure which is at or below threshold, and its gross density is unlikely to be significantly above gross fog level. Note, however, that the presence of gas in the gastric fundus or in the colon may cause local increases in density.

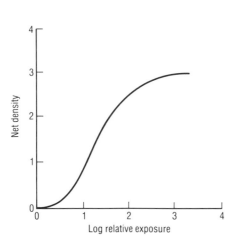

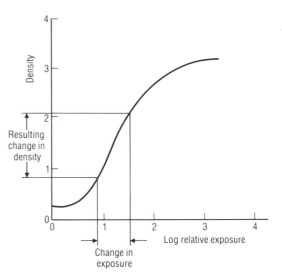

Fig. 4.14 A characteristic curve obtained by plotting *net* values of density. Note that the curve appears to pass through the origin of coordinates.

Fig. 4.15 A characteristic curve showing that on the 'straight line' part of the curve, changes in exposure produce marked changes in density.

4.5.5.2   The region between the toe and shoulder

This is often called the **straight-line part** of the characteristic curve, although it is rarely a straight line in the case of radiographic materials. The most important feature of this region is that changes in exposure cause significant changes in density (see Fig. 4.15). There are two major consequences of this:

(1) Contrast;
(2) Latitude.

(1) Contrast

The exposure variations which constitute **subject contrast** (see section 3.1.1) generate differences in image density and therefore produce contrast in the radiographic image (**radiographic contrast**). Figure 4.16 shows that the same change in log relative exposure (e.g. 0.5) produces different changes in density at different points on the characteristic curve. The greatest density differences and therefore maximum image contrast are generated between the toe and shoulder, where the curve is at its steepest. In fact, the slope or **gradient** of the curve is used as a measure of contrast. The gradient (*G*) at a point on the curve is the slope of the tangent to the curve at that point.

If the angle of slope is *A*, then mathematically:

$G = \tan A$ where $\tan A$ is the trigonometric tangent of A

Gamma The value of gradient varies according to where on the curve it is measured. If the characteristic curve has a true straight-line part, the value of *G* is constant throughout the length of the straight line and is known as **gamma**. Thus, gamma may be defined as the tangent of the angle of slope of the straight-line part of the characteristic curve (Fig. 4.17(a)). For film materials with a suitably shaped curve, gamma is a convenient method for summarizing their contrast properties. However, there is no true straight-line part on an X-ray or

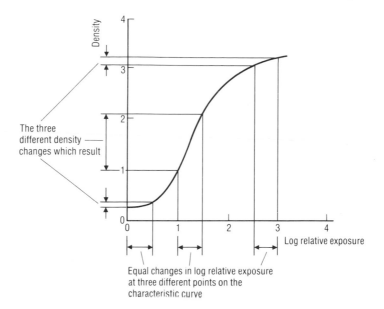

Fig. 4.16 The same change (0.5) in log relative exposure produces different density changes at different points on the characteristic curve. Maximum density change (contrast) is generated on the 'straight line' part of the curve. Note that an increase of 0.5 in the log value represents an increase by a factor of 3.16 × in the actual value (antilog 0.5 = 3.16).

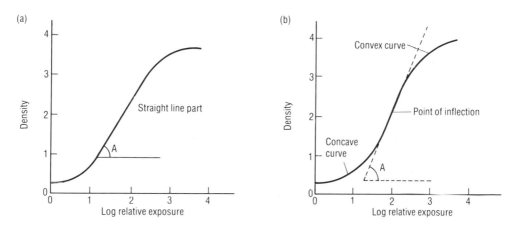

Fig. 4.17 (a) Characteristic curve with a true straight line part. Gamma is the tangent of angle *A*, the slope of the straight line part. (b) Characteristic curve with no straight line part. Gamma is the tangent of *A*, at the point of inflection of the curve.

fluorographic film characteristic curve, so a different definition of gamma is required: **maximum gamma** is the tangent of the angle of slope of the characteristic curve at its **point of inflection**. The point of inflection is the point at which the curve changes from being concave to convex (Fig. 4.17(b)). For some film emulsions, particularly the direct-exposure type, the point of inflection occurs at a density well above the mid-range values most useful in diagnostic imaging. It is therefore common to adopt an alternative method of expressing film contrast, known as average gradient.

Average gradient (Fig. 4.18) Two points are selected, one (X) just above the toe, the other (Y) below the shoulder of the curve, and the average value of G between these limits is taken as representative of the contrast characteristic of the film material. The average gradient is obtained by drawing a straight line between points X and Y and determining the tangent of the angle of slope of this line. The symbol $\bar{G}$ (pronounced 'gee' bar) is used to represent average gradient. Then, from Fig. 4.18:

$$\bar{G} = \frac{D_Y - D_X}{\log E_Y - \log E_X}$$

Although points X and Y are chosen arbitrarily, the manufacturers of radiographic materials have established a convention where X has a net density of 0.25 (i.e. 0.25 above gross fog) and Y has a net density of 2.0. Thus, the expression $D_Y - D_X$ always has the value of 1.75. The net density values 0.25 and 2.0 are said to represent the limits of **useful density**, because they include the density values most frequently encountered on radiographs (Kodak, 1981). Certainly, the densities measured from a correctly exposed antero-posterior radiograph of the abdomen lie within these limits.

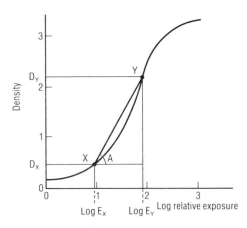

Fig. 4.18 Average gradient. The tangent of A, the angle of slope of the line joining X and Y, is defined as $\bar{G}$ or average gradient. Thus

$$\bar{G} = \frac{D_Y - D_X}{\log E_Y - \log E_X}$$

By convention D_X has a net density of 0.25 and D_Y has a net density of 2.0.

Factors affecting average gradient The contrast characteristic and therefore average gradient of a film or film–screen system depend on several factors:

(1) Film emulsion characteristics, particularly grain size distribution, which are determined during manufacture (see section 4.3.3);
(2) Whether the film is duplitized or single-coated (sections 4.4.1.1 and 4.4.1.2);
(3) Film processing conditions, particularly during development (section 9.2.1.5);
(4) Characteristics of the intensifying screen(s), if used (Chapter 7).

Note that average gradient does *not* depend on the type of subject being radiographed nor on the X-ray tube kilovoltage selected, although of course the contrast of the final image *is* influenced by these parameters.

Average gradient is not the only method available for indicating the contrast of X-ray film systems. Quality assurance programmes commonly use the quantity known as **contrast index**, which is obtained directly from a sensitometric test strip without the need to plot a characteristic curve. We shall describe contrast index in section 18.4.2.

(2) Latitude

Latitude refers to the way a film or film–screen system is able to record successfully a wide range of exposure. It is an expression of the **tolerance** of the system to extreme conditions of exposure. Latitude is considered in two parts: film latitude and exposure latitude.

(a) *Film latitude* This represents the difference between the upper and lower limits of log relative exposure, which produce densities within the useful range (i.e. 0.25–2.0 above gross fog). Referring to Fig. 4.19(a):

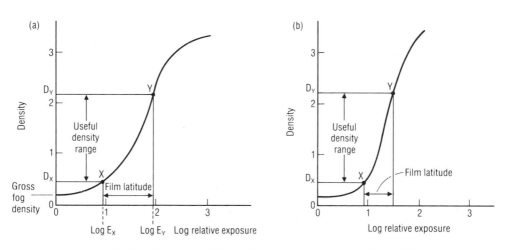

Fig. 4.19 (a) Film latitude is the difference between the upper and lower limits of log relative exposure which produce densities within the useful range (0.25–2.0 above gross fog). Film latitude = $\log E_Y - \log E_X$. (b) The film latitude of this film is reduced compared with that illustrated in Fig. 4.19(a) because the characteristic curve is steeper due to the increased contrast of the film emulsion.

$$\text{Film latitude} = \log E_Y - \log E_X$$

But, in the previous section on contrast, we defined average gradient as:

$$\bar{G} = \frac{D_Y - D_X}{\log E_Y - \log E_X}$$

so

$$\text{Average gradient} = \frac{\text{Useful density range}}{\text{Film latitude}}$$

and

$$\text{Film latitude} = \frac{\text{Useful density range}}{\text{Average gradient}}$$

We also stated that:

Useful density range $(D_Y - D_X) = 1.75$

thus, we can conclude that:

$$\text{Film latitude} = \frac{1.75}{\text{Average gradient}}$$

Figure 4.19(b) shows that as the contrast of a film system increases (represented by a steeper characteristic curve) so the latitude of the system reduces, because the range of exposure required to give the same density range decreases. This reciprocal relationship inevitably leads to a compromise between film contrast and film latitude, since radiographically both high contrast *and* high latitude are desirable characteristics.

Note that film latitude depends on exactly the same parameters as average gradient. It is *not* dependent on X-ray tube kilovoltage.

(b) *Exposure latitude* This represents the tolerance of a film or film–screen system to errors in the selection of the exposure factors (e.g. kVp, mAs, time, FFD, etc.) when the radiographic or fluorographic exposure was made. We know from practical experience that minor errors in exposure selection are not necessarily disastrous. A film may receive a slight over- or underexposure without loss of diagnostic value. Exposure latitude depends partly on the inherent film latitude described above, but it also depends on the **subject contrast** in the X-ray beam which exposes the film.

Consider two aspects of the spread of values of log relative exposure corresponding to the subject contrast or range of X-ray intensities transmitted through the body part being examined:

(1) The **median** of the log exposure values. This represents the value midway between the maximum and minimum log exposure values and depends essentially on the total **quantity** of X-radiation used. For example, the median value increases if we raise the tube voltage (kVp), tube current (mA), exposure time or mAs.

(2) The **range** of the log exposure values. This represents the difference between the maximum and minimum log exposure values. As we saw in section 3.1.1, the range of intensities in a beam depends on a number of factors, including the quality of the X-radiation used. In particular, the magnitude of the spread (and subject contrast) is reduced if we raise tube kilovoltage. But note that adjustment of kVp also alters the median value, since it changes both the quality and intensity of the beam.

By adjustment of exposure factors prior to making an exposure, we can exercise control over both the range and the median of log exposure values.

To image a subject successfully, each value of exposure present should be recorded as a density within the useful density range. To meet this condition, each log exposure value must lie within the limits $(\log E_Y - \log E_X)$ that we established above when we defined film latitude. It is clear from Fig. 4.20(a) that this can only

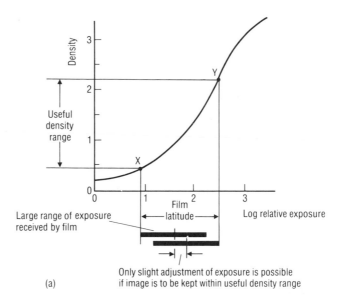

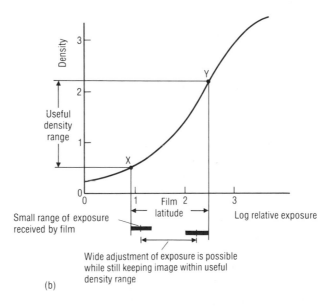

Fig. 4.20 (a) To image a subject successfully each log exposure value must fit within the limits imposed by film latitude. If the range of exposure is only just within film latitude there is little room for manoeuvre when selecting exposure factors; exposure latitude is small.

Fig. 4.20 (b) In this case the range of exposure received by the film is small and easily fits within the film latitude. The exposure latitude is large and the radiographer's choice of exposure factors is less critical.

be achieved if the range of log exposure values is no greater than the film latitude. For a particular body part:

Exposure latitude = film latitude – log exposure range

If film latitude and log exposure range approach each other in magnitude, the selection of exposure factors by the radiographer demands great accuracy and the **exposure latitude** is poor because slight over- or underexposure results in densities outside the useful range.

On the other hand, if conditions are such that the range of exposures in the X-ray beam is well within the film latitude (Fig. 4.20(b)), the radiographer's choice of exposure factors is less critical and the exposure latitude is improved.

Radiography of body parts which possess an extreme range of tissue densities or tissue thicknesses is generally known as **steep-range** radiography, e.g. the antero-posterior projection of the thoracic spine. Exposure latitude problems in such cases may be relieved by the selection of a high kVp, which improves exposure latitude by reducing subject contrast.

Speed and sensitivity

The speed (sensitivity) of a film or film–screen system is an expression of the X-ray exposure required to produce a given image density. A high-speed system requires less exposure to produce a specific density than a slower system. The higher the speed of a system, therefore, the further to the left its characteristic curve appears. In radiography, speed is most frequently quoted as a **relative** value and is defined thus:

The speed of system A relative to system B is the ratio of the exposure required by system B (E_B) to that required by system A (E_A) to give the same density under the same exposure conditions.

In terms of exposure factors:

$$\frac{\text{Speed of system A}}{\text{Speed of system B}} = \frac{\text{mAs for system B}}{\text{mAs for system A}}$$

to give the same density at the same kVp and FFD. The value 100 is commonly assigned to the speed of the reference system (system B in the example above). Thus if the speed of system A was half that of system B, its relative speed would be quoted as 50.

It is a widely accepted convention to assess relative speed at a net density of 1.0 (Pizzutiello & Cullinan, 1993) because this is the most typical density value on radiographic images. The density level at which relative speed is assessed is known as the **speed point**.

How is relative speed assessed from characteristic curves? A value for the relative speed of two film systems can easily be obtained from the characteristic curves of the two systems *provided they share a common log relative exposure axis*. Figure 4.21(a) shows how this is achieved. The log relative exposure values corresponding to a net density of 1.0 are read off and the difference between them is calculated:

$$\log E_B - \log E_A$$

But the mathematics of logarithms states that:

$$\log E_B - \log E_A = \log E_B/E_A$$

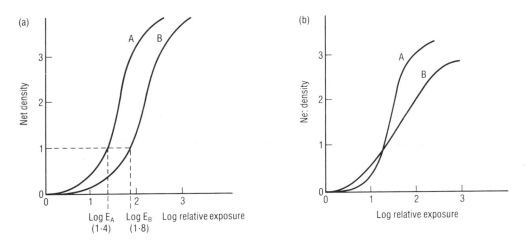

Fig. 4.21 (a) Estimation of relative speed from characteristic curves for systems A and B. Values of log relative exposure to produce a net density of 1 are obtained: $\log E_A = 1.4$; $\log E_B = 1.8$; $\log E_B - \log E_A = 0.4$; therefore $E_B/E_A = \text{antilog}(0.4) = 2.5$. Thus system A is $2\frac{1}{2}$ times the speed of system B and its relative speed value is 250.
(b) Changing the relative speed at different speed points. At densities above 1 system A is the faster; at densities below 1 system B is the faster; at a density of 1 both systems have the same speed.

Thus, obtaining the antilog of log E_B/E_A (e.g. from an electronic calculator) provides us with a value for E_B/E_A which, by definition, *is* the relative speed of the two systems.

Note that the relative speed of the two systems illustrated is different at different density levels. Reference to the intersecting characteristic curves shown in Fig. 4.21(b) emphasizes the importance of establishing an agreed speed point, the density at which the speed assessment is made.

4.5.5.3   The region to the right of the shoulder

This is sometimes referred to as the region of overexposure. There are two aspects of film behaviour which may be demonstrated on this part of the characteristic curve:

(1) Maximum density;
(2) Reversal.

(1) Maximum density
As the film or film–screen system is subjected to greater and greater exposure, a point is reached where *all* of the silver halide grains in the film emulsion are reduced to silver during development (Fig. 4.22). Further increases in exposure cannot then result in any increase in density. Thus, the film achieves a maximum level of density known as D_{max}.

In this region, subject contrast does not produce image contrast and no subject detail can be visualized. The characteristic curve has zero gradient in this region of maximum density, indicating that image contrast is zero.

Numerical value of D_{max} The value of maximum density depends on two major factors:

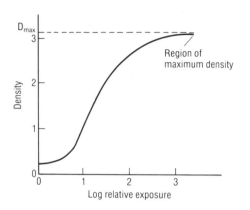

Fig. 4.22 Characteristic curve showing the region of maximum density (D_{max}). Further increases in exposure produce no increase in density.

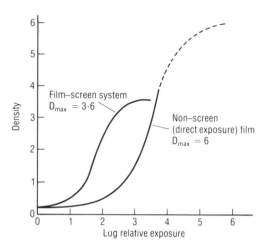

Fig. 4.23 Characteristic curves showing the increased maximum density of direct exposure film. Note that the density axis has been extended to accommodate the high density region. Normally the part of the curve shown with a broken line would *not* be included on the characteristic curve.

(a) **Silver coating weight** – the greater the amount of silver halide per unit area of film, the higher is D_{max}. Thus, a non-screen direct-exposure film has a higher value of D_{max} than a screen-type X-ray film (Fig. 4.23).

(b) **Processing conditions** – changes in developer activity, perhaps due to temperature variations or exhaustion of developing agents, can lead to a failure to achieve the optimum value of D_{max} (see section 9.2.1.5).

The changes in density that *do* occur above the maximum useful density of 2.0 (net value) are generally not noticed if the image is viewed under normal conditions, since they all appear to be 'black'. However, if, as in direct-exposure film, D_{max} is well above a net value of 2.0, there may well be valuable details hidden in this high-density region. The use of a high-intensity light source will reveal image contrast, even here. This technique is often used to obtain maximum information from the images produced during mammography.

(2) Reversal

A film emulsion may exhibit a rather strange phenomenon when subjected to exposures many times greater than that required to achieve D_{max}. It may begin to respond in the opposite way to normal, producing a *reduction* in image density as a result of an *increase* in exposure (Fig. 4.24). This behaviour is known as **reversal** and it is a feature which is absent from the emulsion of the most commonly used X-ray films (Jenkins, 1980).

Testing for reversal properties

A film may be tested for reversal by removing it from its cassette and deliberately exposing it to a bright light for several seconds (e.g. by holding it against an X-ray viewing box for 10 s). The film should then be processed normally. Given such treatment, most X-ray films will appear black, but a film which exhibits reversal will

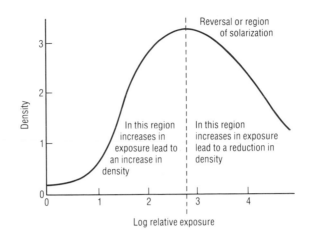

Fig. 4.24 Characteristic curve showing reversal properties. Note that the log relative exposure values in the reversal region range from 3 to over 5. These represent exposures 100 to 10 000 times greater than those normally employed in radiography.

be almost transparent! Such a result is guaranteed to be a source of astonishment and disbelief.

Historically, photographic films were exposed to bright sunlight in order to trigger image reversal. Such films were said to be **solarized** and the use of this term persists to this day. For example, the reversal part of a characteristic curve may be referred to as the **region of solarization**.

Image reversal is an extremely useful characteristic because it provides a means of obtaining an exact copy of a radiograph in a single process (see Chapter 24). Duplicating film has a reversal type of emulsion, but it is given chemical pre-treatment by the manufacturer rather than a heavy pre-exposure to prompt it to react to exposure in this unusual way.

4.5.5.4 Summary

We have now completed our discussion of those aspects of film or film–screen response which a characteristic curve can depict. Let us review these aspects briefly:

(1) Basic fog (section 4.5.5.1);
(2) Contrast and average gradient (section 4.5.5.2);
(3) Film latitude and exposure latitude (section 4.5.5.2);
(4) Relative speed (section 4.5.5.2);
(5) Maximum density (section 4.5.5.3);
(6) Reversal characteristics (section 4.5.5.3).

In radiography, characteristic curves can be used for:

(1) Comparison of film performance (section 18.3.1);
(2) Comparison of film–screen systems (section 18.3.2);
(3) Monitoring of film processing (section 18.4.1);
(4) Calibration of step-wedges (section 4.5.5.5).

4.5.5.5   Calibration of step-wedges

We referred earlier in this chapter to using a calibrated aluminium step-wedge for the production of characteristic curves by intensity-scale sensitometry (see section 4.5.4.1). We shall now describe a practical method for calibrating a step-wedge (Kodak, 1981). There are two stages in the procedure:

(1) A characteristic curve of the relevant film–screen system at a specified tube kilovoltage is produced by time-scale sensitometry, as described in section 4.5.4.1. The characteristic curve produced for this purpose is known as a **calibration curve**. It is common practice to place in the X-ray beam a 0.2 mm copper filter to mimic the filtering effect of the aluminium step-wedge.

(2) The calibration curve is then used to determine the exposure increment (wedge factor) between adjacent steps on the step-wedge at the selected kilovoltage. Using the same film–screen system and tube kilovoltage, but *without* the copper filter, an exposure is made through the step-wedge such that after processing, a density range of about 0.2–3.0 is produced. This film must be processed under exactly the same conditions as the time-scale film. The density of each step should then be measured with a densitometer.

   The two densities (e.g. steps 2 and 10) which are closest in value to those at the top and bottom of the 'straight line' part of the calibration curve are selected and marked on the curve, as shown in Fig. 4.25. The values of log relative exposure corresponding to these densities are read off the calibration curve. The difference between these two values is calculated (e.g. $1.76 - 0.8 = 0.96$) and then divided by the number of steps (e.g. 8) straddled by the two values in order to determine the log relative exposure *per step* ($0.96 \div 8 = 0.12$ in Fig. 4.25).

   The antilogarithm of this value (1.3) is the wedge factor for the step-wedge under the specified conditions. New calibration curves are required to determine the wedge factors for other conditions.

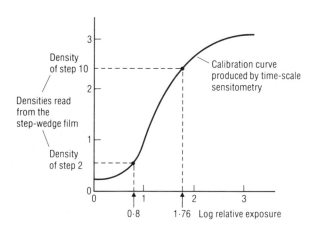

Fig. 4.25 Calibrating a step-wedge. From the step-wedge film, the two steps whose densities match most closely the upper and lower limits of the 'straight line' part of the calibration curve are noted (e.g. steps 2 and 10) and marked on the curve. The corresponding log relative exposure values are read off. From these the wedge factor of the step-wedge can be calculated (see text).

4.5.6 *Spectral sensitivity*

In section 4.4.1.3 we discussed the spectral response of films and indicated that photographic emulsion may be classified as **monochromatic** (blue-sensitive), **orthochromatic** (green-sensitive) or **panchromatic** (red-sensitive). We said that the spectral response of a screen-type X-ray film should correspond to the spectral emission of the intensifying screen phosphors with which it is to be used. Unfortunately, spectral response cannot be shown on a film's characteristic curve. Instead, the spectral sensitivity characteristics of a film are displayed as a spectral response curve on a graph, such as Fig. 4.26, which shows the response of an orthochromatic film.

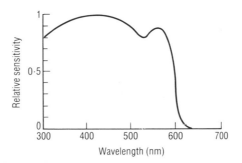

Fig. 4.26 Spectral sensitivity curve showing the response of a typical orthochromatic X-ray screen-type film. The reader should refer to Fig. 4.8 to identify the colours of light represented by different wavelengths.

The graph is a plot of the sensitivity (speed) of the film against the wavelength of light to which it is exposed. Sensitivity is assessed by measurement of the densities produced when a film is subjected to equal exposures of different wavelengths of light. Sensitivity is plotted on a **relative** scale, with the peak sensitivity shown as 1 (or 100%). The wavelength axis is scaled in nanometres.

The spectral response curve is a convenient way of recording this important aspect of a film's behaviour.

Applications of spectral sensitivity curves
The spectral curves have two main uses, which will be referred to in later chapters:

(1) Matching of film spectral response to intensifying screen spectral emission (see section 7.5).
(2) Ensuring the choice of safelight illumination is appropriate to the spectral response of the films being handled in the darkroom (see section 12.5.2.3).

In this chapter we have studied the photographic effect of radiation and the properties of photosensitive materials. We have outlined the sensitometric 'tools' available for describing and comparing the response to exposure of different radiographic recording media. In the next chapter, we shall examine in detail the range of X-ray films and film–screen systems employed in modern imaging departments.

4.6   Key relationships

Transmission ratio $= I_t/I_0$ (section 4.5.1)

Percentage transmission $= 100 \times I_t/I_0$ (section 4.5.1)

Opacity $= I_0/I_t$ (section 4.5.1)

Optical density $= \log_{10}$ Opacity (section 4.5.1.1)

Net density $=$ Gross density $-$ Gross fog (section 4.5.5.1)

Average gradient $= \dfrac{\text{Useful density range}}{\text{Film latitude}}$ (section 4.5.5.2)

$$\bar{G} = \frac{D_Y - D_X}{\log E_Y - \log E_X} \quad \text{(section 4.5.5.2)}$$

Film latitude $= \dfrac{\text{Useful density range}}{\text{Average gradient}}$ (section 4.5.5.2)

Film latitude $= \dfrac{1.75}{\text{Average gradient}}$ (section 4.5.5.2)

Exposure latitude $=$ film latitude $-$ log exposure range (section 4.5.5.2)

$$\frac{\text{Speed of system } A}{\text{Speed of system } B} = \frac{\text{mAs for system } B}{\text{mAs for system } A} \quad \text{(section 4.5.5.2)}$$

Chapter 5
The Recording System: Film Materials

Two main groups of film material may be differentiated in a modern imaging department:

(1) Those films exposed to X-rays alone (**direct-exposure** film) or to a combination of both X-rays and light (**screen – film**). These are both known as **X-ray films**.
(2) Those films exposed to light only. Examples of these are fluorographic, duplicating or polaroid films, as well as the 35 mm roll films which every photographer knows well.

Some of the films in the first group may be **duplitized** (i.e. having a sensitive emulsion on both sides of the base), whilst others may be **single-sided** (one emulsion surface only).

All of the films in group (2) have a single emulsion surface only.

5.1 Film construction

Figure 5.1 shows magnified cross-sections through the structure of duplitized and single-sided films.

A number of distinct layers may be identified: base, subbing layer, emulsion layer, supercoat, etc. Let us now examine each of these in detail.

5.1.1 *Film base*

Nowadays, polyester, which is made from polyethylene terephthalate resin, has almost completely replaced cellulose triacetate as the material used in the manufacture of film base. It is extremely strong, virtually untearable and demonstrates high dimensional stability, even under the most rigorous manufacturing or processing conditions.

5.1.1.1 Function of film base

(1) To provide a support for the emulsion layer.
(2) To transmit light so that an image can be viewed.

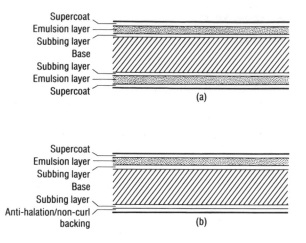

Fig. 5.1 Magnified cross-section through (a) duplitized film and (b) single-sided emulsion film.

5.1.1.2   Desirable characteristics of film base

(1) Transparent, free from any defect or blemish, and uniform in its ability to transmit light.
(2) Strong but flexible:
    (a) So that it can withstand mechanical stress in daylight loading systems and automatic processors for example;
    (b) Strength of material will allow base to be made thinner, important in minimizing unsharpness due to parallax (see section 4.4.1.1);
    (c) Must not be *too* flexible, however, or kinking is likely to occur.
(3) Uniform in thickness, otherwise there will be variations in emulsion layer thickness.
(4) Dimensionally stable throughout processing.
(5) Impermeable to water or processing solutions, thus easier to transport through automatic processors because the base will remain firm when wet.
(6) Non-flammable: film base is therefore sometimes referred to as 'safety base' (on account of this characteristic).
(7) Chemically inactive, otherwise emulsion may be attacked with consequent deterioration of the image.
(8) Uniform in colour; if a colour tone is added during manufacture (common in X-ray type films) it should:
    (a) Show batch to batch consistency;
    (b) Not change in colour with time.

5.1.1.3   What is the thickness of film base?

The answer will depend on the type of film and its use. For example: medical X-ray sheet film needs a film base 0.18 mm thick, whereas fluorographic roll film only needs a film base 0.08 mm thick.

    The physical characteristics of film base are very specific in order to cope with the precise demands made upon it by today's automated handling and processing systems. Moreover, roll film needs to be thinner than sheet film because it spends a greater part of its life rolled up.

5.1.2 The subbing layer

A **subbing** or 'adhesive' layer is required between the base and the emulsion for two reasons:

(1) To ensure that the emulsion layer adheres to the smooth and shiny base material during the coating stage in manufacture;
(2) To prevent any separation of the emulsion layer from the base during processing. This might otherwise occur when the emulsion swells and contracts during the processing cycle. Such movement might well induce parting of the emulsion from the base.

The preparation used is a mixture of gelatin solution and solvent of the film base. In some instances, coloured dyes may also be added to the subbing layers by certain manufacturers to counteract the **crossover** or **transmission** effect (see section 7.12).

5.1.3 The emulsion layer

As we saw in Chapter 4, the sensitive emulsion consists of silver halide crystals suspended in gelatin.

Emulsion technology has made great advances in recent years. Film manufacturers are now able to produce flat-shaped halide grains instead of the older rounded-shaped crystals. Kodak led the field with their 'T-Grain' emulsion. Because of their shape, the grains offer a larger surface area to the imaging source, thus increasing the film's sensitivity and thereby its speed.

The shape of the grains also means that they are able to lie in close proximity to each other and so minimize the amount of light able to pass through the emulsion to the base and produce the crossover effect, a phenomenon which contributes to image unsharpness.

Kodak also add a light-absorbing magenta dye to the surface of the grains, known as an **optical sensitizing dye**, the effect of which is to increase still further the sensitivity of the emulsion as well as absorbing irradiated light within the emulsion.

The end result is a film with the qualities of both speed and sharpness, two features which do not normally go hand in hand!

With all films, the emulsion layer is applied on top of the subbing layer, and in the case of duplitized X-ray film it will be coated on both sides of the base.

5.1.4 The supercoat

This is a thin layer of clear gelatin which is applied to the emulsion.

It has two prime functions:

(1) To protect the sensitive emulsion from the effects of light pressure or abrasion which might occur during use. Such occurrences would result in damaged areas, appearing as dark spots or patches on the processed film. The supercoating is sometimes referred to as the **anti-abrasive** layer.
(2) To provide suitable surface characteristics. Here, the manufacturer has to make a compromise. He must produce a film which is sufficiently glossy to discourage the accumulation of dust, but at the same time not so glossy as to prevent the automatic processor rollers having sufficient grip. In such circumstances, the film would be described as lacking **tooth**.

5.1.5   Non-curl backing

This is present only in single-sided emulsion sheet films. Because the film emulsion layer swells during processing, the film as a whole will have a tendency to curl. In the case of duplitized film, there is no such tendency since the emulsion layers on both sides of the film's base will swell to an equal extent.

In order to prevent or discourage the curling tendency with single-sided emulsion film, the emulsion layer is balanced by coating the base on the opposite side to the emulsion, firstly with a subbing layer and then with a layer of gelatin. The latter layer is not only of similar thickness to the emulsion stratum but also has the same absorbent qualities.

This layer is of course not present in roll film.

5.1.6   Anti-halation layer

When the image is formed by light, some of the light incident on the film will pass through the emulsion layer and reach the base.

Depending on the angle at which this light strikes the film base/air interface at the back of the film, it may either pass out of the base or be totally reflected back towards the emulsion. Such reflected light will produce a diffuse image or 'halo' around the proper image. This phenomenon is known as **halation** (Fig. 5.2) and is a cause of unsharpness in the image.

Although halation is a phenomenon attributable mainly to single-sided emulsion films, it can also occur with duplitized materials.

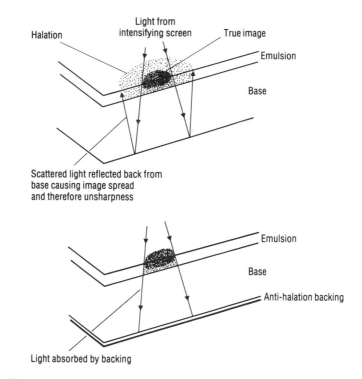

Fig. 5.2 Halation.

Manufacturers use one of the following methods in order to prevent halation occurring:

(1) Adding a dye to the non-curl backing.
(2) Adding a dye to the base.

(1) Adding a coloured dye to the gelatin of the non-curl backing
This is the method preferred for most of the single-sided emulsion films used in the radiography department. Examine some of the single-sided films used in your department. Note how the colour of the dye used in the anti-halation backing varies from one type of film to another, depending on the colour of light which is to be used to expose the film (i.e. intensifying screen emission).

The dye colour selected is always the opposite or 'complementary' colour to the exposing light, consequently the incident light will be absorbed by the backing and not reflected: e.g. a yellow dye will absorb blue light, a red dye will absorb green light, and so on. For example, subtraction film is green/blue for the yellowish tungsten light used with it, whilst duplication film has a dark blue, almost purple, anti-halation backing for the ultraviolet and tungsten light it is exposed to during the copying of radiographs.

These dyes are removed during development.

The anti-halation backing is known sometimes as the **anti-halo layer** or **gel coat**.

(2) Adding a dye to the base itself
This is the case with 35 mm still and cine film, for instance. Such a dye cannot be removed during processing. Its density therefore is very carefully controlled so that whilst it may function adequately as an anti-halation screen, it none the less transmits sufficient light for viewing.

5.1.7 *The crossover effect*

A type of halation known as the crossover effect (see section 7.12) can occur when film is used with intensifying screens. To prevent this, one manufacturer uses coloured subbing layers which effectively absorb the incident light.

Some Kodak X-ray films have a magenta dye added to the surface of the emulsion crystals during manufacture. Magenta is the complementary colour of green (which is the colour of emission of Kodak 'Lanex' intensifying screens). Besides the principal function of increasing the sensitivity of the emulsion, the dye has the effect of reducing light scattering within the emulsion and, at the same time, limiting crossover and thus image unsharpness.

These dyes are removed from the film during processing and thus do not interfere with the image when viewed by transmitted light.

5.1.8 *Irradiation*

The term should not be confused with halation. **Irradiation** is the sideways scattering of light within the emulsion itself as a result of the light striking the grains of silver halide comprising the emulsion (Fig. 5.3).

This scattered light contributes nothing valuable to the image proper and, like halation, is another source of unsharpness (blurring) in the image.

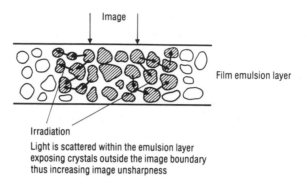

Fig. 5.3 Irradiation.

Irradiation is least likely to occur in thinly coated emulsions, and where there is least irradiation there will also be least risk of halation.

5.2 Films for medical imaging

Films used in medical imaging include:

Duplitized emulsion film

(1) Direct-exposure (non–screen-type) film: intra-oral dental film, kidney surgery film, radiation-monitoring film.
(2) Screen-type film (for use with intensifying screens).

Single emulsion film

(1) Screen-type film (used with a single intensifying screen).
(2) Photofluorographic film: cine film, 70 mm and 105 mm roll film, 100 mm sheet film.
(3) Cathode-ray-tube (CRT) photography: Polaroid film, $10'' \times 8''$ and $14'' \times 11''$ sheet film.
(4) Duplication film.
(5) Subtraction film.
(6) Laser imaging film for use with laser imagers.

5.2.1 *Duplitized X-ray film*

5.2.1.1 Direct-exposure-type film
This is sometimes known as **envelope-wrapped** or **non-screen** film because of its exposure to X-rays only.

Each film is individually folder-wrapped in paper and mounted with a stiff card for support inside a moisture-resistant paper envelope.

We stated in Chapter 4 that direct-exposure film is much slower than a screen–film combination. Nowadays, instead of increasing coating weights as a means of producing greater film blackening for a given exposure, sensitizers are added to non-screen X-ray film emulsions during manufacture. This is a preferable alternative to increasing the thickness of the emulsion, the result of which might make the film impossible to process satisfactorily in a rapid automatic processor.

Non-screen films are used because of their superior resolution compared to a screen–film system. They are sometimes used for extremity radiography where fine bony detail is required, or for mammography when microcalcification may be demonstrated.

As we pointed out in Chapter 4, the comparatively high exposure and thus increased radiation dose associated with imaging using these low-speed materials means that the use of this type of film is only rarely justified nowadays, especially when very good high-resolution screen–film systems are readily available.

Intra-oral dental film
Figure 5.4 shows:

(1) **Periapical** – 31 × 41 mm film for single or groups of teeth.
(2) **Occlusal** – 57 × 76 mm film for imaging mandibles or maxillae in the occlusal plane.
(3) **Bitewing** – a similar film to the periapical but with a custom-made flap which is slid around the film to enable the film to be positioned vertically behind the upper and lower teeth, the patient biting on the flap. Used for demonstrating the crowns.

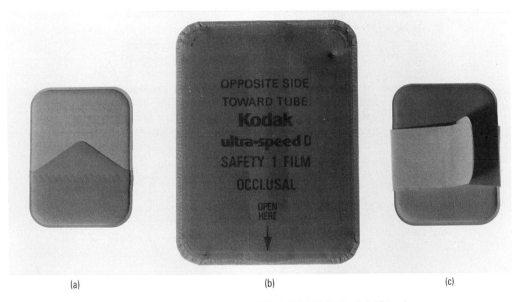

Fig. 5.4 Three types of intra-oral film. (a) Periapical. (b) Occlusal. (c) Bitewing.

The wrappings of a dental envelope package can be seen in Fig. 5.5. The lead-foil insert acts as an attenuator of back-scattered radiation arising from the intra-oral structures, and because of its presence it is essential that the film back be positioned with the correct side facing the tube.

The outer waterproof packet protects the film from moisture, whilst the paper inserts afford some protection from pressure.

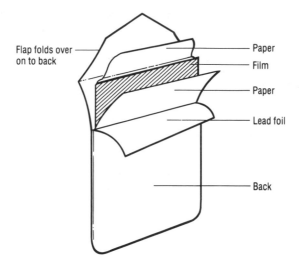

Fig. 5.5 The wrappings of an intra-oral dental film.

Dental film emulsions are a little thicker than in ordinary duplitized film, so this feature along with their size demands specialized processing facilities.

The tube side has an embossed dot. If the film pack is positioned so that the dot is always towards the crowns when carrying out a radiographic examination, it becomes much easier to identify upper and lower teeth and obtain the correct orientation when viewing or mounting the processed films.

Kidney surgery film
This duplitized non-screen film is designed to enable a radiographic exposure of the kidney to be made extra-abdominally during surgery for the removal of renal stones. The shape facilitates easy placement of the kidney and renal vessels (Fig. 5.6).

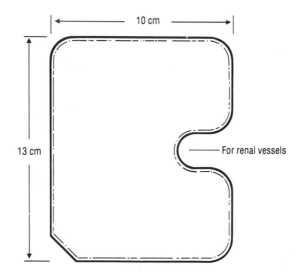

Fig. 5.6 Kidney surgery film. The characteristic shape is to facilitate the placement of the kidney whilst still attached to its renal vessels.

Each packet contains two films, one with a fast emulsion, the other slow. Should a set of radiographic factors result in overexposure of a small calcareous deposit on one film, then the chances are that it will, however, be demonstrated on the slower one. Thus, the two-film feature allows a wider range of renal stone densities to be demonstrated for any given radiographic exposure, and from the radiographer's point of view allows greater latitude in exposure choice.

The films are enclosed in a light-tight, waterproof polythene packet; the whole pack is capable of being cold-sterilized.

The film can be processed in an automatic processor.

Radiation-monitoring film
Outwardly similar to dental film in appearance, this film, although duplitized, has one very important difference. On one side of the base is a high-speed emulsion, whilst on the other side is a slower emulsion (Fig. 5.7). This permits a wide range of exposure levels to be recorded.

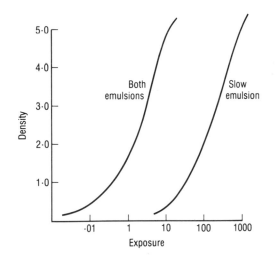

Fig. 5.7 Characteristic curves for radiation monitoring film. The base has a fast emulsion coating on one side and a slow emulsion on the other. After processing, the fast emulsion may be removed to allow measurement of high doses.

A large exposure to radiation may result in complete blackening of the fast emulsion, to the extent that exposure will be unmeasurable. Some of this emulsion can then be removed and radiation exposure estimated from the density of the slower emulsion.

It is to be hoped that only the fast emulsion will ever need to be used when estimating radiation doses received by radiographers!

5.2.1.2 Screen-type film

These films are used in conjunction with pairs of intensifying screens, the latent image being produced mainly by light emission from the screen phosphors (see Chapter 7).

A wide range of different manufacturers' films are available: both blue-sensitive (monochromatic) and green-sensitive (orthochromatic) and varying in speed, contrast, latitude and resolving power. These types of films are sometimes referred to as **contrast amplifiers** because their average gradient is > 1 (see section 4.5.5.2).

However, the choice of film is very much a question of compromise. For example, attendant upon the advantages of a high-contrast film would be a decrease in exposure latitude compared to that of a low-contrast material. Similarly, an increase in speed will probably be gained at the expense of some loss in resolution, and so on.

Each manufacturer produces films to match his intensifying screens, and it is unlikely that the fast film of one manufacturer will exactly match in speed the so-called fast film of another film producer. Consequently, care should be taken when changing from one film type to another to assess first their relative speeds so that correct exposures can be calculated for the new film system. How this exercise is carried out is described in section 18.3.

Sizes of screen-type X-ray films and packing Table 5.1 lists the sizes of screen-type X-ray films available. The last five sizes of film are the most frequently used.

The usual box of films supplied by the manufacturer contains 100 sheets of film, although larger packs containing 500 sheets are available.

Table 5.1 Sizes of screen-type X-ray films.

13×18 cm
15×30 cm
15×40 cm
20×40 cm
18×24 cm
24×30 cm
30×40 cm
35×35 cm
35×43 cm

5.2.2 Single-sided emulsion film

5.2.2.1 Screen-type film

This type of film is used in conjunction with a cassette fitted with a single intensifying screen (see section 7.8). One particular application is mammography.

The films are medium-to-high contrast with high definition, capable of demonstrating microcalcifications in soft tissue.

5.2.2.2 Photofluorographic film

These are films used to record the image produced at:

(1) The output phosphor of an image intensifier tube;
(2) The fluorescent screen of a camera system such as one used to provide miniature radiographs of the chest.

All of the films have a single emulsion and an anti-halation layer.

The emulsions are predominantly orthochromatic, since most image intensifier output phosphors (e.g. zinc cadmium sulphide) have light emissions containing a strong green component.

Although panchromatic emulsions are available for fluoroscopic recording, they are not as popular as orthochromatic materials because of the need to handle them in complete darkness. They do have one advantage in so far as they are comparatively faster because of their extended sensitivity.

We shall now examine some of these fluorographic films in more detail.

16 mm and 35 mm cine film
This is used for making a cine recording (cinefluorography) from the output phosphor of an image intensifier. There is a choice of orthochromatic or panchromatic fine grain emulsions, and the film can be supplied in either 85 or 170 m lengths. The reference to 16 mm or 35 mm is an indication of the width of the film (Fig. 5.8).

Cinefluorography is discussed further in Chapter 21.

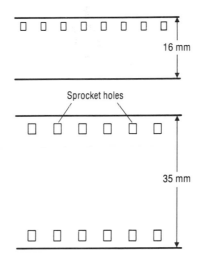

Fig. 5.8 16 mm and 35 mm cine film. The sprocket holes are used for transport purposes.

70 mm and 105 mm roll film
Orthochromatic single-emulsion film of medium-to-high contrast, used for recording images from the output phosphor of an image intensifier. These films are available with either perforated or unperforated edges, depending on the type of camera, and are supplied in rolls 45 m long. They are used in rapid-sequence filming, e.g. up to six frames per second, or for serial ('spot' filming) work.

100 mm cut film (10 × 10 cm)
This film, which is single coated, has an orthochromatic emulsion of medium-to-high contrast. It has a thicker base (0.2 mm) than roll film, the base usually being blue tinted. The film incorporates an anti-curl backing. Its principal application is in camera systems used with image intensifier work.

5.2.2.3 Films for use with a cathode ray tube or TV monitor
These single-emulsion films have applications in the following imaging modalities:

● Ultrasound;
● Computerized tomography;

- Magnetic resonance imaging;
- Nuclear medicine;
- Digital subtraction imaging.

The films are used in conjunction with cathode-ray-tube cameras and multi-formatters, which we look at in greater detail in Chapter 23.

The emulsions are orthochromatic, of medium-to-high contrast, and made to match a wide variety of CRT phosphors whose light emissions are known by their 'P' numbers: e.g. P4 – white; P11 – blue; P20, P31 – green.

The film sizes most commonly used are $10'' \times 8''$ and $14'' \times 11''$, and can be supplied with either a clear or a blue-tinted base.

The films can be processed in a conventional 45-90-s automatic processor, although special processors are available which can be sited in or near the imaging room, so saving on the time that might otherwise be spent conveying films to a centralized processing area.

Polaroid film

Polaroid film has had extensive applications throughout medical imaging departments for many years, particularly for recording ultrasound scan images.

A Polaroid film pack comprises positive and negative film sheets plus a pod of jellified processing chemistry. The photographic sheets are connected by a paper linkage (Fig. 5.9(a)).

After exposure the paper tab is pulled, so bringing the exposed surface of the negative sheet into close approximation with the positive sheet and at the same time bringing the paper leader towards the pair of rollers at the exit of the film magazine (Fig. 5.9(b)).

Once the leader emerges from the rollers, the paper tab is discarded and the leader is pulled firmly but smoothly until the entire film pack clears the rollers.

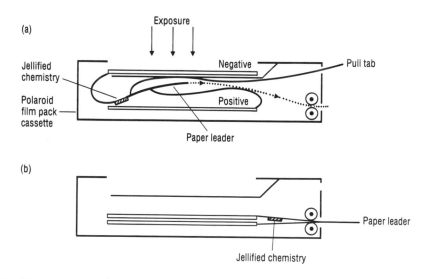

Fig. 5.9 A cross-section through a polaroid film pack (one film only shown). After exposure the effect of drawing on the pull tab brings the paper leader through the roller system. The paper leader is then pulled gently until the two films are clear of the cassette. The pressure from the two rollers spreads the jellified chemistry over the surface of the two emulsions.

The action of pulling the film pack through the roller system bursts the pod containing the processor chemistry and the solution is then uniformly spread between the two sheets of film as they pass between the rollers. On completion of processing, the two sheets can be pulled apart and the positive image viewed.

Formation of the visible image

The latent image is formed in the silver halide emulsion of the negative sheet. During processing by the jellified chemistry, both exposed and unexposed silver halides in the negative emulsion are simultaneously developed.

In those areas of the negative which have received an exposure, black metallic silver is deposited (Fig. 5.10). This is the negative image. Those areas which have not received an exposure have their silver halides reduced also, the silver ions migrating across the reagent where they are reduced to a crystalline silver layer on the positive film. This is the eventual image for viewing, and will be the reverse of that on the negative film. Processing takes about 30 s.

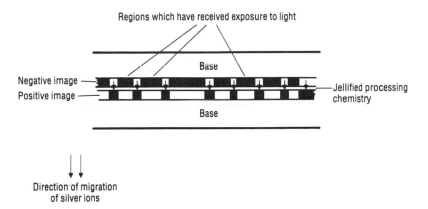

Fig. 5.10 Cross-section through the two film materials comprising the Polaroid film pack. The transfer of silver ions from the unexposed areas of the negative to the positive sheet of film forms the positive print.

5.2.2.4 Duplication and subtraction films

These very specialized films are examined in detail in Chapters 24 and 25.

In Chapter 6 we shall examine in some detail the way in which all these sensitive materials should be handled and stored.

Chapter 6
The Recording System: Film Storage

Film materials are expensive, and all begin to deteriorate to some extent from the time of manufacture. Whilst poor storage conditions will hasten this process, good storage procedures will enable us to use materials in which the ageing process should be of such minor consequence as to be unnoticeable in the final image.

Poor storage conditions and ageing are indicated by a rise in gross fog and a consequent reduction in film contrast.

Due to their greater sensitivity, fast film materials are more susceptible to poor storage conditions than the slower ones, and so too are the panchromatic emulsions in comparison to the monochromatic or orthochromatic types.

6.1 Storage areas

Three principal areas for storage of unexposed film may be identified:

(1) The hospital or X-ray department store (reserve stock);
(2) The darkroom (stock for immediate use);
(3) The imaging room (films inside cassettes awaiting use).

Many of the guidelines that we consider below in connection with the main departmental film store are equally applicable where darkroom storage is concerned.

6.1.1 *The X-ray department store*

Location
Ideally, this room should be purpose-designed and sited within easy access of the department and processing areas that it will need to service.

Care and protection of film
In order to maintain sensitive film materials in perfect condition, consideration needs to be given to protecting them from:

(1) Physical damage;

(2) Light;
(3) High temperatures;
(4) High relative humidity;
(5) Harmful gases and fumes;
(6) X-rays and radioactive sources;
(7) Fire and theft.

Before considering how these factors should be dealt with, three important expressions need to be understood: **expiry date**; **shelf-life**; **stock rotation**.

Expiry date This is a date that the film manufacturer stamps on the film box to indicate the date by which the film should be used. It is an indication of the length of time that a box of films can be kept safely providing they are stored under the manufacturer's recommended conditions.

In the event of a box of films being found to be outside the expiry date, it should be opened and several of the films processed. Gross fog can then be measured using a densitometer. If fog level is unacceptable, the box must be withdrawn from stock and the silver recovered by processing the remaining films.

Shelf-life This is an expression of the period of time for which a box of films may be kept under specified conditions. If those conditions should change, e.g. temperature were to increase in the storage area, then the risk of storage fog increases, and consequently shelf-life can be said to have become shorter.

Shelf-life will be shorter for fast film materials because of their greater sensitivity.

Stock rotation In order to comply with the conditions set out above under 'expiry date' and 'shelf-life', stock rotation should be practised.

All film boxes should be date stamped on receipt and used in strict rotation, so that the oldest box is used first. The level of stock should be monitored carefully to ensure that no over-ordering takes place and that, in particular, only a low level of the little-used film types or sizes is kept in stock.

6.1.1.1 Physical damage
Undue pressure or rough handling can cause **bruising** of the emulsion and lead to artefacts which will be seen in the final image. In order to avoid this one should:

(1) Check all boxes on receipt for signs of damage, since this may be an indication that the film will also be affected.
(2) Handle boxes with care.
(3) Site all shelving, if possible, in the centre of the room with the height of shelving ranging between 30 and 160 cm off the floor, to make handling easier.
(4) Stand boxes vertically upon the shelves, side by side. Stacking boxes on top of each other will expose the emulsion to undue pressure, and consequent damage. Pressure marks or bruising of the unexposed emulsion will be evidenced as areas of increased density on processing.
(5) Stand larger size film boxes on lower shelves in order to facilitate handling. This minimizes the risk of boxes being dropped, with possible damage to film or feet!
(6) Use shelving which is deep enough to accommodate safely the largest size film box.

(7) Individual films should be handled at their corners and kinking of the emulsion avoided otherwise bruising (crimp marks) will occur.

6.1.1.2   Light

It is unlikely that exposure to light will be a problem in the film store, since boxes are rarely opened here for any reason. The darkroom is the appropriate place for such activity when boxes can be opened under safelighting conditions.

6.1.1.3   High temperatures

Room temperatures which fluctuate wildly or are higher than those recommended will cause an increase in gross fog. Film manufacturers generally recommend that the film store temperature be maintained between 18 and 21°C for materials stored up to three months.

Any films stored below 15°C should be allowed to reach room temperature before being used.

Useful points to remember:

(1) Store boxes away from strong sunlight because of its heating effect. Ideally, storerooms should not have any window, especially a south-facing one.
(2) If the storeroom is part of a single-storey building, the roof should be insulated against the heating effect of sunlight.

6.1.1.4   High relative humidity

Film is very susceptible to dampness. Rooms which are prone to this, or rooms which may suffer from sudden changes of temperature with the consequent risk of condensation, should not be used as film storage areas.

In order to protect the sensitive emulsion from possible exposure to moisture, the film is sealed in packaging of foil or polythene following manufacture. This is done under very strictly controlled conditions of between 30 and 65% relative humidity. The film is then 'safe' until opened. However, since the storeroom is rarely, if ever, going to accommodate opened film boxes, the problem of high relative humidity is unlikely to arise. The recommended relative humidity for a film storeroom is 50%.

To these ends, the room should not have any hot water or steam pipes running through it, it should be well ventilated, and the storage shelves should be arranged with adequate air-space above and below them.

6.1.1.5   Harmful gases and fumes

Film fogging may occur if unsealed film packages are exposed to certain gases such as **formaldehyde, ammonia** and **hydrogen sulphide**. In addition, fumes from certain paints, solvents and cleaning materials may also cause film fogging.

It is advisable, therefore, that storage areas be free of such substances, and a general rule adopted that film be stored well away from strong fumes or vapours.

6.1.1.6   X-rays and radioactive sources

Films must be stored away from the effects of ionizing radiations. Sources of these are, for example:

(1) Diagnostic X-ray rooms;
(2) Radiotherapy treatment rooms;
(3) Radioisotope storage areas;
(4) Background radiations.

In so far as radiation sources (1), (2) and (3) are concerned, the best protection is afforded by siting the storeroom at sufficient distance from these areas. Where this is not possible, it will be necessary to ensure that the walls, ceiling, floor and doors of the storeroom have full protection incorporated in them. Walls, for instance, can be protected by coating with barium plaster, or building them with greater thickness. Doors can be lined with lead ply-sheet, care being taken to ensure that any gaps around the door are also shielded.

Monitoring radiation levels

In order to check on the possibility of any damaging levels of radiation within the storeroom, strategically sited radiation-monitoring film may be attached to walls adjacent to X-ray rooms, remembering to fix them so that the front of the film faces the wall. The films are left in place for a week and subsequently processed by the radiation-monitoring service.

An alternative method is to attach thermoluminescent dosemeters (TLDs) to the walls and, as with the radiation-monitoring film, leave in place for a week. They can then be sent to the medical physics department for assessment.

If either of these methods indicates that the room is unsafe, a full radiation survey must then be requested.

Background radiation occurs naturally in the environment. For example, certain elements used in the manufacture of building materials, such as house bricks, may be a source of radiation. A storeroom constructed from these materials may give rise to a level of background radiation which proves unacceptably high. Such a situation is fortunately rare, but it is as well to be aware of it.

Where stock control makes it possible for film to be stored for more than 3 months, background radiation should not exceed 1.29 nC/kg/h.

6.1.1.7 Fire and theft

Film is a very costly product by any standards, and can account for something like 25% of an X-ray department's annual budget. Efficient stock management is therefore essential, with storeroom security a priority consideration.

From the point of view of fire safety, the room should be fitted with an automatic smoke detector connected to the hospital fire-alarm system.

6.1.2 *Darkroom storage*

The same advice relating to handling, temperature control, relative humidity, radiation protection, etc. also applies to darkroom storage. But whereas it should be possible to control the storeroom environment strictly, the darkroom area with its automatic processors, chemical mixers and working personnel, for example, is much harder to control within strict guidelines. Raised humidity can be a problem here if the moist air from the processor is inadvertently allowed into the darkroom. Hence, the need for adequate air-ducting, along with sufficient ventilation to allow at least ten air changes per hour.

Because of these problems, darkroom storage periods should be short, and to this end film stocks should be replenished weekly.

Films not in immediate use should be kept in their original packaging until the time they are going to be needed. The films in immediate use can be stored in a hopper, a light-tight container having several compartments and which can accommodate various sizes of films.

The hopper should have a microswitch incorporated, so that it cannot be opened accidentally while the darkroom white light is still on. (A more detailed description of the hopper can be found in section 12.6.3).

The hopper should not be overloaded, otherwise access to individual films will be difficult and film-handling marks are likely to occur.

Where films of different speeds are required to be retained in the same darkroom, they should be stored in separate hoppers and the hoppers clearly identified.

6.1.3   *The imaging room*

In this environment, the unexposed films will be protected inside cassettes. Care should be taken to ensure that these are well shielded from radiation exposure and preferably stored inside a lead-lined box.

6.2   Stock control

Mention has already been made of the importance of efficient stock control and about some of its aspects, such as date stamping, stock rotation and security.

The methods used for obtaining and maintaining the correct level of film stock are equally important, and it is these that we shall now examine in greater detail.

Before setting about planning a film-ordering policy for a department, several questions need to be considered.

What is the rate of film usage?
In an established department, this can be assessed from statistical information kept by the department.

For a new department, the answer here will depend on the number and type of examinations that it is anticipated will be performed, and the number of projections which will be carried out for each radiographic examination. Moreover, consideration will need to be given to the individual sizes of films that will be required. All this is a necessary but onerous task for the radiographer manager. The data will provide a rough idea of expected film requirements, then, once the department is functioning, ongoing and detailed information-gathering will allow a more accurate assessment of film needs to be made, and film-ordering can be amended accordingly.

Are there seasonal variations?
For example, a hospital sited near a popular coastal resort may experience a large increase in the number of patients, and thus X-ray examinations, during the summer months.

Are any new imaging techniques anticipated?
The introduction of a new imaging modality (computerized tomography, magnetic resonance, etc.) into a department will have repercussions in so far as the type and number of films required are concerned. Sometimes it will mean an increase in the number of films to be purchased. On other occasions, an actual reduction in film requirements may be engendered, e.g. when Polaroid film used in conjunction with a CRT is exchanged for large-format film (10 × 8″) and a video imager to record ultrasound images.

Will staffing levels change?
Generally speaking, additional staff mean that more patients can be examined and thus more films used. This will be particularly true of an increase in radiologists.

How reliable and frequent will deliveries be?
If there is any possibility that deliveries will be infrequent or in any way unpredictable, then extra film stock over and above that which should normally be required will need to be stored in order to help support the department in the event of a delay in delivery.

This is not a satisfactory state of affairs since, as a consequence, large fluctuations in the level of stock may arise from time to time and the job of maintaining an adequate supply of film will be made more complicated. Such a situation should be avoided if at all possible by using an alternative film supplier.

Do all sizes and types of film share equal availability?
This information needs to be obtained from the manufacturer so that those film types or sizes less frequently supplied by the manufacturer and therefore possibly harder to obtain quickly, can be ordered well in advance.

What discounts are given against bulk ordering?
This information will dictate the amount of film ordered at any one time and therefore the frequency with which orders need to be placed with the supplier.

What storage capacity does the film store have?
Naturally there will be a limit to the amount of film which can be held in stock, defined by the space available in the department's film store. In any case, over-ordering will result in some film boxes eventually exceeding expiry dates.

All of the above considerations will have a bearing on the level of stock that the department needs to hold from week to week or from month to month, as well as the amount and frequency with which certain stock items need to be reordered.

6.3 Film-ordering methods

Three principal reordering methods may be considered:

(1) Fixed amount of film, delivery day varied;
(2) Fixed amount of film, delivery day fixed;
(3) Ordering according to need, delivery day fixed.

(1) Fixed amount, delivery day varied
For example, it may be decided that when the number of 24×30 cm film boxes falls to 10, reordering of that size must take place. Similar reordering levels are decided for all the other film sizes. In order to avoid the possible multiplicity of orders as, one by one, the different film sizes reach their reordering levels, a safety margin is built into the system so that replenishment of individual sizes can safely wait until a number of them reach reordering levels.

This sort of scheme is not an easy one to manage, since it requires that a large proportion of time be spent on stock-control duties. Only in this way can the regime run efficiently and economically.

(2) Fixed amount, delivery day fixed

This is a much simpler method than the previous one, but less accurate. The film usage rate for the various film sizes is calculated from statistical information gathered over, for example, the previous 12 months.

If storage capacity allows for one month of storage, then the average monthly usage rate is calculated from past evidence, and this number of films is ordered monthly.

This ordering system has a major drawback in so far as it means that the stock level of certain film sizes will increase over and above that required, whilst other sizes may well be exhausted.

(3) Ordering according to need, delivery day fixed

This system is the most accurate, since the amount ordered varies according to usage and thus the stock level is always being brought back to a maximum level.

This method, in common with the others, requires an ongoing monitoring of film usage if it is to run efficiently. However, since the quantity of film can be varied according to need, it does mean that the superintendent radiographer can anticipate changes in film usage and reflect this in the film-ordering regime very quickly.

Chapter 7
The Recording System: Intensifying Screens

In Chapter 4 we looked at the principles involved in X-ray imaging and examined briefly the use of intensifying screens for producing a radiographic image.

Because X-rays are so penetrative, only about 1% of them are absorbed by the emulsion layers. Thus, when X-rays alone are used to create radiographic images (non-screen radiography), most pass straight through the film without causing any film blackening. In order, therefore, to create adequate radiographic density, comparatively large exposures have to be made.

An intensifying screen works by converting X-ray energy into light energy. As X-ray photons pass through the phosphor layer of the screen, they are absorbed by the phosphor crystals which then become excited and fluoresce, emitting ultraviolet and/or visible light (Fig. 7.1).

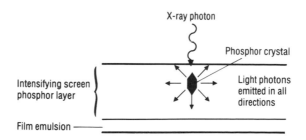

Fig. 7.1 The interaction of an X-ray photon with a screen phosphor crystal results in the emission of light in all directions. That light travelling towards the film emulsion is absorbed by the film's silver halide crystals producing the latent image.

For every X-ray photon absorbed, hundreds of light photons are emitted by the screen, so the screen can increase the effect of a beam of radiation emerging from a patient by creating a very large number of light photons for a relatively small number of X-ray photons incident upon the screen. This feature, in addition to the fact that film is more sensitive to light than X-radiation anyway, means that the screen is effectively intensifying the photographic effect of the beam. As a consequence, radiographic exposures can be reduced considerably over those required for non-screen imaging.

We have already used the word 'fluoresce' to describe what happens when X-rays interact with the phosphor material of intensifying screens. Before we examine intensifying screens in any more detail, this and another word, **luminescence**, need to be explained briefly.

7.1   Luminescence

The emission of light from a substance bombarded by radiation is termed luminescence and includes two effects: fluorescence and phosphorescence.

Fluorescence, which is the light emission we described earlier, lasts only as long as the radiation exposure. **Phosphorescence**, on the other hand, is afterglow, i.e. light continues to be emitted for some time even after radiation exposure has ended.

Phosphorescence is an undesirable phenomenon in X-ray imaging. The consequences of afterglow occurring in intensifying screens would make the use of a rapid film changer, for example, impossible.

7.2   Intensifying screens and unsharpness

In Chapter 4 (section 4.4.1.1) we explained the advantages of using duplitized emulsion films. In order for a satisfactory image to be produced in each emulsion layer, intensifying screens are used in pairs as Fig. 7.13 illustrates.

The use of intensifying screens inevitably means that a certain degree of unavoidable unsharpness will be introduced into the image in comparison to that obtained where non-screen film material is used. This unsharpness is due to light divergence.

Diffusion of light
Because light spreads outwards in all directions from its source, any point of light arising within the intensifying screen will no longer be a point by the time it reaches the film emulsion (Fig. 7.2). Even the phosphor crystals at the surface of the screen are not in contact with the film owing to the supercoat, and this is a reason why the transparent supercoat is made as thin as possible. The further away each source of fluorescence is from the film, the greater the degree of light divergence and thus the greater the unsharpness.

However, the advantages of using screens far outweigh the disadvantages resulting from this small loss of definition. As we examine screen construction during the course of this chapter, we shall see how screen manufacturers constantly strive for maximum sharpness and system speed, two features not always easy to reconcile.

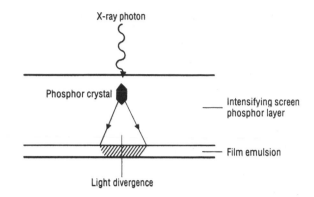

Fig. 7.2 Light emitted from a phosphor crystal diverges on its way to the film. The further away each source of fluorescence is from the film, the greater the degree of light divergence and thus the greater the unsharpness..

Another cause of unsharpness, but one which is avoidable, arises when a cassette becomes damaged and the close and uniform contact between the film and the screen is lost. When this happens the light arising in the screen phosphor as a consequence of an X-ray photon interaction is allowed to spread to too great an extent (Fig. 7.3), and the image so produced is unsatisfactory.

Poor film/screen contact generally arises from the misuse of X-ray cassettes, and in the event of there being suspicion that poor contact has occurred, the test described in section 18.2.1 should be carried out.

Radiographic unsharpness which arises as a consequence of using film and screen materials is referred to as intrinsic or **photographic unsharpness**, in contradistinction to geometric and movement unsharpness which we looked at in Chapter 3.

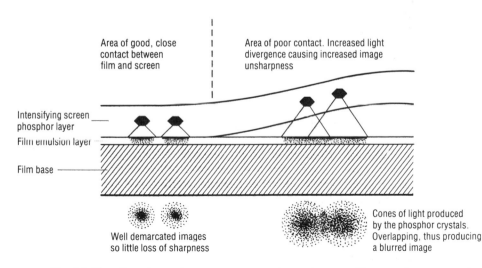

Fig. 7.3 The effect of poor film/screen contact on image sharpness. The area of poor contact has resulted in the increased spread of light and the subsequent blurring of image boundaries.

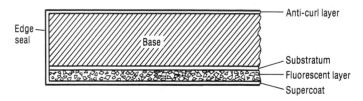

Fig. 7.4 A magnified cross-section through an intensifying screen.

7.3   Screen construction

A magnified cross-section through an intensifying screen is shown in Fig. 7.4.

7.3.1   *Base*

Screen base is made from paper, cardboard, or more usually a clear plastic such as polyester, the function of which is to provide a strong, smooth, but flexible support for the fluorescent layer. The thickness of the base is about 0.18 mm.

Additional characteristics required of screen base are that it should:

● Be chemically inert;
● Be uniformly radioparent;
● Be moisture resistant;
● Not discolour with age or on exposure to X-rays.

The base sometimes incorporates a light-reflective pigment such as **titanium dioxide** (e.g. Kodak Lanex screens). This has the same function as the 'reflective layer', to be described later.

7.3.2   *Substratum layer*

This is a bonding layer between the base and the phosphor layer. It may be reflective, absorptive or simply transparent in nature, depending on the manufacturers' intended characteristics for the screen.

Use of a reflective substratum layer
The function of a **reflective** layer is to maximize the effect of the screen by reflecting light which would otherwise be lost through the base, back towards the film emulsion (Fig. 7.5).

To give the screen this characteristic, a highly reflective white pigment, **titanium dioxide**, is added to the substratum layer.

A reflective layer thus increases the speed of the screen since, for a given X-radiation input, the screen produces a proportionately greater blackening effect on a film than will a similar screen without a reflective layer. The reflected light, however, extends the real image boundary, so leading to an increase in photographic unsharpness.

Use of an absorptive substratum layer
An absorptive layer has a directly opposite effect to a reflective layer. Any light travelling backwards towards the screen base is prevented from being reflected by the base/phosphor interface, and is instead absorbed (Fig. 7.6).

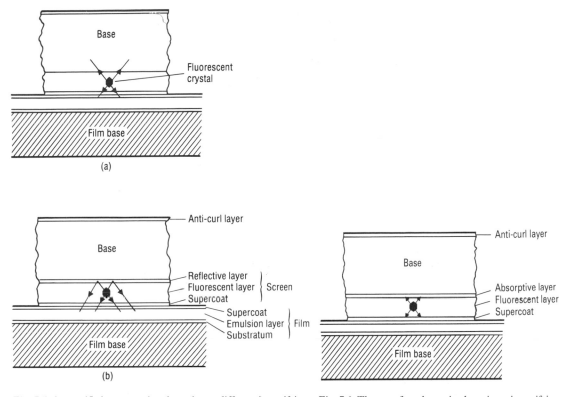

Fig. 7.5 A magnified cross-section through two different intensifying screens. (a) No reflective layer so light is lost through base of screen. (b) The use of a reflective layer maximizes the intensifying effect of the screen by reflecting light back towards the film.

Fig. 7.6 The use of an absorptive layer in an intensifying screen. Light travelling backwards is effectively absorbed.

A screen with an absorptive layer is thus slower than a screen with a reflective layer, but has less photographic unsharpness. The substratum layer is made absorptive by adding a coloured dye to it.

7.3.3 *Phosphor layer (fluorescent layer)*

This is the active layer of the screen. It consists of fluorescent crystals which emit light when struck by X-radiation. They are suspended in a transparent binder such as **polyurethane**. The binder material effectively holds the fluorescent crystals together and, because many phosphors are hygroscopic, polyurethane is an ideal choice because it prevents any moisture penetration which would otherwise cause reduced luminescence.

In addition to the phosphor crystals, the binder in a high-resolution screen may also contain **carbon granules** or a **coloured pigment** (known as an 'acutance' dye). The function of both of these is to absorb any laterally scattered light within the fluorescent layer (irradiation) which, if it were to reach the film, would contribute to image unsharpness.

Light which has the longest travel distance (i.e. the oblique rays) will stand more chance of being absorbed by the medium and thus fail to reach the film emulsion.

The use of carbon granules thus minimizes photographic unsharpness but reduces the speed of the screen.

The type of phosphor used, the thickness of the layer and the density with which the crystals are packed, are all variable properties which will determine the nature and quality of a particular screen's performance in terms of speed.

The term **coating weight** is often used in connection with screen phosphors. It is an expression of the quantity of phosphor grains incorporated in a phosphor layer, and will therefore depend on:

(1) Grain size;
(2) Coating thickness.

In other words, the greater the number of grains, the greater is said to be the coating weight.

7.3.4 Supercoat

This has a protective function and is made from acetate. It helps to resist surface abrasion and may include anti-static qualities, a valuable characteristic where the film is to be used with rapid sequence exposure equipment, for example.

The coating must be thin ($\sim 8\,\mu m$) in order to reduce the distance between film and phosphor layer and thus minimize photographic unsharpness. It must be transparent, so that the light produced in the fluorescent layer may reach the film, and also waterproof in order to protect the sensitive phosphor crystals.

The supercoat is extended around the edges and back of the screen, where it is effective both in minimizing edge wear and providing a **non-curl** backing.

With such a thin supercoat, great care should be taken when handling and cleaning screens in order to prevent damage to the sensitive phosphor layer.

The complete screen is attached to the front or back of the cassette by double-faced adhesive tape.

7.4 Types of phosphor

Materials which convert invisible radiation into luminous radiation are known as phosphors, and whilst a number of such substances exist, only a few of them have applications in radiography.

Two qualities common to the selected phosphors are:

(1) They are very efficient at X-ray absorption;
(2) They fluoresce strongly, with little afterglow.

Examples of some of the phosphors available are: calcium tungstate; barium fluorochloride; barium lead sulphate; barium strontium sulphate; gadolinium oxysulphide; lanthanum oxysulphide; lanthanum oxybromide; yttrium oxysulphide; yttrium tantalate. The last five named are commonly known as **rare earth** phosphors.

7.4.1 The rare earths

In the late 1960s and early 1970s, new phosphors were developed from the rare earth series of elements, i.e. those elements with atomic numbers between 57 (lanthanum) and 71 (lutecium). These phosphors have *two* important physical attributes which give them an advantage over conventional phosphors such as calcium tungstate:

(1) They are more efficient at absorbing X-ray photons (**absorption efficiency** or **quantum detection efficiency**);
(2) They are more efficient at converting X-ray photons to light (**conversion efficiency**).

(1) Quantum detection efficiency (QDE)

Rare earth screens are generally more efficient at absorbing incident radiation than are conventional screens of calcium tungstate. This absorption property is known as the screen's QDE.

The QDE depends not only on the type of phosphor but on the thickness and coating weight of that phosphor, an increase in either resulting in an increase in the QDE.

In addition to these three factors, the QDE is also dependent upon the photon energy of the incident beam, as Table 7.1 shows. It can be seen that for a 60 keV beam some 51% of the incident photons are absorbed by the rare earth screen phosphor, as opposed to only 13% by calcium tungstate. As beam energies increase, so the difference between the absorption abilities of the two screens diminishes.

Table 7.1 Comparison of the absorption characteristics of calcium tungstate and gadolinium oxysulphide phosphors at various photon energy levels. (Data from *Electromedica* 56, 2/88, p. 64.)

Phosphor	X-ray absorption (%) at photon energy level		
	40 keV	60 keV	80 keV
Calcium tungstate	33	13	27
Gadolinium oxysulphide activated with terbium	37	51	28

However, whilst absorption differences may decrease, conversion differences, i.e. the ability of the rare earth screen to convert X-ray energy to light energy, remain far superior.

Summarizing, we can say that a screen which is said to have a high QDE will therefore be faster than a screen with a low QDE.

(2) Conversion efficiency

The rare earths are more efficient at converting X-ray photon interactions into light, e.g. 15–20% light conversion efficiency compared to calcium tungstate 3–5%. This means that for a given radiographic exposure much more light is produced with rare earth screens and so exposure factors can be reduced considerably when using them.

7.4.1.1 Use of activators

Rare earth phosphors are invariably used in conjunction with **activators** which are small quantities of some foreign element added to the phosphor during manufacture.

The choice of phosphor–activator combination not only determines the intensity of luminescence obtainable from the screen but also the colour of the light emitted.

Table 7.2 lists some of the more common rare earth phosphors and activators, along with the colour of light they emit.

Table 7.2 Common rare earth phosphors and activators.

Phosphor	Activator	Emission
Gadolinium oxysulphide	Terbium	Green
Lanthanum oxysulphide	Terbium	Green
Yttrium oxysulphide	Terbium	Blue
Yttrium tantalate	Niobium	Blue
Lanthanum oxybromide	Thulium	Blue

7.5 Matching film to intensifying screen

In order to obtain optimum speed from a film–screen system, i.e. to obtain maximum film blackening for the least radiographic exposure, it is vitally important that films are matched to the colour of intensifying screen emission. For instance, a screen phosphor emitting light towards the green end of the spectrum is best matched with an orthochromatic film (Fig.7.7(a)). This will mean that the film's maximum sensitivity matches the screen's maximum light emission and consequently optimum performance, in terms of speed, will be obtained from that film–screen combination. If the same screen were inadvertently mismatched with a monochromatic film (Fig. 7.7(b)), then the light emission from the screen would have a much diminished effect on the film. In other words, for the same exposure, less film blackening occurs (i.e. system speed is decreased).

Figure 7.8 is another example of a correctly matched film–screen combination; in this case, calcium tungstate (blue emitter) and a monochromatic film.

A comparison of the screen emission pattern in Figs 7.7 and 7.8 shows another significant difference between the older-type phosphors, such as calcium tungstate, and the rare earth phosphors. In the latter type, luminescence is concentrated in a number of narrow bands of wavelengths, quite unlike the continuous spectrum of calcium tungstate emission.

Because of this, phosphors such as calcium tungstate are sometimes known as **broad-band emitters**, whilst the rare earth phosphors are referred to as **line emitters**.

7.6 Types of screen and their applications

In radiographic imaging, intensifying screens are commonly used in pairs.

All screen manufacturers produce at least **three** types of screen of differing speed. The common grades are shown in Table 7.3.

Screen manufacturers are able to produce a variety of screen speeds by the choice of phosphor and size of phosphor grain, the addition/exclusion of absorptive/reflective layers, and by varying the amount of reflective/absorptive material used in screen construction.

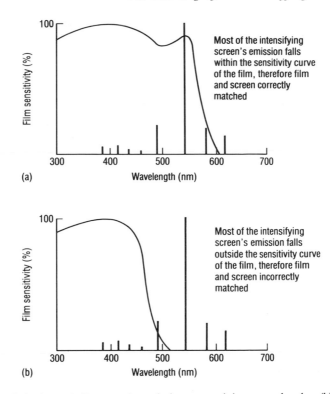

(a)

(b)

Fig. 7.7 (a) Orthochromatic film correctly matched to green emitting screen phosphor. (b) Mismatching of film and screen. A monochromatic film emulsion has been used (maximum sensitivity around 420 nm) whilst the screen's greatest emission is in the 540 nm wavelength range.

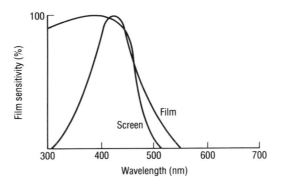

Fig. 7.8 This time the monochromatic film has been correctly matched. Note the continuous spectrum of emission here compared to the type of luminescence seen in Fig. 7.7 – known as line spectra.

7.6.1 High resolution ('Detail')

High-resolution screens are manufactured by making the substratum layer absorptive, as we saw earlier.

Slow-speed screens can be used when the fine detail is required, when radiation dose is less important and when the body part being radiographed does not necessitate a high tube loading (e.g. extremity radiography).

Table 7.3 Common screen speeds

Screen	Speed
High resolution	Slow
Regular or standard	Medium
Fast	Fast

These screens may require exposures two or three times greater than those used with 'regular' screens. Their use will therefore be contraindicated where there is a risk of patient movement, unless effective immobilization can be applied.

7.6.2 *Regular*

This is a medium–speed screen which aims to give the radiographer the best of both worlds (adequate speed and sharpness). It is suitable for most general radiographic applications, and often provides the base from which, in practice, the speeds of other intensifying screens are calculated.

7.6.3 *Fast*

These screens produce greater film blackening for a given radiographic exposure than do 'high-resolution' or 'regular' screens. However, detail sharpness will be diminished, due to the presence of the reflective layer and/or the larger size phosphor grains used in their construction.

These screens are chosen for radiographic examinations where the risk of unsharpness from movement is high, e.g. paediatric radiography. They are also ideal where there is the need to image dense body parts and yet maintain as low a patient dose as possible. The abdomen is a good example.

7.7 Variation in speed of front and back screen

Since most types of X-ray films are duplitized, intensifying screens are commonly used in pairs, with each emulsion surface being placed in close contact with the effective surface of one intensifying screen.

It has been accepted practice in the past to try to obtain equal film blackening on both emulsion surfaces, by increasing the speed of the back screen of the cassette. Were this not to be done, radiation which had traversed the first screen, first emulsion, film base and second emulsion would naturally have been attenuated by the time it reached the fluorescent layer of the back screen. The diminished intensity of radiation will naturally produce a decreased fluorescence in the second screen, resulting in unequal film blackening of the two emulsions.

To get around this problem, the manufacturer can either provide a greater coating weight for the back screen (making it relatively faster) or he can add a pigment to the supercoat of the front screen, the effect of which will be to absorb a proportion of the light being emitted by its fluorescent layer and thus effectively make it slower than the back screen.

Nowadays, however, it is becoming usual to ignore the relatively minor disadvantage of having unequal film blackening, and to purchase pairs of screens which are identical in speed.

7.8 Single-screen radiography

Although intensifying screens are nearly always used in pairs, one exception is in mammography where a single-screen cassette is used in conjunction with a single-coated emulsion film. Eliminating the extra screen and emulsion reduces photographic unsharpness.

If you examine one of these cassettes you will see that the screen is placed at the back, rather than at the front of the cassette as might at first be expected. The reason for the use of a back intensifying screen can be seen in Fig. 7.9.

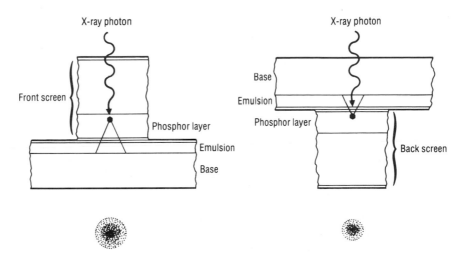

Fig. 7.9 The advantage of a back screen arrangement. Because the photon is absorbed early in its travel through the fluorescent layer a front fitted screen affords more opportunity for the lateral spread of light and therefore increases image unsharpness. A back screen, however, means a reduction in light divergence and therefore a sharper image.

The greatest intensity of light emission arises amongst those phosphor crystals with which the X-ray beam first comes into contact. In the case of a front-fitted screen, it will be those crystals furthest away from the film. Consequently, there will be greater light divergence and more opportunity for irradiation to occur. A back screen, however, results in light being produced in those phosphors nearest the film and therefore there will be less light divergence, less irradiation and a sharper image produced.

7.9 Other less common types of screen

7.9.1 Graduated

This is a screen where the speed gradually decreases across the screen from edge to edge, and is indicated on the screen by '+' and '−' signs.

It is achieved by adding to the supercoat a pigment of gradually increasing density across the screen. Applications for this screen lie in pelvimetry and orthodontics. The fast 'end' of the screen being placed adjacent to the densest part of the patient (the vertebrae in the case of the pelvimetry), whilst the slower part of the screen is sited adjacent to the less–dense anterior abdomen. Thus, a large range of tissue densities can be accommodated on the one film. In orthodontics, it could usefully be employed for a lateral projection in order to demonstrate the relationship of soft tissue and bony structures on the one radiograph prior to, or following, corrective treatment.

7.9.2   Screens for multisection cassettes

Because the radiation is progressively attenuated as it passes through the several pairs of screens of a multisection cassette, the bottom pair of screens will receive less radiation than the top pair, and the film thus exposed at this level will be under-exposed in comparison to the uppermost films in the cassette.

In order to obtain similar film blackening on all films in the cassette, the screen pairs are arranged in increasing speed from top to bottom, the film thus furthest away from the X-ray tube being exposed by the fastest pair of screens. The manufacturers produce these varying screen speeds by either adding varying amounts of pigment to the supercoat or by gradually increasing the coating weight of each fluorescent layer.

7.10   Intensification factor (IF)

The intensification factor is the number by which one must multiply an exposure (mAs) used with screens, in order to produce a film of similar density if exposing the same type of film without screens.

$$\text{Intensification factor (IF)} = \frac{\text{Exposure without screens}}{\text{Exposure with screens}}$$

For example, if the exposure required to give a density of 2.0 on a film used without screens is 150 mAs, and 10 mAs when used with screens, then:

$$\text{IF} = \frac{150}{10} = 15$$

The intensification factor for these screens would therefore be 15.

In practice, the intensification factor is seldom referred to by radiographers. There are three principal reasons for this.

(1) The IF only has meaning when assessing *one* particular type of film which is to be used either *with* or *without* the benefit of screens. It should not be used to compare screen type with non-screen-type film, nor should it be used to contrast different types of screen-type film.
(2) The IF changes with kV (Fig. 7.10). An increase in kV (over the range of kilovoltages used in diagnostic imaging) results in an increase in the intensification factor. **This is the reason why IF must always be quoted in conjunction with a given kV.**
(3) The IF is not constant for all densities. Look at the characteristic curves in Fig. 7.11. They represent a screen type emulsion which has been exposed with and without screens. To obtain the density 1.00 on radiograph B has required more

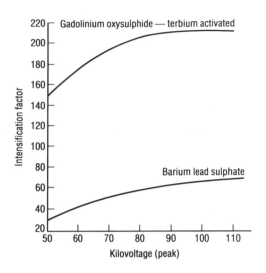

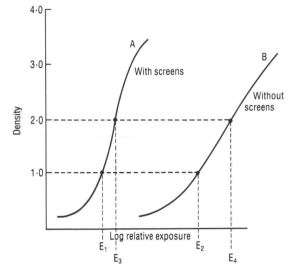

Fig. 7.10 A graph to show how intensification factor varies with increasing kilovoltage for two different screen phosphors.

Fig. 7.11 The curves represent a screen type emulsion which has been exposed (A) with and (B) without screens. It can be seen that the intensification factor is not constant for all densities. At density 2.0 the exposure difference required to produce comparable densities on film A and B is greater. Therefore intensification factor will also be greater.

exposure than it did on radiograph A, the difference in log relative exposure values ($E_2 - E_1$) being representative of the intensification factor for the screens at that density. Consider now density 2.00. The log exposure difference ($E_4 - E_3$) necessary to obtain this density on film B is noticeably larger than at density 1.00. So the IF has not remained constant, but can be seen to be variable throughout the range of densities.

From the foregoing, we can see that the intensification factor for a given screen is only meaningful when considering one particular density and one particular kV value. Were we to examine the IF in the context of another density level or a different kV setting, then the IF (even though it would be for the same screen) will probably not have an identical value.

Little surprise, then, that the IF is very rarely considered by the practising radiographer. (See also *speed class*, section 17.2.2.4).

7.11 Quantum mottle

We explained earlier (section 3.1.3) how the X-ray beam can be thought of as a stream of particles (quanta or photons) of radiation energy. The more photons per square centimetre or the higher the density of photons present in the transmitted beam, the greater will be its information content. If the photons are spread too thinly, the gaps between them may become significant, and lead to a grainy or mottled appearance.

In the ordinary course of events, the number of light photons produced within the phosphor layer from one X-ray photon interaction is many-fold. However, if a situation arose where the number of X-ray photons interacting with the screen phosphor were very few, or the energy of the individual photons was low, then the number of light photons produced would be fewer. Indeed, a situation could arise where the number of light photons produced would fall to a level incompatible with producing a recognizable image. Our film would take on a spotty appearance.

Any factor which contributes to a fall in X-ray absorption by the screen, e.g. increasing kV, poor absorption efficiency, or the combination of fast film–screen and low radiographic exposure, will lead to a fall in the number of X-ray quanta used to create the image, so the light photons produced by the screen will be less and the risk of producing a radiograph of non-uniform density with a mottled appearance will be increased.

Remember! Quantum mottle is a function of neither film nor screen grain size but a product of fast radiographic systems and very small radiation exposures.

7.12   Factors of screen construction affecting speed and sharpness

Earlier in this chapter we described how a certain degree of unsharpness was unavoidable when using intensifying screens due to the diffusion of light (section 7.2).

Now seems a good time to bring together some of the points relating to screen construction which have a bearing on an intensifying screen's performance in terms of speed and sharpness.

Phosphor grain size
Larger crystal sizes mean increased light emission (so an increase in speed) but increased light divergence, the latter factor contributing to loss of sharpness. The smaller the particle size, the greater the amount of light scattering within the phosphor layer leading to greater light absorption by this layer (Eastman Kodak, undated). In other words, light emission is diminished and image sharpness improved.

Thickness of intensifying screen
Consider three different screen thicknesses (Fig. 7.12).

The greater the screen thickness, the greater will be the vertical distance between many of the phosphor grains and the film emulsion, and therefore the greater the lateral spread of light by the time it reaches the film (Fig. 7.12(a)).

Although the cone of light emitted by each screen phosphor in the illustration has the same cone angle θ, the area of density on the film represented by the base area of the cone varies, being greater where the grain is furthest away (Fig. 7.12).

Consequently, with all other factors being equal, there will be more unsharpness with screen (a) than with screen (b), and similarly screen (b) will be less sharp than screen (c).

Nature of substratum layer
We considered the way in which **reflective** and **absorptive** layers influenced screen sharpness and speed earlier in this section (section 7.3.2).

Presence/absence of carbon granules or pigment dye in binder
See section 7.3.3.

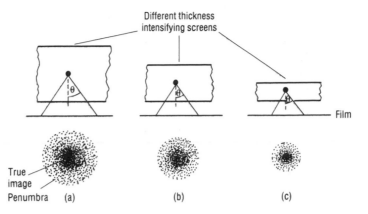

Fig. 7.12 Effect of screen thickness on sharpness. The thicker the intensifying screen, the greater will be the lateral spread of light before it can reach the film and consequently the greater will be image unsharpness.

Crossover effect

Crossover is image degradation caused by light produced in one intensifying screen passing through the film base and producing an image in the opposite emulsion layer (Fig. 7.13 (a)). Crossover thus produces increased blurring because of the longer path taken by the light in reaching the opposite emulsion and the consequent lateral spread of such light. Screens incorporating a reflective layer aggravate this problem.

As we saw with film construction (section 5.1.2), some film manufacturers put an absorbing layer into their films between the base and the emulsion to prevent crossover (Fig. 7.13(b)).

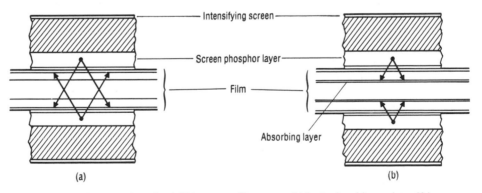

Fig. 7.13 Crossover in an intensifying screen–film system. Light produced in one intensifying screen passes through film emulsion and base to produce a latent image in the opposite emulsion. Such extended light travel results in increased divergence and thereby increased image unsharpness. In (b) the addition of an absorbing layer in the film helps to prevent crossover.

Film emulsions are very efficiency at absorbing UV light in particular, so screens of barium lead sulphate which emit strongly in the UV region of the spectrum are able to minimize crossover because most of the light emitted by the individual screens is absorbed in the adjacent emulsion.

Table 7.4 Features of screen construction which affect speed and sharpness.

Feature	Speed	Sharpness
(1) Crystal size	Increases	Decreases
(2) Phosphor layer thickness	Increases	Decreases
(3) Reflective layer	Increases	Decreases
(4) Absorptive layer	Decreases	Increases
(5) Carbon granules or binder pigment	Decreases	Increases
(6) Crossover	Negligible effect	Decreases
(7) QDE	Increases	No effect
(8) Conversion efficiency	Increases	No effect

Table 7.4 summarizes those screen features which affect screen speed and sharpness.

An understanding of the close relationship which exists between speed and sharpness is important. As we have seen, increasing the speed of an intensifying screen can sometimes mean a concomitant decrease in the resolving power of the screen. It should not be forgotten that whilst unsharpness is an undesirable feature in radiographic imaging, the benefits of speed far outweigh the disadvantages of such unsharpness arising from the use of such screens (at least in most instances).

Some radiographic problems will demand that sharpness be the overriding criterion, whilst other types of situation, e.g. the restless infant, will necessitate that speed be the essential feature.

With the advent of rare earth phosphors and the ongoing development of screen technology, screen manufacturers are able to offer increased speed with little or no loss of sharpness when compared to the older phosphors such as calcium tungstate.

7.13   Assessing the relative speed of a new film–screen system

We pointed out earlier that one manufacturer's 'fast' screen will seldom match precisely the 'fast' label attached to another manufacturer's product.

It is necessary, therefore, when replacing old cassettes and screens to be able to assess what difference in speed there is between the old film–screen combination and the new system, so that compensatory adjustments can be made to exposures. Such a test is described in section 18.3.

7.14   Care and maintenance of intensifying screens

An intensifying screen damaged in any way is irreparably damaged. Since screens are often sold in pairs correctly matched, the only remedy is to replace both. A very expensive exercise.

Finger marks, stains, dust or other foreign fragments will all adversely affect the screens' fluorescent emission. The radiographic evidence will be of sites of reduced density, owing to the inhibition of normal fluorescence in the affected areas.

The following rules will help to eliminate many of these hazards:

- *Do not* open cassettes in the vicinity of chemicals or other liquids.
- *Do not* leave cassettes open on the bench, exposed to contamination.

● *Do not* store cassettes near sources of heat such as radiators (cassettes may warp and film/screen contact will be lost).

7.14.1 Mounting intensifying screens

Manufacturers provide their intensifying screens with special adhesive tape, usually already in position on the back surface of each screen, ready for mounting. A protective layer of paper or thin plastic material is removed from the tape before the screens are positioned in the cassette.

The screens should be handled only at the edges. The front screen is mounted first. It may be identified by the manufacturer specifically as 'FRONT', in which case it should be mounted as such. The prepared screen is dropped carefully into the well of the cassette, with its active surface facing the operator. Similarly, the back screen has its protective pieces removed from the adhesive strips and is placed on top and aligned with the front screen so that the active surfaces face each other. The cassette is then closed and fastened, this manoeuvre being sufficient to give the adhesive adequate hold.

In order for the cassette to be used with some sort of actinic marker, a thin lead blocker is mounted in relation to the front intensifying screen and corresponding in size and position to the window of the photographic marker, usually the lower left or upper right-hand corner. A piece of the new front screen is carefully excised in order to accommodate this lead strip.

A small identification letter or numeral can be placed along one edge of one of the screens so that its image will appear on all radiographs. The outside back surface of the cassette is marked with the same numeral so that a cassette containing dirty screens may be identified easily from a radiograph. Finally, the type of screens that the cassette contains and the date of commissioning is entered on the external surface of the cassette.

7.14.2 Cleaning screens

Should screens require cleaning, the following procedure should be adopted using a mild liquid detergent or proprietary screen cleaner:

(1) Moisten (not saturate) some cotton wool with the solution and gently wipe the screen surfaces. At no stage must the screen be allowed to become excessively wet, nor must water reach the back or edges of the screen.
(2) Wipe the screen free of soap or cleaner with fresh cotton wool.
(3) Wipe dry.
(4) Stand cassette on edge, partly open, and allow to dry completely.
(5) Record date of cleaning on back of cassette.

7.14.3 Checking a screen for artefacts

Should a visual examination fail to identify which of the two screens in a cassette is the faulty one, a piece of black paper the same size as the film is placed inside the cassette, and positioned between the front screen and the film. The film is then exposed. The exercise is repeated, this time placing the paper between the film and the back screen.

Examination of both films should identify which is the faulty screen.

7.15 Advantages of using intensifying screens

In comparison with the use of non-screen film materials, these advantages can be summarized as follows:

(1) Lower exposure factors may be used, thus allowing for reduced patient dose, more frequent use of fine focal spots, the successful use of low-output equipment and less wear and tear on the X-ray tube.
(2) Permits the use of very short exposure times, which is useful where movement unsharpness may pose a problem.
(3) Higher contrast image compared to non-screen imaging.

Chapter 8
The Recording System: Film Cassettes

A film cassette is a container for exposed or unexposed film and this chapter examines not only those types of cassette commonly known as **X-ray cassettes**, and which are used to hold unexposed X-ray film and intensifying screens in close and uniform contact with one another, but also a large variety of other types of cassette, all with very particular applications.

8.1 X-ray cassettes

8.1.1 Functions

(1) To hold intensifying screens and protect them from damage.
(2) To exclude all light from entering the cassette and fogging the film.
(3) To maintain a close and uniform contact between the film and screens.
(4) To exclude dust and dirt from the sensitive screens.

8.1.2 Features of the ideal cassette

(1) Strong and rigid to withstand daily wear and tear.
(2) Lightweight to facilitate easy handling and carrying.
(3) Easy to open and close, under low light conditions.
(4) No sharp edges or corners which might injure patients or staff.

(5) The cassette front must provide minimal beam attenuation, be of uniform thickness and have no irregularities which might be visible on a radiograph.

(6) Have a sliding aperture for use in patient identification systems (see section 14.2.2.2).

(7) Internal rear surface must have an adequate layer of lead foil attached in order to minimize the amount of radiation passing through the cassette and thus reduce the risk of back-scatter.

(8) Cassette design and construction to include features contributing to close contact between film and screen(s), e.g. foam sponges, etc.

(9) Vinyl (or some similar material) covered front providing 'warmth to the touch'.

(10) Availability in range of film sizes.

(11) Be sold with some guarantee of quality.

8.1.3 Construction

The cassette essentially consists of a front and a back hinged at one long edge. Attached to the inside back of the cassette is a thin sheet of lead foil and attached to this a plastic foam pressure pad and an intensifying screen (Fig. 8.1).

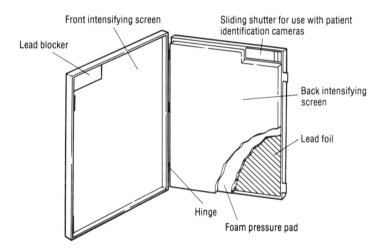

Fig. 8.1 X-ray cassette construction.

The recessed front of the cassette, sometimes referred to as the 'cassette well', contains the front intensifying screen and a short lead blocker along one edge which produces a small unexposed area on the film. This is used for patient identification.

Some cassettes incorporate an additional foam pressure pad underneath the front intensifying screen, e.g. Kodak 'X-Omatic' cassette.

The back of the cassette may incorporate, in one corner, a recess and sliding aperture for use with patient identification cameras (see section 14.2.2.2).

Various manufacturers use a range of locking methods for their cassettes, from spring clips to sliding locking bars, but all serve the dual purpose when in the locked position of helping to exclude all light and, together with the foam pressure pads, maintaining close and uniform contact between film and screens.

All internal metal or plastic surfaces are given a black coating in order to prevent the possibility of internal light reflections.

NB A further design feature aimed to ensure good screen/film contact is a slightly curved cassette back. This assists in providing additional pressure when closed. The importance of good films/screen contact was explained in section 7.2.

8.1.4   Materials used in cassette construction

Since the tendency nowadays is for lightweight cassette design, a large number of synthetic materials are used in their construction.

Cassette front
The front should be of uniform thickness and density and have no irregularities which might be made visible on the radiograph.

   In order to minimize beam attenuation, cassette fronts should conform to British Standards (BS 4304/1968). This recommendation states that the cassette front, if metal, should have an Al equivalent of no more than 1.6 mm when used at 60 kVp or, if plastic, no more than 0.2 mm Al equivalent.

   Metal (e.g. aluminium), plastic laminate or carbon fibre are materials commonly used in cassette front construction.

   All these materials share the following advantages:

(1) Strength and stiffness;
(2) Light in weight;
(3) Low beam absorption.

   The use of carbon–fibre cassettes in particular can mean a significant reduction in patient dose because of their lower beam attenuation, especially at low kilovoltages.

Cassette back
The cassette back may also be of metal or plastic construction and lined with lead foil in order to protect the film from radiation scattered backwards from a bucky tray or other surface. The BS recommendation states that it should have a lead equivalent of at least 0.12 mm when used with equipment operating at 150 kV constant potential.

Cassette fittings
Clips or fasteners –usually stainless steel.
Hinges – metal or plastic.
Pressure pad – plastic foam sponge.

8.2   Types of X-ray cassette available

8.2.1   Single-screen cassette

Some cassettes have a single intensifying screen and are designed to be used with single-sided emulsion film (see section 5.2.2). Their principal application is in mammography (section 8.7.1).

8.2.2   Curved cassettes

Two types of curved cassette are available (Fig. 8.2).

The first type (Fig. 8.2(a)) is used when the necessary close object/cassette contact cannot be achieved with a conventional flat cassette, e.g. intercondylar projections of the knee with the joint flexed.

The second type of curved cassette (Fig. 8.2(b)) is used to obtain panoramic views of the mandible and maxilla in orthodontic radiography (orthopantomography).

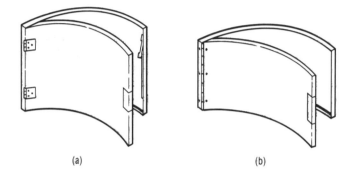

(a)   (b)

Fig. 8.2 Two types of curved cassette; (a) is used where the necessary close contact between object and cassette cannot be achieved with a conventional flat cassette, e.g. intercondylar views of the flexed knee joint; (b) is used to obtain panoramic views of the mandible (orthopantomography).

8.2.3   Gridded cassette

These cassettes have a stationary, secondary radiation grid incorporated in the front well of the cassette, between the front intensifying screen and the front of the cassette. The cassette is used for radiography where a conventional bucky system is unavailable, e.g. in ward mobile work.

Details of the grid, such as its grid ratio, should be identifiable on the outside of the cassette. Gridded cassettes are supplied in most of the usual cassette sizes but have a limited choice of grid ratios.

8.2.4   Multisection cassettes

The most common use for these cassettes is in tomography where they are used to produce, with one radiographic exposure, a set of films each bearing an image of a different layer height within the body. Moreover, the layer images so produced will be representative of body sections equal distances apart.

These cassettes may be designed to hold 3–7 films, with their respective intensifying screens and spacers. The spacers may be 5 or 10 mm in thickness and made of radiolucent foam sponge. Films which are separated by 5 mm spacers will produce images of body sections 5 mm apart. Similarly, films which are separated by 10 mm of spacing material will bear images of separate body layers 10 mm apart.

The cassette in Fig. 8.3 holds four 24 × 30 cm films, with their intensifying screens and 10 mm spacers.

We discussed the types of intensifying screens used in multisection cassettes in section 7.9.2. Multisection cassettes have another application in a technique known

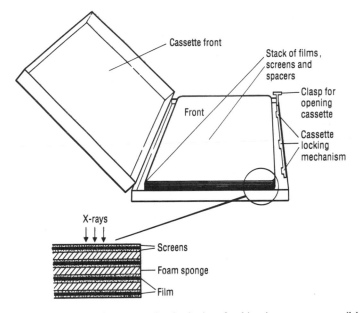

Fig. 8.3 A multisection cassette for tomography. A selection of multisection cassettes are available with a choice of spacer thickness and number of screen pairs.

as **multiple radiography**. In this procedure the cassette is loaded with a set of films and varying speed intensifying screens, but no spacers. Thus, with one exposure a set of films is produced each with a different density range and contrast due to the variation in intensifying screen speeds used. The intensifying screen–film combinations can thus be chosen in order to give the desired range of image densities, e.g. from bone to soft tissue.

8.3 Cassettes and automatic exposure devices

Where cassettes are to be used with a phototiming device placed behind the cassette, the back of the cassette must have no lead present and be as radiolucent as the front. This is in contradistinction to the situation where ionization chamber devices are being used, when, because of their placement between the source and the film, they may be used with any conventional X-ray cassette.

8.4 Care of X-ray cassettes

Treated with care, X-ray cassettes will survive many years of hard work. Careless handling sooner or later leads to cassette damage and problems such as poor film/screen contact or light leakage.

Note the following points:

(1) Treat cassettes gently.
(2) Limit the number of cassettes carried at any one time. Carry securely between body and arm, with the fingers holding their bottom edges.
(3) If cassettes are stored on edge, ensure that cassettes are as near vertical as

possible. Damage can ensue if cassettes are stored at an angle, with other more weighty ones leaning against them.

(4) Where cassettes may need to be placed directly under a patient (not in a Potter bucky), the use of a cassette tunnel should be considered in order to prevent undue pressure on the cassette itself.

(5) Avoid contact with fluids. Protect the cassette with some sort of plastic waterproof cover when necessary.

8.5   Cassette maintenance

In order to provide both a check on a cassette's lifespan and contribute to the efficiency of maintenance, the following procedures should be carried out:

(1) Record on the cassette the date it was introduced into the department.
(2) Identify each cassette with a letter or numeral placed on one edge of an intensifying screen and the same on the outside of the cassette. The image of such a numeral will then appear on the exposed film and any subsequent film fault is thus easily traced to the relevant cassette.
(3) Keep a record of cassette maintenance, e.g. when inspected, when cleaned, when tested for light leakage, etc.

Cassettes and screens should be inspected regularly for signs of damage and withdrawn from service if necessary.

If radiographs show evidence of either light fogging or poor film/screen contact, the tests described in section 18.2 should be carried out.

8.6   Loading and unloading a cassette

The normal, useful life of intensifying screens depends to a large extent on the care taken during film loading and unloading, for it is at this time that the sensitive screen surfaces are exposed to the possibility of dust contamination and the danger of insensitive handling.

Unloading
Under safelights, the cassette is placed face downwards on the bench and the locking clip released. The cassette is then turned over and the front of the cassette tipped so that the film falls from the cassette well. The film is removed with the free hand and the cassette closed.

Loading
Under safelights, the cassette is placed face downwards on the bench and, as before, opened from the back. The unexposed film, lightly gripped at its edge, is lowered gently into the cassette well. The cassette is closed by bringing over the back and engaging the locking clip.

8.7   Other types of cassette

8.7.1   *Vacuum cassette*

These cassettes (which are supplied with a vacuum pump) are made from flexible vinyl material and have a valve attached at one edge. Inside is a removable plastic folder containing a single intensifying screen (Fig. 8.4).

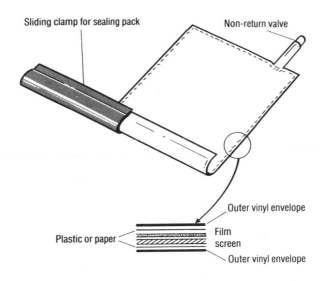

Fig. 8.4 A vacuum cassette. Once the film has been inserted and the sliding clamp replaced, all air is extracted via the non-return valve thereby bringing film and screen into intimate contact.

To prepare the cassette for use, a single-sided emulsion film is inserted inside the folder, with its emulsion surface facing the intensifying screen. The entire folder is placed inside the cassette and the cassette sealed by applying pressure along the edges of the opening. A sliding clamp is then drawn over the sealed edges.

The vacuum pump is attached to the valve and air expelled, thus bringing the intensifying screen and film into very close contact. In this position they are held by uniform distribution of atmospheric pressure.

Although primarily developed for use in mammography, vacuum cassettes have other applications in radiography where their inherent flexibility can be used to advantage in positioning, e.g. under a flexed joint.

The cassettes are available in a range of sizes, 18 × 24 cm and 24 × 30 cm being the most popular.

8.7.2 Formatter cassette

This type of cassette is used for imaging from cathode ray tubes (CRT) and TV monitors in ultrasound, nuclear medicine, computerized tomography (CT), digital subtraction angiography (DSA) and magnetic resonance imaging (MRI). It is used in conjunction with a formatter or video–imager (section 23.4).

The cassettes consist of a frame designed to hold two single-sided emulsion films by their edges, and two removable slides which protect the films from light exposure when not in use (Fig. 8.5). They do not contain intensifying screens.

The cassette is loaded under safelight conditions by removing the two slides and sliding the individual films, emulsion side facing outwards, into either side of the frame, carefully ensuring that they are securely held in the side channels of the frame by their long edges (Fig. 8.5). This is very important, otherwise when the slide is removed the film will sag when in the imager. Finally, the slides are inserted.

When required for use, the cassette is inserted into the multiformat imager and

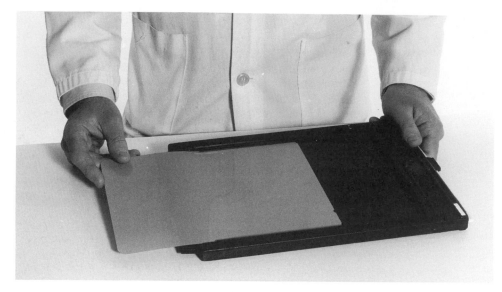

Fig. 8.5 A formatter cassette being loaded.

the slide nearest the film to be exposed is removed. The film is now ready for exposure. Once imaging is complete, the slide is returned to the cassette, the cassette withdrawn from the imager, turned over and reinserted. The second slide is removed, thus making the second film available for exposure.

The cassettes are available in Imperial sizes $10 \times 8''$ and $14 \times 11''$, and several manufacturers produce cassettes which are compatible with daylight loading/unloading systems.

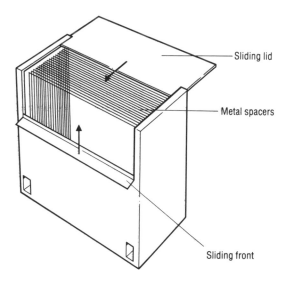

Fig. 8.6 The AOT film supply cassette. Individual films are inserted between the metal spacers and sliding front raised to lock with the sliding lid. The cassette is then inserted in the AOT film changer.

8.7.3 *Angiography cassettes*

Siemens Elema AOT system

The film feed or supply cassette will hold up to 30 sheets of unexposed films, size 35 × 35 cm, each positioned between metal spacers (Fig. 8.6).

After loading and sliding shut the two panels under safelight conditions, the cassette can be inserted in the AOT equipment. The take-up cassette (Fig. 8.7), with its sliding lid open, is also inserted in the AOT.

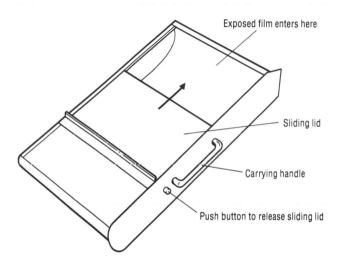

Fig. 8.7 The AOT film take-up cassette.

On completion of an imaging sequence, the exposed films will have been transferred via the exposure area of the AOT apparatus to the take-up cassette. A button on the front of this cassette is pressed, closing the sliding lid. The take-up cassette can then be withdrawn and conveyed to the darkroom, where the exposed films are removed and processed.

Puck system

Whilst the particular details of construction may be different from the Siemens AOT system, the basic principles are nonetheless the same, i.e. during an angiographic procedure 35 × 35 cm films are rapidly conveyed from supply to take-up cassette (Fig. 8.8).

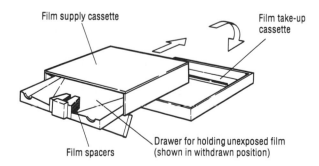

Fig. 8.8 The puck rapid film changer cassettes.

8.7.4   *Photofluorography cassettes*

Photofluorography, or the recording of images from the output phosphor of an image intensifier tube, is usually carried out on 70 mm or 105 mm roll film, or on 100 mm sheet film. All these various film formats have their individual cassette systems. We examine them in more detail in Chapter 21.

So far, we have looked at how images are produced and the recording system itself. Now we turn to the next important aspect of image production, film processing.

Chapter 9
Radiographic Processing – Principles

In Chapters 4 and 5 we described the essential features of the photosensitive emulsions used in modern X-ray films. We stated that the effect on such materials of exposure to light or X-ray radiation is to produce an invisible **latent image** within the emulsion. The emulsion of X-ray films must be chemically processed to render visible and permanent the information recorded in the latent image. The purpose of this chapter is to describe the principles employed in the processing of film in modern X-ray departments, while in the next chapter we discuss the applications of these principles.

The processing of X-ray films by hand (**manual processing**) is now undertaken only in exceptional circumstances. By far the most common method of X-ray processing is to use automatic, wholly mechanized processors. We shall therefore concentrate mainly on automatic processing and consider manual processing in outline only, at the end of each section.

Film processing involves a number of complex chemical reactions whose activity and efficiency are influenced by various factors, including the temperature and acidity or alkalinity of the chemical environment in which the reactions take place. Thus, it is essential to have at our disposal methods of describing these factors quantitatively. Temperature (in the UK) is quoted in Celsius (°C) and acidity/alkalinity is expressed using the pH scale. Because of the importance of pH in photographic processing, we have outlined below the basic concept of pH. (Readers who are familiar with pH may omit this section.)

9.1 The pH scale

The pH scale is used to express the degree of acidity or alkalinity of a solution. It is based on a measure of the concentration of the positively charged hydrogen ions in a solution.

In water the H_2O molecule dissociates into a hydrogen ion (H^+) and a hydroxyl ion (OH^-). In a neutral solution, such as pure water, these ions are present in equal numbers at a concentration of 10^{-7} mol/l (moles per litre, where the mole is a fundamental unit of matter). If added to water, some substances cause an increase in the concentration of hydrogen ions to $> 10^{-7}$ mol/l. The solution is then said to be acidic. The addition of other substances to water may result in a reduction in the concentration of hydrogen ions to $< 10^{-7}$ mol/l and the solution is then alkaline.

As a solution becomes more acidic, its hydrogen ion concentration rises; for example, in gastric juice, which contains hydrochloric acid, the H^+ concentration is $\sim 10^{-1.7}$ mol/l. An alkaline solution has a reduced H^+ concentration, e.g. $\sim 10^{-7.4}$ mol/l, for blood plasma. The logarithm of the H^+ concentration provides a convenient figure on which to base a scale of acidity and alkalinity.

For gastric juice, for example:

$$\log_{10} (H^+ \text{ concentration}) = \log_{10} 10^{-1.7}$$
$$= -1.7$$

the pH of gastric juice is then said to be 1.7.

For blood plasma:

$$\log_{10} (H^+ \text{ concentration}) = \log_{10} 10^{-7.4}$$
$$= -7.4$$

the pH of blood plasma is then said to be 7.4.

Thus, pH can be defined as the negative logarithm (to the base 10) of the hydrogen ion concentration of a solution. A solution with a pH of 7 is neutral, pH of > 7 is alkaline and pH < 7 is acidic. Figure 9.1 shows a scale of pH with some typical examples included. Note that the developers used in radiography are alkaline, while the fixing solutions are acidic.

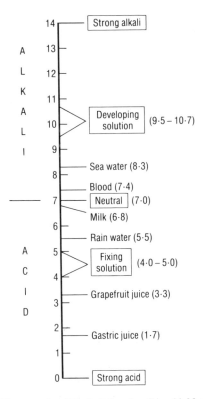

Fig. 9.1 The pH scale. A pH greater than 7 is alkali, less than 7 is acid. Note that even unpolluted rain water is acidic, due to the effects of dissolved carbon dioxide.

It is important to remember that because pH is a logarithmic quantity, a change of 1 in a pH value represents a *tenfold* change in hydrogen ion concentration (Plummer, 1989). A doubling of the hydrogen ion concentration is expressed as a fall of only 0.3 in pH. Thus, what may appear to be quite small changes in pH can represent very significant changes in acidity or alkalinity.

9.2　The processing cycle

In automatic processing the complete processing cycle comprises four main stages:

(1) Development;
(2) Fixing;
(3) Washing;
(4) Drying.

The object of the whole cycle is to produce a dry radiograph carrying a high quality image which can be stored for a number of years without deterioration. We shall now consider each of the stages in the processing cycle in more detail.

9.2.1　Development

Development is the first stage in processing. Its primary purpose is to convert into visible form the invisible latent image produced when the film was exposed. During development, the silver halide grains in the emulsion which were affected by exposure are reduced to metallic silver, while those which were unaffected by exposure remain largely unchanged.

In practice, the developer is not completely successful in differentiating between the exposed and unexposed silver halide grains. Given sufficient time, the developer will reduce *all* the silver halide to silver. A good developer is highly selective in that it acts far more quickly on exposed grains than on unexposed ones. A poor developer (or a good developer working under adverse conditions) will act on unexposed grains and produce **chemical fog**.

NB *The reader may wish to review the action of exposure on silver halides and the process of latent image formation described in Chapter 4 before studying the next section.*

9.2.1.1　Chemical action of developer
Development is a process of chemical reduction. The reduction is achieved by the developer donating electrons to the silver ions in the exposed silver bromide (and iodide) grains, converting them to atoms of metallic silver. The mode of action of developers is not fully understood but the existence of electric charge barriers around the halide grains is thought to be involved (John, 1967).

Charge barriers
Both exposed and unexposed silver bromide grains are surrounded by a negative charge barrier of bromine ions created by the excess of potassium bromide employed in the synthesis of silver bromide during the manufacture of emulsion (see section 4.3.3). The charge barrier normally protects the silver bromide from attack by electrons in the developing solution (Fig. 9.2).

Exposed silver bromide grains possess a weakness in the charge barrier caused by the presence of neutral silver atoms which have collected at the sensitivity speck.

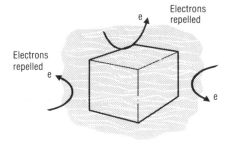
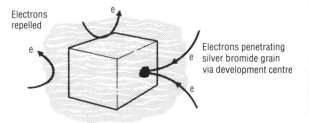

Fig. 9.2 A silver bromide grain in developing solution. The grain is protected from attack by electrons (e) because of the presence of a complete negative charge barrier around the grain.

Fig. 9.3 An exposed silver bromide grain in developing solution. The presence of neutral silver atoms at the sensitivity speck constitutes a development centre which enables electrons from the developer to penetrate the grain and reduce it completely to silver.

This **development centre** enables electrons from the developer to penetrate the grain and reduce all its silver ions to metallic silver (Fig. 9.3).

If a film spends too long a time in the developer, or if the developer is hyperactive, e.g. due to elevated temperature, excessively high concentration, or raised pH, the charge barrier around unexposed grains may be unable to prevent electron penetration, and unexposed grains will be reduced to silver. Chemical fogging will be the result.

By-products of development

As the development process continues and exposed silver halides are reduced to silver, the developer becomes depleted of electrons: it is said to be **oxidized**. Even if no development takes place, reaction with atmospheric oxygen occurs, causing **aerial** oxidation of the developer. Thus, the supply of reducing agent in developer is gradually exhausted.

Additionally, the negative bromine ions which remain when exposed grains are developed may combine with positive hydrogen ions from developer solution to form **hydrobromic acid**. Hydrobromic acid begins to accumulate in the developer causing its pH to fall. The activity of the reducing agents in developer depends greatly on pH and on bromine ion concentration; thus developer activity is adversely affected.

If not corrected, these chemical changes which occur in working developer will cause it to become progressively less effective.

We have described the primary function of developer: to act as a selective reducing agent. But to fulfil this function and maintain it with constant activity is no easy task; many extra chemical constituents are needed to achieve this objective. We shall now examine the most important of the constituents which make up a developing solution.

9.2.1.2   Constituents of developing solution

The developing solutions used in automatic rapid-cycle processors are different in several important respects from those used for manual processing. The description which follows is based on the solutions used in automatic processing, but where relevant we will point out how manual systems differ (M&B, 1976).

Replenisher and starter solutions

The solution which is fed into the developing section of an automatic processor when it is actively processing films is known as **developer replenisher**. It is the developing solution used in greatest quantities in X-ray departments today. When a processor has been drained of its chemicals, perhaps during cleaning or servicing, the developer replenisher in the developing section of the processor has extra ingredients added in the form of a **starter solution,** to modify its activity until a number of films have been processed and the developer activity has settled down.

Manual processing does not use a developer starter. Indeed, the philosophy of manual processing is quite different from that of automatic processing. Radiographers of an older generation may feel that working developer is the solution which should be described first. Current practice suggests that it is the developer replenisher which should enjoy this privilege. We shall therefore describe the constituents of developer replenisher first.

9.2.1.3   Developer replenisher solution

Developer replenisher consists of:

(1) Solvent.
(2) Developing agents.
(3) Accelerator.
(4) Buffers.
(5) Restrainers.
(6) Preservative.
(7) Hardener.
(8) Sequestering agent.

Let us consider each of these constituents in turn.

(1) Solvent

Water is the solvent used in radiographic processing. It acts as the carrying medium in which the developer constituents are dissolved. It also provides a means of controlling developer activity by diluting its effects. It has a softening effect on the film emulsion gelatin, thus allowing the developing chemicals to penetrate the emulsion and act on the silver halides.

Tap water is cheap and universally available, at least in the developed countries of the world. It usually contains dissolved mineral salts, the exact nature of which varies in different regions; calcium salts are particularly common. If present in the high concentrations found in hard-water areas, such minerals may precipitate out of solution, forming a chalky deposit or scum on the surface of films processed in the solutions. Manufacturers anticipate this tendency by including water-softening agents (**sequestering agents**) in their processing solutions, so that only in extreme cases is precipitation a problem.

More serious would be contamination of the solvent with dissolved metals, such as iron or copper. The presence of only a fewer parts per million of copper could cause chemical fogging. In practice, such effects are extremely rare, even though water is commonly supplied to processors through copper piping.

The water used for developer solutions must be clean and free from insoluble deposits, such as grit or rust particles, which could scratch the delicate film emulsion or damage the processing equipment.

(2) Developing agents

Developing agents are the reducing agents which carry out the primary function of supplying the electrons that convert the exposed silver halide grains to silver. The reducing agents in developer must exhibit certain characteristics:

(1) They must be selective and distinguish effectively between exposed and unexposed grains;
(2) They must be of sufficiently high activity to allow complete development of the film in a relatively short time, e.g. 20–30 seconds, giving a total processing time of $1\frac{1}{2}$–2 minutes. Note that selectivity and activity tend to be antagonistic properties: an agent with high activity generally has low selectivity, and vice versa;
(3) They must be as resistant as possible to the presence of bromine ions in solution.

There is no single reducing agent which satisfies all of these requirements. Modern X-ray developers use a combination of two developing agents: **Phenidone** and **hydroquinone**. A developer based on this formulation is known as a PQ developer ('P' from Phenidone and 'Q' from quinol, an alternative name for hydroquinone).

Phenidone Phenidone is the trade name given by Ilford Ltd to the chemical 1-phenyl-3-pyrazolidone, which was developed in their laboratories early in the 1950s. Phenidone is a quick-acting reducing agent, capable of developing *all* exposed silver halide grains. However, its selectivity is low and if used alone would result in high fog levels. It is mildly sensitive to bromine ion concentration.

Hydroquinone Hydroquinone requires a strongly alkaline medium in which to act. It is more selective than Phenidone but it does not begin development as quickly. Once it has begun to reduce the exposed halide grains, development proceeds vigorously although lightly exposed grains are not affected by hydroquinone. Hydroquinone therefore tends to produce a high-contrast result.

Advantages of PQ developers When Phenidone and hydroquinone act together in a PQ developer their characteristics complement each other. PQ developers offer several advantages over other developing agent combinations:

(1) Tolerant of increases in bromine ion concentration;
(2) High selectivity and therefore low chemical fog;
(3) Adequate activity even in low concentrations;
(4) Available in liquid concentrate form (some developers can only be purchased in the less convenient powder form);
(5) Fast acting, permitting complete development in 20–30 seconds;
(6) Adequate contrast characteristics;
(7) Super-additive effect. The presence of hydroquinone increases the effectiveness of Phenidone by regenerating some of the Phenidone which has become oxidized during its reaction with silver halide. Thus, the reducing effect of the combination of Phenidone and hydroquinone is much greater than the sum of the effects they produce when used separately. Figure 9.4 shows that for a given exposure, the image density produced by a PQ developer is greater than the sum of the densities which would result if the developing agents were used separately. This effect is known as **super-additivity** and is a major advantage of PQ developers over other formulations (John, 1967).

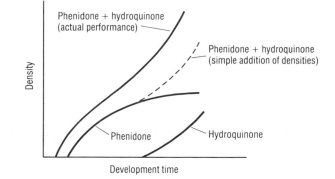

Fig. 9.4 Superadditivity effect obtained with a PQ developer. The effect obtained from the Phenidone–hydroquinone mixture is far greater than the simple arithmetic sum of their separate effects (see text).

(3) Accelerators

PQ developers need an alkaline medium in which to operate. The alkalinity of the solution is established by the inclusion of a strong alkali such as potassium carbonate or potassium hydroxide, whose high solubility makes them particularly suitable in liquid concentrate preparations. The alkali is known as an **accelerator**, since its effect is to accelerate the developing process.

The pH of the developing solution has a marked effect on its activity and on image contrast. If pH is too low (weakly alkaline) the developing action is sluggish; if pH is too high (strongly alkaline) the developer is overactive and uncontrolled, resulting in unacceptable chemical fogging. The range of pH values for different radiographic developer solutions is about 9.8–11.4. Note, however, that for a specific developer the pH must not vary.

(4) Buffers

A buffer is a chemical compound which has the effect of maintaining the pH of a solution within close limits. The presence of buffering agents in developing solution prevents the undesirable effects of changes in pH due to aerial oxidation of developer and the acidic by-products of the development process (see section 9.2.1.1). Normally, adequate buffering action is provided by the carbonates used as accelerators and the sulphides acting as preservatives. Thus, no *additional* buffering chemicals are necessary in most developing solutions.

(5) Restrainers

The action of a restrainer is to modify the behaviour of developing agents so that they become more selective in their action. The effect is to reduce the tendency to convert unexposed silver halide grains to silver and therefore to prevent chemical fogging. Restrainers act by increasing the negative charge barrier which surrounds the silver halide grains. The development process itself produces as a by-product **potassium bromide**, which is a very effective restrainer. A working developer solution therefore contains potassium bromide as a natural consequence of the passage of films through the solution. Thus, the developer replenisher which we are describing does not need to include potassium bromide among its constituents. However, it is usual to provide in PQ developers a quantity of a powerful organic restrainer or **anti-foggant**, such as **benzotriazole**, since the amount of potassium bromide otherwise required would be so excessive as to cause staining of the image. Developer replenisher therefore contains such an anti-foggant.

(6) Preservatives
These chemicals have two functions in developing solution:

(1) Developing agents are easily oxidized and readily combine with atmospheric oxygen. If nothing is done to check this, the consumption of developer replenisher will be increased. A **preservative** is therefore included, which reduces the oxidation of developing agents.
(2) The preservatives permit more efficient regeneration of Phenidone by hydroquinone, by preventing the hydroquinone oxidation products from interfering in the regeneration process.

Potassium sulphite is a commonly used developer preservative.

(7) Hardeners
The gelatin in a film emulsion swells and softens when it absorbs water. The effect is even more pronounced in an alkaline solution, such as developer. In an automatic processor, excessive swelling must be prevented in order that the film can be transported successfully, without jamming or being damaged by the roller mechanism of the processor. Swelling is minimized by a pre-hardening process during film manufacture (see section 4.3.3) and by the inclusion of a hardener in the developer. Powerful organic hardeners, such as **glutaraldehyde**, may be employed because they are effective in the alkaline developer. However, manufacturers are increasingly using alternatives to glutaraldehyde because of its undesirable allergenic effects (HSE, 1992; Kodak, 1993). If the emulsion is over-hardened, the speed with which the developing agents penetrate to the silver halide grains is reduced, resulting in inadequate development. Developers formulated for manual processing may not include a hardening agent.

(8) Sequestering agents
Sequestering agents are chemicals which prevent the precipitation of insoluble mineral salts, which tends to occur in 'hard-water' areas. They act by combining with the minerals to form soluble compounds which do not react with the developer chemicals. Compounds based on EDTA (ethylene-diamine-tetra-acetic acid) are commonly included in developer for this purpose.

Other constituents of developer replenisher
In addition to the eight constituents described above, developer replenisher solution also contains bactericides and fungicides to inhibit the growth of organisms in the solution and in its containing vessels. Such organisms can lead to unpleasant effects, such as the formation of a slimy coating on the walls of the developer tank in the processor.

9.2.1.4   Starter solution
The manufacturer supplies developer replenisher for automatic processors in a concentrated liquid form, which requires dilution before it can be used in a processor. Additionally, it contains no potassium bromide restrainer and even after appropriate dilution it has a higher pH than is required for a working developer situation. When it has been in use for some time and a number of films have been developed, the pH will have been reduced and potassium bromide will have been

created as a result of the effects of the development process. Initially, however, when the developer tank has been refilled, e.g. after emptying for cleaning purposes, the developer replenisher will be overactive and the first few films to be processed will be overdeveloped, resulting in chemical fogging, excessive density and reduced contrast. To prevent these undesirable effects, a **starter** solution is added to the fresh replenisher in the developing tank. Starter solution is basically an acidic restrainer. When added to developer replenisher, it reduces the pH to its normal working value and it provides a supply of potassium bromide restrainer until such time as the films being developed generate their own. Thus:

Developer replenisher + Developer starter = Working developer

Developers for manual processing do not use starter solutions. The basic developer solution provided by the manufacturer for manual processing contains potassium bromide restrainer and when diluted is of the correct pH. It is already a working developer. A differently formulated solution (replenisher) needs to be added to the working developer to maintain its activity when films are being processed.

9.2.1.5   Factors affecting development
The conversion of the invisible latent image into a visible radiographic image takes place during the developing stage in the processing cycle. The production of optical density and radiographic contrast can be used as a measure of the efficacy of development (Pizzutiello & Cullinan, 1993). The factors which influence the quantity and quality of development may be described under three headings:

(1) Constitution of developing solution.
(2) Developer temperature.
(3) Development time.

Let us study each of these factors in more detail.

(1) Constitution of developing solution
The image density produced depends on the amount of metallic silver formed in the film emulsion. For a particular level of exposure this depends both on the emulsion characteristics and on **developer activity**. It is the effect of developer activity which is the subject of this description. Developer activity is influenced by:

(1) Choice of developing agents and their relative proportions. This affects what we might term the **inherent characteristics** of the developer. X-ray film developers are **high-energy, high-contrast** developers.
(2) Concentration of developing agents in solution. This is established as the liquid concentrate supplied by the manufacturer is diluted with water when the solution is mixed ready for use. In general, higher concentrations result in greater activity but eventually lead to increased chemical fog. For this reason, the dilution recommended by the manufacturer must be adhered to in order to achieve optimum results.
    As more films are processed the supply of developing agents becomes exhausted. Unless they are replaced, this leads to a reduction in their concentration and a decrease in developer activity. Even if *no* films are developed, the **aerial oxidation** of developing agents will result in their gradual exhaustion. If carried out at the correct rate, developer replenishment main-

tains a constant developing agent concentration and thus optimum developer activity.

(3) pH of the developer solution. The by-products of development are acidic and the pH of the developing solution tends to fall. Developer activity is heavily dependent on solution pH and development is inhibited if pH decreases. Buffers can stabilize pH to an extent but replenishment of the alkaline accelerator is essential if developer activity is to be maintained. Again, the *rate* of replenishment is critical. The addition of too much replenisher will result in the developer becoming too alkaline and cause an increase in chemical fog. The absence of developer starter from a newly filled developing tank has a similar effect because the pH of fresh replenisher solution is too high for it to be used as a working developer (see section 9.2.1.4).

(4) Concentration of restrainer and anti-foggant. As we have seen, potassium bromide restrainer is released continuously into a working developer as a by-product of developing activity. The organic anti-foggant, however, needs to be replaced if chemical fog and a reduction in image contrast are to be avoided. Proper developer replenishment ensures that the correct concentration of anti-foggant is maintained.

Thus, it is clear that without replenishment the activity of a developing solution inevitably falls and image quality suffers. Developer **exhaustion** occurs. Activity can only be maintained if the lost chemicals are replaced by adding developer replenisher at the correct rate.

Factors affecting developer replenishment rate The volume of replenisher required to maintain developer activity depends on a number of factors:

(1) Area of film processed: e.g. processing a 35×43 cm film uses more developer than an 18×24 cm film because more emulsion and therefore more silver halide is present. The volume of replenisher required is approximately proportional to the area of film processed. Note that a single-coated film has only half the emulsion area of a duplitized film of the same size, and thus needs less replenishment.

(2) Type of emulsion: a direct-exposure film consumes more developing agent than a screen-type film of the same size because it has a higher silver halide coating weight. The replenisher requirement is therefore greater for direct-exposure film.

(3) Types of image: a heavily exposed film contains more exposed silver halide grains than a similar film which has received less exposure. Thus, more development takes place and more replenishment is needed for a darker image: for example, an abdominal radiograph of a barium-filled colon uses less developing agent than the same abdomen with no barium present; a radiograph for which the beam has been collimated well inside the edges of the film uses less developing agent than a similar radiograph with no obvious collimation (M&B, 1976).

(4) Aerial oxidation: developing agents exposed to atmospheric oxygen become oxidized. The rate of aerial oxidation (and thus the need for replenishment) is reduced if the area of the surface of developer solution exposed to the air can be minimized, e.g. by the use of a lid. The effect of aerial oxidation is more significant if the developer tank is shallow rather than deep (see Fig. 9.5). This is because the ratio of exposed surface area to volume of solution is greater in the case of shallow tanks.

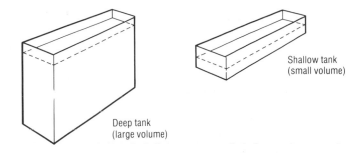

Deep tank
(large volume)

Shallow tank
(small volume)

Fig. 9.5 Aerial oxidation is more significant in shallow developing tanks because for the same exposed surface area the shallow tank contains a much smaller volume of developing solution.

The rate of aerial oxidation also depends on developer temperature, because chemical activity increases with temperature.

Maintenance of developer volume Without replenishment, the volume and therefore the level of developer solution in the developing tank of a processor will fall. The loss occurs due to:

(1) Carry-over. Each time a film leaves the developer tank it carries with it a small but significant volume of developing solution. This **carry-over** of solution consists of:
   (a) Developer solution which has been absorbed into the gelatin of the film emulsion. Its volume depends on the film throughput of the processor: specifically, on the area and thickness of the emulsion and on the extent to which it has been hardened.
   (b) Developer solution adhering to the surface of the film. Its volume depends on film throughput: specifically, on the surface area of the film. In automatic processors, rollers with a **squeegee** action remove most of the surface solution and allow it to drain back into the developing tank (see section 10.1). In manual processing, a few seconds are allowed for some of the surface adherent solution to drain naturally from the film back into the developing tank. Other than this, no positive steps are taken to reduce carry-over of developer during manual processing.
(2) Evaporation. A small amount of solution volume will be lost due to evaporation from the exposed surface of developer in its tank. The volume lost increases with the area of exposed surface and with developer temperature. The use of a lid minimizes evaporation losses.

An incidental, but important function of developer replenishment is to replace the *volume* of solution lost due to carry-over and evaporation. To prevent a fall in developer solution level, the volume replenishment rate must be *no less than* the volume loss rate and must be matched to the film throughput of the processor.

Having completed our discussion of the effects on development of the constitution of the developer solution, we shall next examine the influence of developer temperature.

(2) Developer temperature
Most chemical activity is temperature-dependent, and photographic development is no exception. In general, developer activity increases with temperature.

Consequently, the image density and contrast produced when a film is processed can only be standardized if developer temperature can be maintained constant. Temperature control is therefore an essential feature of processor design (section 10.5.2).

High-temperature development In the early days of rapid automatic processing, developer temperatures of up to 42°C were necessary to permit 90 s processing cycle times. At such temperatures it was difficult to control chemical fogging, aerial oxidation rate was high and emulsions softened unduly. More recently, manufacturers have been able to overcome these problems and offer in their range of processing chemicals **high-temperature** developers, which are used at temperatures in the range 38–42°C and which enable 90 s or even faster cycle times to be operated.

Low-temperature development However, **low-temperature** developers for automatic processing are also available, which operate at around 30°C and can still produce very rapid results. Such low-temperature chemistry offers the advantages of reduced energy consumption, reduced wear and tear on the processing machine and cooler, more pleasant working conditions around the processor. Some developers are extremely versatile and can be used over a range of temperatures, requiring different processor cycle times, e.g. a 7 min cycle at 20°C but a 90 s cycle at 30°C.

Medium-temperature development Most modern developers operate within a mid-range of temperatures (e.g. between 37 and 33°C) offering dry-to-dry processing cycle times of 90 to 160 seconds, depending on the particular processor model concerned (Pizzutiello & Cullinan, 1993).

Effects on the image of increased developer temperature (Fig. 9.6). A *slightly* raised temperature (e.g. 0.5°C) without a compensating reduction in development time results in:

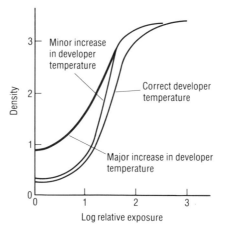

Fig. 9.6 Effect of increased developer temperature. At a temperature several degrees above normal the image suffers increased density, increased fog and reduced contrast.

(1) Increased image density for the same exposure (and thus increased film speed);
(2) Slightly increased chemical fog;
(3) Increased image contrast.

A more severe rise in temperature (e.g. several degrees) initially leads to:

(1) Gross increase in density;
(2) Unacceptable increase in chemical fog;
(3) Reduction in contrast (due to increased fog).

NB If the temperature rise is left uncorrected, the developer becomes exhausted, resulting in *low*-density, *low*-contrast images.

Effects on the image of reduced developer temperature (Fig. 9.7) A *slightly* lowered temperature results in:

(1) Decreased image density for the same exposure (and thus reduced film speed);
(2) Slightly reduced chemical fog;
(3) Reduced image contrast.

A more severe fall in temperature leads to:

(1) Gross overall reduction in density;
(2) Loss of contrast (due to reduced D_{max}).

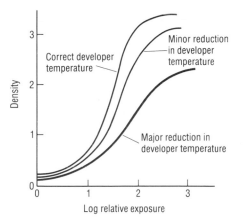

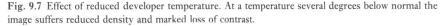

Fig. 9.7 Effect of reduced developer temperature. At a temperature several degrees below normal the image suffers reduced density and marked loss of contrast.

Developer temperature in manual processing Manufacturers of developers for manual processing recommend a temperature of only 20°C for optimum results. These developers can give acceptable results at temperatures two or three degrees above or below this figure, but in such cases the developing time must be adjusted to prevent over or under development.

(3) Development time
Development time may be defined as the time interval which elapses between the entry of a specified part of a film (e.g. its leading edge) into the developing solution and the exit from the developing solution of the same part of the film. During this

period the film emulsion must absorb developer, the developer must penetrate to the silver halide grains, and the chemical reduction of the exposed grains must be completed to the point where optimum image density and contrast is achieved.

As Table 9.1 shows, development time varies according to the full cycle time of the processor. In radiography, the cycle time is designed to be as short as possible, consistent with achieving a satisfactory image quality. Short processing times offer a number of practical advantages, e.g.

(1) Patient waiting times in the X-ray department can be minimized;
(2) Examination times can be decreased, possibly reducing the risk to the patient, e.g. by reducing anaesthetic time in the operating theatre;
(3) Patient throughput can be increased and waiting lists reduced.

We should thus examine the factors which determine development time in order to see how minimum development time may be achieved.

Table 9.1 Variation of development time with total processing cycle time. The figures quoted are fairly typical but may vary slightly between individual auto processors.

Cycle time	Development time (s)
7 min	130
$3\frac{1}{2}$ min	68
110 s	30
90 s	26

Factors determining development time The development time required to produce optimum image quality is determined by:

(1) Developer activity. Clearly, an active developer solution is (by definition) capable of achieving a given image density more rapidly than a less-active solution. We have seen in section 9.2.1.5 that the activity of developer depends on:
   (a) Constitution of the working developer;
   (b) Developer temperature.
   Thus, the inherent properties, the condition and temperature of the working developer are major influences on development time. In manual processing, the relatively low-activity developers employed require 4 min to achieve optimum development at the recommended temperature of 20°C. Attempts to reduce this time may well result in loss of image quality.
(2) Type of film emulsion. Developing solution takes longer to penetrate a thick emulsion than a thin one. Direct-exposure (non-screen) X-ray films therefore tend to require longer processing times than screen-type X-ray films. To enable rapid processing to be achieved, emulsion thickness must not be excessive.
(3) Agitation of developer solution. It is important that the solution in a developing tank is vigorously agitated in order for the exhausted developer and by-products of development which are formed to be carried away from the surface of the film emulsion and replaced by fresh developer. Without such agitation the development process would slow down and development time

would need to be extended. Agitation is not a problem in automatic processors because:
(a) The film is always in motion;
(b) The rotation of the film transport rollers induces circulation currents in the solution;
(c) Forced circulation forms part of the developer replenishment and temperature control systems (section 10.5.1);
    However, lack of agitation is a common feature of poor processing technique in manual processing and may lead to incomplete and uneven development.

We have now completed our study of development – the first stage in the processing cycle – and the next task is to consider the second stage: fixing.

9.2.2　Fixing

Fixing (or **fixation**) is the second stage in automatic processing. It has four major functions:

(1) To stop any further development;
(2) To **clear** the image by removing the remaining silver halide from the emulsion;
(3) To **fix** the image, i.e. to render it chemically stable so that it undergoes no further changes and is no longer photosensitive;
(4) To complete the process of hardening of the film emulsion.

(1) Stopping further development
This function is achieved by making the fixing solution acidic (pH between 4.0 and 4.5). PQ developing agents only operate in an alkaline environment, thus any further development is inhibited as the film enters the fixing solution.
    NB In manual processing an intermediate rinsing stage between developing and fixing partially fulfils this function. The addition of an acid to the rinse (the acid **stop-bath**) improves its efficiency.

(2) Clearing the image
In a typical radiographic image, only about 40% of the silver halide in the film emulsion is converted to silver during development (M&B, 1976). The remaining 60%, representing the unexposed silver halide grains, if not removed, will have an obscuring effect on the image, impeding the transmission of light through the radiograph and giving the image a milky, opalescent appearance. During the process of fixation, the unexposed halide grains are converted into soluble compounds, which then dissolve out of the emulsion into the fixing solution. Thus, the unexposed parts of the image become transparent and the milky appearance is lost.

Clearing time The time taken for the image to lose its milky appearance is known as the **clearing time**. It provides a useful indicator of the condition of a fixing solution, particularly in manual processing.

The chemical agents in fixing solution which convert silver halide to soluble compounds are known as **fixing agents**.

(3) Fixing the image

When the clearing action described above is complete, the emulsion should no longer contain any silver halides. No photosensitive agents remain in the emulsion and it is no longer sensitive to light or radiation. The metallic silver image is now stable. Thus, the process of clearing the image is also the process of fixing the image. As one process is accomplished, so is the other. The fixing agents fulfil both functions. We shall identify an example of a fixing agent and describe its specific action when we discuss the constituents of fixer in section 9.2.2.1 below.

(4) Hardening the emulsion

The process of hardening of the gelatin in the film emulsion was partly achieved in the developer (section 9.2.1.3). The process is continued and completed in the fixer. This ensures that the gelatin does not absorb too much water and thus minimizes drying time (section 9.2.4.1). Hardening also toughens the emulsion and protects it from mechanical damage during the washing and drying stages of processing.

Having described the functions of fixer we shall now examine the constituents which make up a fixing solution.

9.2.2.1 Constituents of fixing solution

As with developing solution, the activity of the fixer in an automatic processor is maintained by controlled replenishment of its constituents. Unlike developer, we do not distinguish between a working fixer and a fixer replenisher, other than to note that a working fixer contains the by-products of the fixing process whereas fixer replenisher does not.

Fixer replenisher solution
Fixer replenisher consists of:

(1) Solvent.
(2) Fixing agent.
(3) Acid.
(4) Hardener.
(5) Buffer.
(6) Preservative.
(7) Anti-sludging agent.

Let us consider each of these constituents in turn.

(1) Solvent Water is the solvent and diluent used in fixing solution. It acts as a carrying medium for the active constituents in fixer. It provides a means of controlling the activity of fixer by diluting its effects. Most of the points relating to developer solvent, identified in section 9.2.1.3, apply equally to a fixer solvent.

(2) Fixing agent A fixing agent is a chemical which combines with the largely insoluble silver halide (bromide or iodide) in the film emulsion to form soluble compounds which can diffuse and be washed out of the emulsion. Fixing agents must not affect the silver image. Although most fixing agents *do* dissolve metallic silver, no significant loss of image density occurs within the normal fixing time.

Although a variety of silver halide solvents are known, the fixing agent used in radiographic auto processing is **ammonium thiosulphate**. Ammonium thio-sulphate offers several advantages over alternative fixing agents, e.g.:

(1) High solubility, thus it is available in convenient liquid concentrate form;
(2) High activity, thus fixing can be accomplished rapidly, e.g. 15 s in a 90 s processing cycle;
(3) The highly soluble by-products of fixation are more readily washed out of the film emulsion.

When ammonium thiosulphate reacts with silver bromide, two soluble compounds are formed:

(1) Ammonium argento-thiosulphate (commonly known as an ammonium 'silver complex');
(2) Ammonium bromide.

(The reaction with silver iodide is very similar, but produces ammonium iodide instead of ammonium bromide.)

The soluble ammonium compounds which form are unstable. If they are not completely washed from the emulsion during processing, the radiographic image will be prone to staining and deterioration during storage.

Unlike developing agents, fixing agents are relatively insensitive to changes in solution pH, but the pH of fixer must be stabilized for other reasons (see below).

(3) Acid Fixer solution is made acidic for two reasons:

(1) To ensure that development ceases when a film enters the fixer. If development is allowed to continue in the fixer, staining of the image may occur. In particular, **dichroic fog** may be produced. This gives a characteristic yellow–green–blue-tinged stain when the image is viewed by reflected light, while the stain is tinged pink when viewed by transmitted light (Longmore, 1955; Horder, 1958; Jenkins, 1980). It is caused by a deposit of very fine silver particles, which diffract the light and produce the strange colour effects described.
(2) To provide a suitable environment for the hardening agents in fixer (see the section on hardeners below).

The weak acid, **acetic acid**, is included to provide a pH of between 4.0 and 4.5. A solution which is too acidic (pH < 4.0) causes breakdown of thiosulphate, which decomposes to an insoluble precipitate of sulphur (**sulphurization**). If the solution is insufficiently acidic (pH > 4.5), the hardening will be inadequate.

(4) Hardener As we have seen, emulsion hardening to limit water uptake by the emulsion is essential in automatic processing:

(1) It reduces drying time;
(2) It prevents physical damage (e.g. scratches) to the emulsion surface.

Aluminium chloride and aluminium sulphate are commonly used hardening agents in fixing solutions. They work rapidly and most effectively within the rather narrow pH range of 4.1–4.4. Manufacturers sometimes provide hardener in a separate container from the fixer replenisher, to which it is added when the fixer is prepared for use. This improves the storage characteristics of fixer and extends its shelf-life.

(5) Buffer Precise control of pH of fixer is important in order to:

(1) Prevent sulphurization;
(2) Ensure neutralization of developer;
(3) Maintain optimum hardener activity.

For these reasons, fixing solution must be chemically buffered, particularly against the neutralizing effects of alkaline developing solution carried over by films from the developing tank. **Sodium acetate** is commonly included to act as a buffer, in conjunction with the acetic acid.

In manual processing, the intermediate rinse reduces the problem of developer carry-over into the fixing solution but creates an additional problem of water carry-over which tends to dilute the fixer.

(6) Preservative The preservative in fixer retards the decomposition of thiosulphates and thus delays the onset of sulphurization. Its presence is particularly important in liquid concentrates. The **sodium sulphite** commonly used is an effective preservative unless the fixer becomes too acidic.

(7) Anti-sludging agent The aluminium salts used as hardeners have a tendency to produce insoluble aluminium compounds. These may precipitate out of solution and form a sludge, which adheres to the films and to the sides of the fixing tank. To reduce the formation of sludge, **boric acid** is included as an anti-sludging agent in the fixer formulation.

9.2.2.2   Factors affecting fixation

The process of fixing a film material occurs in three stages:

(1) The fixing solution diffuses into the film emulsion;
(2) The fixing agent reacts chemically with the silver halides in the emulsion;
(3) The resulting soluble silver complexes and halides dissolve and begin to diffuse out of the emulsion.

The emulsion hardening process takes place concurrently with all three of the above stages.

The factors which influence the quantity and quality of fixation may be described under three headings:

(1) Constitution of fixing solution.
(2) Fixer temperature.
(3) Fixing time.

Let us study each of these factors in more detail.

(1) Constitution of fixing solution
At a given temperature, the activity of a fixer depends on a number of aspects relating to the chemical composition of the fixing solution:

(1) Choice of fixing agent. This affects what we might term the *inherent characteristics* of the fixer. X-ray film fixers invariably use ammonium thiosulphate, which gives a rapid-acting, high-energy fixer.
(2) Concentration of fixing agent in solution. This is established as the liquid concentrate supplied by the manufacturer is diluted with water when the solution is mixed ready for use. In general, activity increases with concentration

but the best results are obtained by using the dilution level recommended by the manufacturer. As films pass through the fixing tank, fixing agent is used up in the reaction with silver halides. Fixing agent is also lost due to carry-over of fixing solution during the transfer of films to the wash tank. In automatic processing, squeegee action minimizes the losses from fixer carry-over. The supply of fixing agent in solution must be replenished if its concentration is to be maintained.

(3) Presence of hardeners. The presence of hardener slows down the fixing process but speeds up the drying process. However, hardener must *not* be omitted from the fixer in an attempt to accelerate fixation, because emulsion damage and inadequate drying will result. The amount of hardener employed is adjusted to ensure that both fixing and hardening are completed in the same time. As films are processed, the supply of hardening agents in the fixer becomes used up. They must be replaced if adequate hardening is to be maintained.

(4) Presence of soluble silver complexes. As films are fixed, ammonium argento-thiosulphates (silver complexes) accumulate in the fixing solution. They release silver ions into the solution, which retard the action of fixing agent. High concentrations of silver complexes are difficult to remove from film emulsion during the washing stage and lead to the eventual staining of the image. It is recommended that the concentration of silver in the fixing solution should not exceed 6 g/l in a 90 s cycle processor (section 11.2). The accumulation of silver complexes is prevented by the removal of some of the contaminated solution and its replacement with controlled amounts of fresh fixer replenisher. In some circumstances, a process of **electrolytic silver recovery** may be carried out on contaminated fixer, to restore it to a condition where it may be reused (section 11.3.1.5).

(5) Presence of soluble halides. Soluble ammonium halides also accumulate in the fixing solution. Their presence slows down the action of the fixing agents. Fixer replenishment provides a means of controlling the concentration of such contaminants and thus maintaining fixer activity.

(6) pH of fixing solution. As we have seen, the activity of the fixing agent is not affected by changes in pH, but for other reasons it is vital that pH does not vary. The carry-over of alkaline developing solution as films enter the fixing tank tends to neutralize the acid fixer, causing pH to rise. Buffering chemicals resist this tendency but they need replacing if pH is to be kept constant. Accurately controlled replenishment ensures a stable fixer pH.

Thus, it is clear that without replenishment the activity of a fixing solution inevitably falls. Such **fixer exhaustion** results in partially cleared and inadequately dried films, with surface damage and poor storage characteristics. Properly controlled fixer replenishment ensures that lost chemicals are replaced, contaminants are removed and optimum quality films are produced.

Factors affecting fixer replenishment rate The volume of replenisher required to maintain fixer activity depends on a number of factors:

(1) Area of film processed: as with developer, the volume of replenisher required is approximately proportional to the area of film and therefore depends on the size and number of films processed.

(2) Type of emulsion: more fixing agent is needed to process a direct-exposure X-ray film than a screen-type film because the emulsion has a higher coating weight.

(3) Type of image: a lightly exposed film (or a tightly collimated film) contains more unexposed silver halide grains than a similar film which has received a greater exposure (or been less well collimated). Thus, after development there is more silver halide to be cleared, more fixing agent is used and more fixer replenisher is necessary. Compare this with the corresponding requirement for developer replenisher described in section 9.2.1.5.

Maintenance of fixer volume A small volume of fixing solution is lost due to carry-over whenever a film leaves the fixing tank, and a similar volume of solution is *gained* due to carry-over on films entering the fixing tank from the developer. The *net* change in volume from carry-over is therefore not significant. Other fluid losses occur, however, due to evaporation and the deliberate bleeding off of solution to remove contaminants. Fixer replenishment must make good these losses.

(2) Fixer temperature
The activity of fixing agents increases with temperature and at higher temperatures diffusion processes are more rapid and the emulsion gelatin, though more permeable, is softer and susceptible to damage. However, the working temperature of fixer solution does not require such fine control as that of the developer. Too great a difference in temperature between developer and fixer may result in films suffering emulsion damage, known as **reticulation** as they enter the fixer.

(3) Fixing time
During the time taken for a film to pass through the fixing solution, the developer in its emulsion must diffuse out, fixing solution must diffuse in and the processes of clearing and hardening must be completed.

In a 90 s processing cycle, about 15 s is available for the fixing stage, while in manual processing the fixing time may be as long as 5 min.

Factors determining fixing time The time needed to fix a film depends on three major factors:

(1) Fixer activity. The higher the fixer activity, the shorter is the required fixing time. We have seen that fixer activity depends both on the constitution of the fixing solution and on its temperature. In automatic processing the high-energy fixing agent and quick-acting hardeners, used in conjunction with controlled replenishment and relatively high temperatures, facilitate the very short fixing times required without loss of quality.

(2) Type of film emulsion. Rapid-process films incorporate thin emulsions which can be penetrated rapidly by the processing chemicals. Direct-exposure film, which has a thicker emulsion, may cause problems during a rapid fixing stage. The problem is exacerbated by the increased proportion of silver iodide which may be included in its emulsion. Silver iodide reacts more slowly with fixing agent than silver bromide and it may be necessary to use a cycle time of 3 or $3\frac{1}{2}$ min rather than 90 s to process such film successfully. The phasing out of direct-exposure film has largely eliminated this problem.

(3) Agitation of fixing solution. As with development (section 9.2.1.5), vigorous agitation accelerates fixation by speeding the removal of by-products from the film emulsion and their replacement with fresh fixer. Only in manual processing is inadequate agitation likely to be a problem.

This completes our discussion of the fixing stage in processing and we next examine the third stage: washing.

9.2.3   *Washing*

When a film leaves the fixing tank its emulsion is saturated with fixing solution contaminated with silver complexes and ammonium halides. If such chemicals are not removed, the emulsion will gradually acquire a yellow-brown sulphur stain during storage. Additionally, dissolved salts may crystallize out onto the surface of the film. To avoid such effects the film is passed through a washing stage, in which these soluble chemicals diffuse out of the emulsion. Tap water is a satisfactory washing medium for automatic processing.

9.2.3.1   Diffusion
The transfer by diffusion of chemicals from the emulsion gelatin to the wash water can only occur in the presence of a **concentration gradient**, i.e. the concentration of contaminants must be lower in the water than in the emulsion. This is best achieved by arranging that the emulsion surfaces are exposed to a continuous flow of uncontaminated water during the washing stage, either by a spray mechanism or by a rapidly flowing fresh water-bath.

9.2.3.2   Washing efficiency
The washing process is never 100% efficient. Whatever washing method is chosen, it is not possible to guarantee that *all* the residual salts are removed, but it is sufficient to reduce the level of contamination to the point where no image staining occurs in the maximum likely storage time of the radiograph (e.g. 10 years). In a 90 s cycle processor, about 15 s is allowed for the washing stage, while in manual processing a minimum of 10 min is generally advised.

9.2.3.3   Factors affecting washing efficiency
There are a number of factors which determine the efficacy of the washing process:

(1) Film emulsion. The amount of contaminant held in an emulsion depends on the emulsion thickness and on the degree of hardening which has been employed. A thick emulsion therefore takes longer to wash than a thin one. Hardening of emulsion inhibits diffusion but also shortens the diffusion path by reducing emulsion thickness.

(2) Condition of fixing solution. We noted earlier that a fixing solution which contains a high concentration of silver complexes causes problems in the washing stage. To avoid inadequate washing it is therefore important to maintain the fixer in optimum condition by correct replenishment.

(3) Condition of wash water. To maintain the necessary concentration gradient we must ensure that the wash water itself does not become contaminated. The carry-over of fixing solution from the fixing tank as films are transported into the wash tank occurs both within the film emulsion and on its surface. Squeegee rollers again minimize carry-over in automatic processors. For a rapid washing process the wash water must be replenished frequently with fresh supplies and the contaminated water bled off.

(4) Agitation. Vigorous agitation ensures that fresh water is being forced against the emulsion surface and contaminated water is carried away. This helps to maintain the concentration gradient needed for efficient diffusion. In manual

processing it is common to use less dynamic washing conditions. In such cases the washing process is not as efficient and the storage properties of the radiographs may be less satisfactory.

(5) Temperature of wash water. Washing efficiency increases with temperature because the **surface tension** of the water is reduced and its penetration into the emulsion is accelerated. However, if the temperature is too high, the emulsion softens and may even become detached from the film base.

(6) Washing time. This is the time taken for the level of residual contaminants in a film emulsion to be reduced to an acceptable level. Its value depends on the conditions outlined in 1–5 above and on the length of time for which the radiograph is to be stored. Normal storage would not be expected to exceed 10 years. However, if a radiograph is being kept in an archive or X-ray film 'museum', perhaps because it demonstrates a rare pathology, its storage time will be much longer. Experience shows that the washing efficiency of well maintained automatic rapid processors can satisfy even these demands. In the future however, the storage of images in digital form may eliminate the need for original radiographs to have the property of archival permanence (section 15.2.1.4).

9.2.3.4   Measurement of washing efficiency

It is possible to detect the presence of and to measure the level of the contaminants remaining in a film emulsion after it has been processed. The normal method is to check the concentration of residual ammonium thiosulphate with a chemical indicator and use this as a measure of the general level of emulsion contamination (section 18.4.1.4). A thiosulphate level of $< 3\,\mu g/cm^2$ is recommended for archival storage purposes.

9.2.4   Drying

The final stage in the processing of a radiograph is to remove *all* of the surface water and *most* of that retained in its emulsion. Some moisture must remain in the emulsion to prevent it from becoming too brittle. In the days when manual processing was the rule rather than the exception, it was common for radiologists and medical staff to view the *wet* radiographs (or 'wet plates') of casualty patients in order to save time. This was extremely inconvenient since, to avoid damage, a wet film must be handled very carefully because its emulsion is so soft. By the use of ultrarapid drying methods, modern processors have eliminated the need to handle wet films.

In automatic processing, surface water is removed by squeegee rollers, while **evaporation** removes the water from within the emulsion. A 90 s processing cycle allows about 25 s for the drying stage.

9.2.4.1   Factors affecting drying time

The time required to dry a radiograph adequately by evaporation depends on two major factors:

(1) The wetness of the emulsion. This is the volume of water retained in the emulsion per unit area of its surface. It depends on two factors:
  (a) Hardness of the emulsion: a hardened emulsion retains less water than a soft emulsion and therefore can be dried more quickly;
  (b) Emulsion thickness: a thin emulsion retains less water than a thick one.

Direct-exposure X-ray film may therefore take longer to dry than screen-type X-ray film.

(2) The drying conditions. The drying medium is air. The speed with which it can evaporate moisture from the emulsion depends on:

(a) Air humidity: dry air (of low humidity) accelerates the evaporation process and reduces drying time. Generally, the atmosphere within a hospital environment is dry, although local variations may be experienced. Relative humidity should not be greater than 60%.

NB 100% relative humidity represents a state in which air is *saturated*, i.e. it can hold no more water in its gaseous form, and condensation occurs.

(b) Air temperature: heated air can retain more moisture than cold air and is therefore a more effective drying medium. However, the excessive use of heat may damage the film emulsion. Air temperatures between 40 and 65°C are commonly used. Some processors employ radiant (infrared) heating, which raises the temperature of the film emulsion and only indirectly heats the air (section 10.8.2).

NB Hot air is not necessarily any drier than cold air: hot air saturated with moisture is just as ineffective a drying medium as saturated cold air.

(c) Air circulation: as moisture evaporates from the emulsion, the air around the emulsion becomes more humid and retards further evaporation. It is necessary, therefore, to replace this humid air with drier air by employing an air circulation system. The rate of change of air is the prime reason why drying can be achieved so rapidly in automatic processing.

In the next chapter we discuss how the principles we have just described are applied to the X-ray film processing methods and equipment used in modern X-ray departments.

Chapter 10
Radiographic Processing – Practice

The processing of photographic/X-ray film is almost entirely done nowadays by machine, with the film being fed in at one end and received, processed and dried at the other.

Whilst the size, design and capacity (i.e. the number of films a processor can handle in a given time) may vary from one manufacturer's machine to another, the basic steps involved in processing by machine remain the same, irrespective of which piece of equipment is used.

In most machines, a system of rollers moves the film through the various processing sections (Fig. 10.1). It is this transport system that we shall examine first.

10.1 Film transport system

The film to be processed is placed on the input tray and gently advanced until taken up by the entry rollers. It is then automatically transported via a system of rollers and/or guide plates in and out of developer, fixer, wash and drying sections of the processor in turn, to be delivered finally to the output tray, dry and ready for viewing.

The individual solution tanks (developer, fixer, and wash) may hold up to 18 litres of solution, depending on the type of processor.

The rollers are arranged in racks which can be removed easily from the tanks for cleaning. The individual rollers may be in either a face-to-face or staggered (zig-zag) configuration (Fig. 10.2).

Where the film needs to undergo a severe change in direction, e.g. through 90°, rollers alone are inadequate and a system of guide plates is used.

These roller/guide-plate configurations are found at the bottom of the proces-

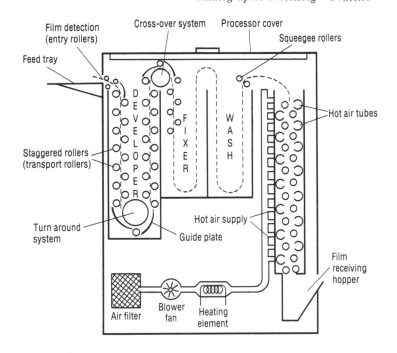

Fig. 10.1 Automatic processor.

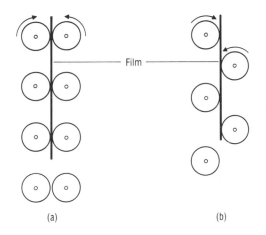

Fig. 10.2 Automatic processor roller configurations (a) Face to face. (b) Staggered.

sing tanks and at the junction between two adjacent tanks, known as **turn-around** and **cross-over** assemblies, respectively (Fig. 10.3). The cross-over rollers may, in some machines, form part of the larger roller racks, whilst in others they may be capable of being removed as separate units.

The rollers are driven through a system of gear wheels or cogs by either a main drive shaft or chain, power being provided via a d.c. motor.

In the interests of safety, the processor lid operates a switch in the roller drive circuit so that when the lid is removed the roller drive becomes inoperative.

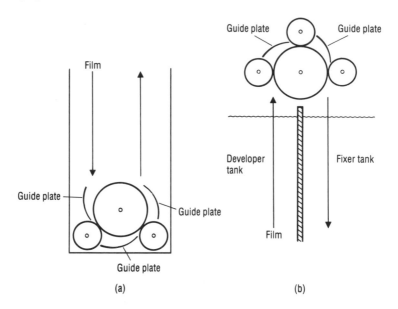

Fig. 10.3 (a) Turn around and (b) cross-over roller assemblies from an automatic processor.

The rollers may be made from PVC or rubber, depending on their situation in the machine. Where extra grip on the film is required, such as at the base of the tank where the film has to undergo a change of direction, rubberized rollers tend to be used. Similar roller material is used for **squeegee rollers**, which are sited between the tanks. These help to remove solution from the emulsion as the film leaves one tank and enters another.

A harder PVC type material is usually satisfactory for the majority of rollers, whose function is to guide rather than change the film's direction.

10.2 Processing cycle time

This is an expression of the time that it takes a film to travel from its dry unprocessed condition on the input tray to the dry processed state in the output tray; sometimes referred to as the **dry-to-dry cycle**. The measurement is usually taken from the time the leading edge of the film enters the first pair of rollers to the time when the trailing edge emerges from the last pair of rollers.

The processing cycles most commonly used in medical imaging departments lie between 90 and 115 s, referred to as **rapid cycle**. Machines with longer processing cycles are available (e.g. up to 9 min).

An example of the length of time that a film will spend in each part of the processor during a 90 s processing cycle is as follows: developer, 26 s; fixer, 15 s; wash, 15 s; drier, 24 s; travel time 10 s; total time 90 s.

Some processors offer the user a choice of one or two processing cycles, a facility afforded by varying the rate of film travel. This feature may come in useful if on occasion it is desired to change the type of developer or film being used, or to carry out the processing at a different developer temperature. In most instances, however, once a machine has been installed and a processing cycle set, there is seldom a requirement to alter it.

10.3   Processor capacity/production capacity

Processor or production capacity is a measure of a processor's ability to process a given number of films in a given time and is expressed by manufacturers in any one or a combination of the following ways:

(1) As the number of single-size films (usually 35×43 cm) capable of being processed in 1 h.
(2) As the number of films of mixed sizes capable of being processed in 1 h.
(3) Film feed time: the speed of the film through the processor (in cms/s or m/h).

In addition, manufacturers will also state the total time taken to process any single film, e.g. 90 s.

To a prospective purchaser who is perhaps replacing an old machine, information about the film feed time is probably the most useful. For example, when purchasing a processor for a department which has to cope with large numbers of films in short bursts of activity – an Accident and Emergency Unit is one instance – it might be pertinent to know how quickly one could 'dispose' of a large number of cassettes all possibly arriving simultaneously.

Below are examples of the sort of capacities one can expect from automatic processors working on a 90 s processing cycle. They are taken from two different manufacturers' brochures:

High-capacity processor	250 (35×43 cm) films/h or
	450 of mixed sizes
Low-capacity processor	70 (35×43 cm) films/h or
	125 of mixed sizes

10.4   The film feed section

When no films are being processed, an automatic processor is normally in what is known as a **stand-by** condition, with certain system functions such as the roller drive inactive.

As a film is fed to the processor, so the cycle of events listed below is initiated:

(1) Drive motor energized (to turn the rollers).
(2) Safelight above feed tray extinguished.
(3) Developer and fixer replenisher pumped into tanks.
(4) Drier heater energized.
(5) Wash water flow rate boosted.
(6) Film signal delay timer activated (audible signal which will sound 1–3 s after the trailing edge of the film has passed the entry rollers, to let the operator know that the next film can be fed to the processor).

10.4.1   *How are all these activities triggered?*

(1) Entry roller detection system
In the type of processor employing this system, the act of pushing the film against the entry rollers causes the top entry roller (see Fig. 10.4) to move upwards,

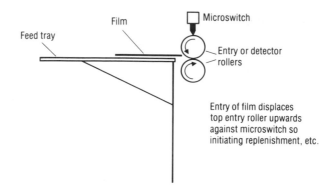

Fig. 10.4 Entry roller detection system on an automatic film processor.

actuating a set of film detector microswitches (usually three), which set in train the sequence of events listed above.

Once the entire length of film has negotiated the entry rollers, the top roller returns to its original position and the microswitches, now no longer engaged, halt replenishment and allow the safelight above the feed tray to be illuminated. The drive, heater and water systems remain 'on'.

(2) Infrared detectors

An example of an infrared film detection system can be seen in Fig. 10.5.

The infrared beams remain 'broken' for as long as it takes the film to pass into the processor, so film length can be calculated. Furthermore, the wider the film, the greater the number of individual beams which will be involved, and from this the processor recognizes film width.

Consequently, film area can be calculated by the microprocessor circuitry, and replenishment appropriate to film area can be dispensed accurately.

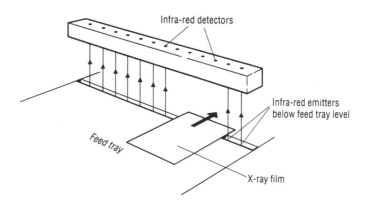

Fig. 10.5 An infra-red detector system used with an automatic processor. The passage of a film interrupts (or breaks) the infra-red beams thus providing evidence of film width. This information along with a knowledge of film length will subsequently be used by the microprocessor to calculate film area and thereby dispense accurate volumes of replenisher solutions.

10.5 The developer section

This incorporates the following subsystems:

- Recirculation;
- Temperature;
- Replenishment;
- Drainage.

10.5.1 Developer recirculation

Adequate agitation of solution is important in achieving satisfactory mixing of the chemical solution and thereby obtaining correctly processed films. Whilst the actual movement of the rollers does provide some movement of the solution, the principal contributor is the recirculation system, which ensures that developer solution is continuously on the move (Fig. 10.6).

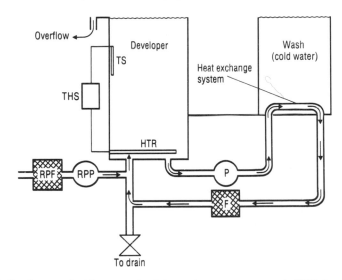

Fig. 10.6 Developer replenishment, recirculation and temperature control. HTR heating element (immersion heater); THS thermostat; TS temperature sensor; P pump for developer recirculation; F filter; RPP replenishment pump; RPF replenishment filter.

Such a system typically incorporates an inlet and outlet pipe from the tank, an electric pump (P) and a filter (F). Solution is continually drawn by means of the pump through the filter and back to the tank via the inlet pipe. The filter ensures that dirt or large particles are safely extracted from the developer so that they will not become embedded within the soft emulsion.

The recirculation system also incorporates the means by which developer temperature is controlled.

10.5.2 The control of developer temperature

We explained in Chapter 9 the influence of temperature on film processing, and stressed the importance of being able to control accurately such a temperature setting within very narrow limits ($\pm 0.5^\circ$C) if image quality is to be maintained from one radiograph to the next. A typical temperature value for automatic processor developer is 35°C.

One control system commonly employed in automatic processors, and illustrated in Fig. 10.6, includes the following:

(1) Immersion heater;
(2) Thermostat;
(3) Heat exchanger.

Consider now the way in which these three function together. The explanation given is for a **cold-water** processor (i.e. one which has only a cold-water supply and which has an immersion heater, thermostat and heat exchanger sited in the developer tank).

The immersion heater applies heat to the developer solution. When the desired temperature is reached, as dictated by the thermostat, the immersion heater is automatically shut off. However, just as with any electric heating element, heat will still be emitted for a short time afterwards, even though the heater is no longer energized. Consequently, solution temperature will continue to rise above that set by the thermostat. This is where the **heat-exchange** system comes into its own, because it effectively moderates against this climb in temperature by taking some of the heat away from the solution.

A typical heat-exchange system used in an automatic processor such as the one described above might be one where part of the developer recirculation piping is routed through the bottom of the cold-water wash tank, the presence of this cold water allowing an exchange of heat between the cold water and the developer in the pipe, thus effectively moderating against the tendency of the developer to rise in temperature.

This process of immersion heater pushing up temperature, and heat exchange pulling it back (known as a **push–pull** system), combined with the continuous movement of developer solution, ensures that a state of equilibrium is reached whereby developer temperature can be maintained within ± 0.5°C of the thermostatic setting.

Other methods of heat exchange which are sometimes used by processor manufacturers are:

(1) Routing the cold-water supply through the base of the developer tank;
(2) Using a fan to play air at ambient temperature onto the external surfaces of the developer tank (this is a similar principle to the combination of cooling fan and radiator used in a car);
(3) Using a separate heat-exchange unit (Fig. 10.7). This is simply a device which allows the conduction of heat between the hot developer solution circulating in a coil and an outer jacket of cold water.

We are dealing here with what are known as cold-water processors, i.e. processors which only have a cold water supply. Therefore, whilst fluctuations may well occur in mains cold-water supply temperature, they do not have any effect on the temperature of the developer.

The introduction of microprocessor control of automatic processors in recent years has meant even more accurate control of temperature. Temperature regulation of ± 0.1°C is now possible.

10.5.2.1   The use of *two* immersion heaters in a developer solution

Some processors employ *two* immersion heaters in the developer tank in order to

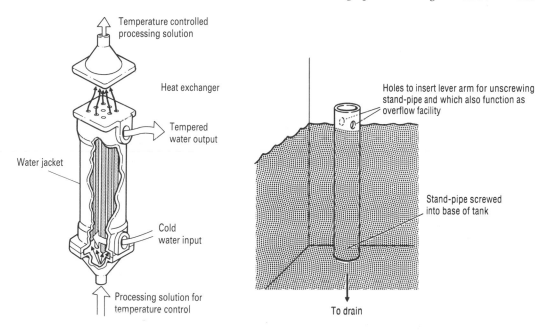

Fig. 10.7 A heat exchanger.

Fig. 10.8 A stand-pipe. It acts as an overflow route and can be unscrewed to provide rapid drainage of a processing tank.

achieve operating temperature quickly from start-up, e.g. first thing in the morning. Once the correct temperature has been reached, only one of the heaters will remain on stand-by in order to maintain solution temperature throughout the day.

10.5.3   Replenishment of developer

The developer tank is connected via a pipe to the developer replenishment tank, which is external to the processor.

Where automatic chemical mixing equipment (automixers) is installed, the replenishment tank forms part of such equipment (see section 10.11). Fresh developer solution is pumped from this tank into the main developer tank within the processor.

The principles of replenishment will be dealt with in greater detail later in this chapter.

10.5.4   Developer drainage

All processing tanks possess a means by which they may be emptied for cleaning purposes. The opening to the drain is at the bottom of the tank and is controlled by either a tap or **stand-pipe** (Fig. 10.8).

10.6   The fixer section

10.6.1   Temperature control

Because fixer activity is less temperature-sensitive than developer, temperature control is not so critical; in the case of a processor supplied by a mixture of hot and

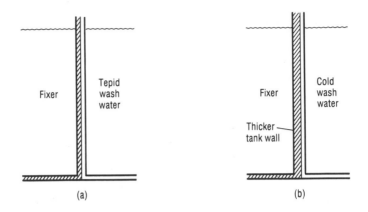

Fig. 10.9 The presence of cold wash water in processor (b) necessitates providing the fixer tank with a thicker wall in order to prevent heat loss.

cold water for the wash tank, heat for the fixer may be obtained by conduction from the adjacent developer tank (Fig. 10.9(a)).

The temperature of the fixer is thus the mean of the temperatures of both developer and wash.

In the so-called **cold-water processor**, where all the water that the processor requires is provided from the cold supply, the wash tank will thus contain only cold water, and conduction in the manner described above would be unsatisfactory since the fixer would adopt too low a temperature. An immersion heater is therefore employed for the fixer tank, and the wall of the fixer tank nearest the cold-water wash tank is made thicker in order to insulate the warmer fixer solution from the cold wash water (Fig. 10.9(b)).

10.6.2   *Fixer recirculation*

A circulation system is provided for the same reasons as for developer, one pump usually serving both developer and fixer systems.

10.6.3   *Fixer replenishment*

Fresh fixer is supplied to the main tank within the processor from an external replenishment tank, which may form part of an 'automixer' installation.

10.6.4   *Fixer drainage*

Used or excess fixer solution is drained from the tank via a stand–pipe or drain valve, either to a holding tank ready for subsequent silver recovery or directly into a silver recovery unit (see section 11.3.1.2).

10.7   The wash section

As the film leaves the fixer solution, squeegee rollers help to remove most of the residual fixer from the surface of the film. The film now enters the washing section of the processor.

We shall describe two very different washing methods which may be found in various types of cold-water processor:

- A spray wash;
- Tank immersion.

10.7.1   Spray wash

Lying between the transport rollers in the wash section of this particular type of processor are a series of water pipes containing perforations through which the water is forcibly sprayed onto each surface of the film as it passes by. Water flow rate in such a processor can be as high as 10 l/min. In the stand-by mode, however, flow rate is reduced in order to economize on water consumption.

10.7.2   Tank immersion

In such a cold-water processor, the water is fed to the wash tank via a developer/ heat exchanger. Sufficient conduction of heat from the developer takes place to ensure that the wash water will be warm enough to be used as a washing solution. The water flow rate in a typical processor using such a scheme is between 4 and 7 l/min when not in the stand-by mode.

10.8   The drying section

In order to facilitate rapid film drying, squeegee rollers situated between the wash and drier sections first remove excess water from the emulsion surface, after which the film is transported through the drier section (typical temperature range for automatic processors is 40–65°C) where the film is commonly dried in one of two ways.

10.8.1   Hot-air drying

Dust-free hot air is blown onto the surface of the film. This is achieved by using a series of cylindrical tubes located behind and between the transport rollers on either side of the film (Fig. 10.10) and through which hot air is blown onto the film as it passes by.

The temperature of this hot air is thermostatically controlled and is usually around 55°C. The hot, moist air is collected; some of it is recycled, reheated and blown back onto the film, whilst the remainder is evacuated by ducting to the outside atmosphere. This ducting away from the processor environment is very important, in order to prevent excessive temperatures and humidity building up in the processing area and causing problems for film storage.

10.8.2   Infrared drying

In a processor using this method, the drying section contains a range of electrically heated elements arranged so as to radiate heat onto both film surfaces as it passes through the heater section. The water vapour produced by the drying process is blown away with the cold air produced by a fan.

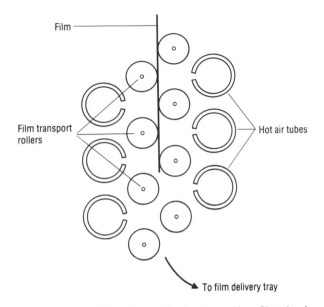

Film

Film transport
rollers

Hot air tubes

To film delivery tray

Fig. 10.10 Cross-section through drier rack assembly showing position of hot air tubes.

The advantages of such a heating method are that it is not only quieter but cooler in operation, in so far as less heat is transferred to surrounding areas.

In both of the drying methods described above, the presence of an air-circulation system is the prime reason why drying can be achieved so rapidly in automatic processors.

10.8.3   *Successful film drying*

The success or otherwise of the film drying process depends not only on the correct temperature of the drier but to a large extent on there having been adequate hardening of the film emulsion in the developer and fixer.

Incorrect levels of hardener constituent in either of these solutions will mean that excess fluid is taken up by the emulsion leading to inadequate drying.

10.9   Stand-by facilities

In order to prevent unnecessary wastage of valuable resources when the machine is idle, a stand-by mode exists on automatic processors. This means that whilst heating of the solutions remains 'on', all other systems (water supply, drier elements, etc.) are either cut off or at least substantially reduced.

Once a film has left the machine, and providing no further film is processed, the stand-by condition will be arrived at within 20–30 s of the film exiting the processor.

This condition may last for 8–10 min before the processor automatically switches itself on again in order to maintain drier temperatures and to agitate developer and fixer solutions. It then switches itself off again for another 10 min. So the cycle continues until interrupted by a radiographer feeding a film. Then, the normal processing cycle is restored.

10.9.1 *Advantages of a stand-by facility*

- Reduction in electrical power consumption.
- Reduction in mains water used.
- Reduction in processor wear and tear.

10.10 Automatic processor replenishment

In Chapter 9 we discussed replenishment solutions and their purpose in automatic processing. We can summarize the latter as follows.

10.10.1 *The purpose of replenishment*

(1) To maintain consistent developer and fixer solution activity.
(2) To maintain a constant volume of developer and fixer solution.

In automatic processors there is little carry-over of chemical solution from one tank to the next because of the effectiveness of the squeegee rollers sited between solutions. Thus, the principal reason for replenishment in an automatic processor is point (1) above; in this respect, the volume of replenisher added is determined in relation to the area of film processed rather than to a fall in solution level. This is of course in contradistinction to manual processing, where due regard has to be taken of the fall in solution level occasioned by a significant carry-over of solutions.

Each time a film is fed into the processor, the entry roller detection system (see section 10.4.1) triggers off the replenishment pumps, and replenisher solutions are pumped to the developer and fixer tanks in the processor. The fresh solutions are rapidly and thoroughly mixed with 'old' chemistry, partly due to the action of the rotating rollers but in particular due to the recirculation activity.

Excess developer and fixer solution overflow to drain and silver recovery system, respectively. Thus both solution activity and solution level are maintained.

10.10.2 *How do we determine the amount of replenishment to be carried out?*

The volume of developer or fixer replenisher pumped to the respective tanks each time a film is fed into the processor is either measured in millilitres per unit length of film or in millilitres per unit area of film. When we talk of replenishment 'rate', we are really referring to the volume of developer or fixer that is moved from the replenishment tanks to the processor in response to a film being fed. It may be advisable to adjust this volume up or down, depending on a variety of factors which we shall examine later, and we refer to this as adjusting the replenishment 'rate'.

You will remember that in Chapter 9 we described those factors which affect the replenishment rate. We list them again:

(1) Area of film processed.
(2) The type of emulsion.
(3) The type of image.
(4) Aerial oxidation.

There is a fifth factor which it is now appropriate to introduce.

(5) Orientation of film.

10.10.2.1   Orientation of film on entry to the processor

This factor applies only to those machines where the volume of replenisher dispensed depends on the length of film fed (entry roller/microswitch detection system).

The movement of a film through the entry rollers initiates developer and fixer replenishment, and in this way the volume of solution added is proportional to the length – and thus to the surface area – of the film being processed. In those machines which have replenishment activated by movement of the entry rollers against a set of microswitches, then replenishment will only last for as long as the film is between the entry rollers. Thus, the length of the film will dictate the duration of replenishment.

Such a simplistic method of replenishment has its drawbacks. For example, it is possible to obtain the same replenishment volume for both a 35 × 43 cm film and an 18 × 43 cm film, by feeding their shorter edges in first! Clearly, this means over-replenishment in the latter case, and is to be avoided. Manufacturers usually issue advice to the effect that films should always be fed to the processor with their longer edges leading. Smaller films may be placed side by side and fed simultaneously. Such protocol will prevent wasteful over-replenishment.

This problem of replenishment by length means that if roll film has to be processed then the microswitches governing replenishment should be isolated, or over-replenishment will occur.

In the case of a processor which employs infrared detectors, there is no problem, since film area is accurately calculated and replenishment is accurately dispensed in true relation to the film's surface area, irrespective of which film edge is leading.

Where roll film material is being processed, the processor with infrared detection can suspend replenishment until it has calculated that an equivalent area of 35 × 43 cm has been taken up by the machine.

10.10.3   *Checking replenishment rates*

Periodically, it is necessary to check the replenishment rates of both developer and fixer, either in response to a suspected malfunction or prior to replenishment rate adjustment.

The check is more easily carried out with the assistance of a second person.

Equipment required

● Two measuring flasks.
● Two 35 × 35 cm films.

The processor lid is removed and the developer replenisher inlet pipe (Fig. 10.11) is lifted out of the developer tank and placed inside a measuring flask. With the processor cover removed, the roller drive and replenishment pumps will be inoperative and so, before a sample of replenisher solution can be collected, the microswitch will need to be engaged by hand. Once this has been done, a 35 × 35 cm film is fed into the processor and the replenisher sample is taken.

The volume, in millilitres of solution collected, is noted and the solution carefully emptied from the flask back into the developer tank in the processor.

The test is repeated for the fixer section using a clean flask.

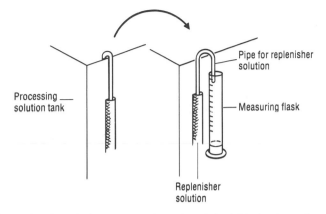

Processing — solution tank

Pipe for replenisher solution

Measuring flask

Replenisher solution

Fig. 10.11 Measuring the replenishment rate. The U-shaped pipe is lifted and turned out over the side of the tank and inserted inside a measuring flask. It is held in this position whilst an assistant feeds a 35 cm × 35 cm film into the processor. The collected replenisher solution is then measured and recorded.

10.10.4 *Adjustment of replenishment rate*

On many machines, adjustment can be carried out by turning the appropriate knob, located on or near the replenishment pump. Turning in one direction has the effect of increasing the flow rate through the pump, whilst rotating the knob in the opposite direction has the opposite effect.

Adjustment is usually a matter of trial and error since the only markings on the pump may be a plus and minus sign, indicating the two options available.

Table 10.1 gives a list of some recommended replenishment rates issued by Kodak Ltd. Note how the busier the processor, the lower needs to be the required replenishment, as aerial oxidation losses are then less significant.

It is important to appreciate that there are no hard and fast rules as to what exact replenishment rates are appropriate for specific processors. The superintendent radiographer is certainly guided by the recommendations of replenishment manufacturers (Table 10.1), but is free to adjust those figures both in light of experience based on the factors we have outlined earlier, and perhaps on the results of a processor monitoring programme (section 18.4).

Table 10.1 Some recommended replenishment rates issued by Kodak Ltd.

Films processed per day	Replenishment rate (ml) per 35 × 43 cm film
Developer	
25–50	90
76–100	75
126–150	65
Fixer	
24–100	115
101–150	100
>150	85

10.11   Automixers

The efficient functioning of an automatic processor depends upon there being sufficient replenishment solutions available at all times.

These fresh solutions are stored in large tanks (capacity around 35–40 litres) near the processor and connected to the processor's replenishment pump by flexible tubing.

Whereas in the past it was always necessary to make up and mix fresh solutions by hand, nowadays **automixers** (Fig. 10.12) do these tasks automatically. They have a similar storage capacity incorporated within them.

Automixers are of two types.

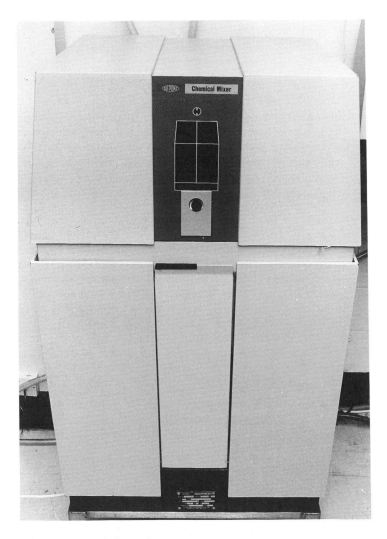

Fig. 10.12 The Dupont chemical automixer.

Fully automatic Fresh boxes of replenisher are placed inside the lid of the mixer by the operator at any time, and these will be automatically punctured by the equipment when fresh solution is required for mixing.

Semi-automatic Boxes are only placed in the mixer in response to some sort of audible or visual alarm indicating a shortage of solution. The box is not automatically punctured but needs to be forcibly pushed down onto some type of perforating device.

For the purposes of describing how an automixer works, we shall consider a fully automatic type (Fig. 10.13). Inside each replenishment storage tank are four sensors:

- A **common** sensor, providing an electrical circuit with the other three;
- An **empty** sensor;
- An **alarm** sensor;
- A **full** sensor.

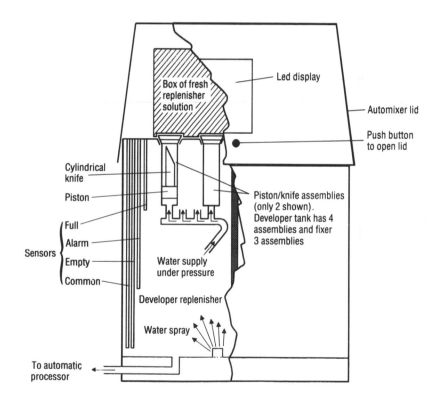

Fig. 10.13 The Dupont chemical automixer.

When the solution in the tank falls below the level of the alarm sensor, an audible alarm sounds, warning the radiographer of the need to place a fresh box of replenisher in the automixer.

When the solution level falls below the level of the empty probe and providing that a full box of replenisher solutions is in situ beneath the automixer lid, the water solenoid is activated and water under pressure (20 psi) enters the manifold and into each of the piston assemblies driving the knives upward to puncture the chemical pack. The chemicals drain into the tank and, at the same time, water enters the pack flushing out the chemical. Simultaneously, water enters under pressure through fine jets at the base of the tank, forming a spray which is met by the incoming chemicals. In this way, adequate mixing of the fresh solution is able to take place.

Water continues to flow in this way until the level of the solution in the tank reaches the full sensor, when the water solenoid is then shut down and an LED on the automixer lid shows that the box is empty. The box is then taken out and immediately replaced with a full pack in readiness for the next needed mix.

Inside the lid is a microswitch and the act of replacing the empty pack with a fresh one resets the circuit so that the cycle of events described above can occur again when required.

Each pack of solution is colour-coded, red for acid (fixer) and blue for the developer. Those parts of the box where the knives will penetrate are made weaker to facilitate easier penetration. The developer pack has four puncture sites, the fixer has three. The arrangement of 'knives' in the top of the automixer mirrors this difference (Fig. 10.14).

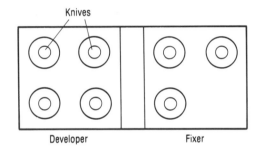

Fig. 10.14 Plan view of knife arrangement on the Dupont automixer.

10.11.1 *Advantages of using an automixer*

(1) Cleaner. No spillage or splashes. No skin contamination.
(2) Convenient. Providing the automixer is regularly checked to ensure that full packs are always in place, the equipment runs itself and makes no demands on precious radiographer time.
(3) Time saving.
(4) Accurate mixing. Correct ratio of replenishment solution to water is made up. A satisfactory mixing of solution is achieved by water entering at very high pressure at the bottom of the tanks through fine jets.
(5) Minimum maintenance required. It is recommended that the automixer be flushed through with clean water once a year to prevent a build up of crystallized solids. This sort of exercise should, if possible, be timed to coincide with an occasion when the tank solutions are low, resulting therefore in little wastage.

10.12 Microprocessor control of automatic processors

The development of microprocessor-controlled automatic processors has made processing more efficient and processor monitoring a great deal easier. In a typical processor of this type, the microprocessor constantly monitors all of the processor's systems and in the process identifies any malfunctions, indicating them by illuminated LED displays and/or audible alarms.

Here are some of the functions which are monitored:

(1) Developer temperature. Accurate control possible within ± 0.1°C.
(2) Developer and fixer replenishment, accurately based on the area of film being processed.
(3) Developer and fixer recirculation.
(4) Wash water flow rate.
(5) Drier temperature.
(6) Roller rotational speed, electronically monitored and speed variable if required.

10.13   Automatic processors for special purposes

10.13.1   *Roll film/100 × 100 mm cut film processor*

Such a processor is capable of processing all types of roll film, from 35 mm to 105 mm. Moreover, with a special adaptor it will also accept 10 × 10 cm cut film. An example of this type of processor is illustrated in Fig. 10.15.

Roll film still in its take-up cassette is removed from the X-ray room and placed inside a special processor-loading cassette (Fig. 10.16), the lid closed and the film advanced until a few centimetres protrude from the end of the loader. This is done by turning a knob on the side of the loading cassette. The loader is finally inserted into the roll film processor, where the entry rollers grip the protruding film and proceed to unwind and process the exposed film.

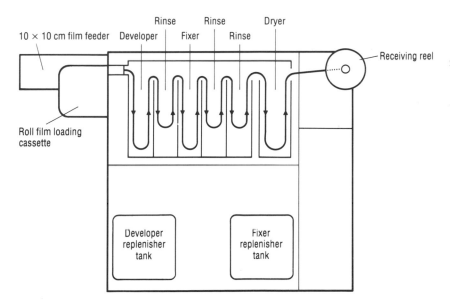

Fig. 10.15 The Scopix 12 roll film processor. The processor is capable of processing all roll films from 35 mm to 105 mm, and with a special feeder will also process 10 × 10 cm film sheets. (Courtesy of Agfa Gevaert.)

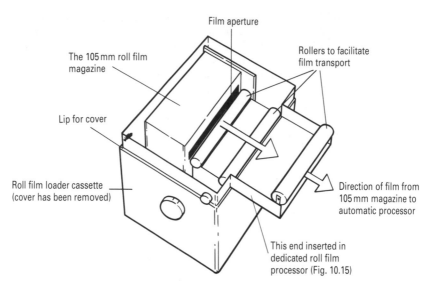

The 105 mm roll film magazine

Film aperture

Rollers to facilitate film transport

Lip for cover

Roll film loader cassette (cover has been removed)

Direction of film from 105 mm magazine to automatic processor

This end inserted in dedicated roll film processor (Fig. 10.15)

Fig. 10.16 A special processing loader cassette for processing 105 mm roll film. The cassette can be attached to the processor shown in Fig. 10.15. The example illustrated is supplied by Philips Medical Ltd.

When the processed film begins to emerge, a buzzer sounds and the operator feeds the first few centimetres into a take-up spool. The reeling mechanism then automatically winds the film onto the spool ready for viewing. A special adaptor allows 100×100 mm cut film processing.

Some machines have a variable processing time facility in order to suit different types of film.

10.13.2 *Dental film processor*

Mini versions of the conventional large film processors are available for processing small films, such as those used in dental radiography.

10.14 Care and maintenance of automatic processors

A manufacturer always provides a manual of instruction with each processor which is sold. This will include a section on the construction of the processor, a 'troubleshooting' guide and advice on the daily, weekly and perhaps monthly maintenance routines to be followed.

Whilst operating procedures may differ in some details for different processors, the main principles outlined below are common to most machines.

10.14.1 *Operating procedures*

10.14.1.1 Start-up procedure

(1) Before switching on, check:
    (a) Solution levels in the processing tanks;

(b) Solution levels in developer and fixer replenisher tanks;

(c) Correct installation of roller racks (developer/fixer/wash), cross-over roller assemblies, processor cover, and drier thermostat setting.

(2) Open the water supply valve.

(3) Turn on the mains electrical power at the mains isolator, together with the processor 'power switch'. Check that the neon indicator lights come on.

(4) Check developer temperature.

(5) Feed two or three obsolete films through the processor to clean those rollers which are above solution level and which may have accumulated dirt particles during the shut-down period. Check the resultant films for surface damage. Check, at the same time, that replenisher pumps are functioning.

10.14.1.2 Shutting the processor down

(1) Check that there are no films in transit through the processor. (Wait a couple of minutes!)

(2) Turn off the processor 'power switch' and the mains isolator.

(3) Turn off the water supply valve(s).

(4) Remove the processor cover.

(5) Remove the cross-over roller assemblies and clean the rollers with warm water and non-abrasive cloth. Wipe dry. Replace assemblies carefully.

(6) Remove any visible chemical deposits from inside the processor.

(7) Replace processor cover but leave slightly open to allow a free flow of air and thus help to prevent condensation problems.

10.14.2 Maintenance procedures

Whilst procedures may differ in some details for different processors, the main principles outlined below are again common to most units.

10.14.2.1 Daily maintenance

(1) Remove cross-over roller assemblies or guide plates. Rinse under warm running water ($\sim 38°C$). Wipe dry. *Do not use the same cloth for developer and fixer.*

(2) Wipe down the entry rollers with a damp cloth. Wipe dry.

(3) Wipe off all chemical deposits in the processing section.

(4) Wipe all top rollers above solution level.

10.14.2.2 Weekly maintenance

(1) Repeat the daily cleaning programme.

(2) Put splashguard between the developer and fixer tanks to prevent contamination from splashes and then remove the deep racks. Rinse and wipe with cloth using a different cloth for developer and fixer.

(3) Operate each rack manually to check for correct tension on chains/gears, that they move freely, and that all rollers rotate correctly. Check gear wheels for missing teeth, broken or missing springs, and any other evidence of trouble.

(4) Re-install racks, being very careful to:

(a) Allow them to drain to prevent dilution of chemicals;

(b) Use splashguard and lower racks in slowly to prevent contamination of solutions.

(5) Replace cross-over assemblies. Check that each component is correctly positioned.
(6) Inspect and change, if necessary, any filters in:
    (a) The water supply;
    (b) The recirculation system.
(7) Remove drier section air tubes and clean by vigorous agitation in warm water. Take care to replace correctly.
(8) Clean drier rollers with a damp cloth.

10.14.2.3   Monthly maintenance

(1) Carry out weekly and daily maintenance schedules.
(2) Drain main tanks and clean with sponge and running water.
(3) Close drain valves.
(4) Fill both developer and fixer tanks with water, replace processor cover and switch on mains power and processor 'on' switch. This activates the solution circulation pumps and flushes the systems through with water.
(5) Turn off the processor and mains isolator. Remove the processor lid.
(6) Drain tanks and refill with fresh chemistry.

Chapter 11
Silver Recovery

In a photographic context, the term 'silver recovery' means the reclamation of silver after it has been used for its intended photographic purposes.

There are two main sources of recoverable silver in a medical imaging department:

(1) Used fixer solution.
(2) Discarded or scrap films.

Within such departments, the recovery of silver is only attempted from the used fixer solutions, it being more convenient to sell in bulk the scrap film to a firm who specializes in refining silver from such material.

A typical departmental silver recovery process, efficiently run, can expect to reclaim some 98% of total silver from used fixer solution.

11.1 Reasons for silver recovery

Profit
Used fixer typically carries some 5–7 g/l of potentially recoverable silver, and being a precious metal fetches a high price on the bullion market.

Economic
Monies received from the sale of recovered silver can be offset against a department's annual film and chemical bill. Furthermore, depending on the method of silver recovery used, the fixer can be recycled and used again once silver recovery has been carried out.

Anti-pollution
A reduction in the amount of silver going down the drains can only assist in the subsequent purification of effluent.

Conservation
Silver as a natural resource is becoming scarcer.

Efficiency
As the concentration of silver in the fixer solution increases, so the activity of the fixer falls and fixers become less efficient at providing image permanence because film hardening is less effective. Films may emerge from the processor damp and/or stained. Sodium thiosulphate fixers are more sensitive than ammonium thiosulphate fixers to the presence of silver complexes in solution.

11.2   Factors affecting the amount of silver in fixing solutions

Type of film used
Duplitized screen film has less silver in its emulsion than non-screen film.

Replenishment rates
If these are too high, the concentration of silver in the used fixer solution will be correspondingly small, and vice versa. Monitoring silver content by the use of silver estimating papers (see section 11.3.2.3) can be a very useful way of helping to determine an appropriate fixer replenishment rate. For example, assume that on monitoring it was discovered that the silver concentration of the fixing bath was consistently around 2 g/l. In these circumstances one could well afford to decrease the fixer replenishment rate, which would in turn have the effect of raising the concentration of silver in solution. Providing that this concentration did not exceed 5–6 g/l, fixer activity would not be compromised, and a saving in the amount of fixer replenisher used would thus be made. Such a practice only makes sense, however, by assuming that the department's silver recovery equipment is capable of efficiently recovering these levels of silver in solution.

Type of procedure and radiographic technique used
Chest radiography produces a greater concentration of potential silver for recovery than, for example, does orthopaedic or skull work. This is not just because of the larger film size which is generally used, but also because a larger percentage of the film area is unused during the formation of the chest image, the unexposed silver being removed during fixation.

Another aspect of the radiographic technique which influences the amount of silver in solution is beam collimation. Greater collimation means less of the silver halides are used in creating the image and therefore a greater number of unexposed silver halides eventually find their way into the fixer solution.

It has been estimated that only some 30–40% of the available silver halides on a 35×43 cm film are used in the formation of a chest image. Indeed, most other radiographic procedures only use, on average, 40% of a film's silver content. The remainder ends up in the fixer.

11.3 Methods of recovering silver from used fixer solution

Two methods are commonly encountered by radiographers:

(1) Electrolysis.
(2) Metallic replacement.

11.3.1 Silver recovery by electrolysis

11.3.1.1 Principle of electrolysis

Used fixer contains silver thiosulphate complexes which are negatively charged and some silver ions which are positively charged. These two exist in an electrochemical balance or equilibrium (Fig. 11.1).

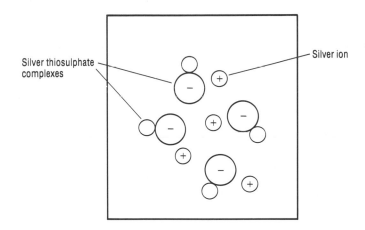

Fig. 11.1 Used fixer solution containing silver thiosulphate complexes and silver ions. The two exist in an electro-chemical balance.

If two electrodes, an anode and a cathode, are placed in the solution and a d.c. current passed between them, the positively charged silver ions will be attracted towards the negatively charged cathode where they will be deposited as metallic silver (Fig. 11.2(a)). This means, however, that because the chemical equilibrium is disturbed, the balance is restored by some of the silver thiosulphate ions dissociating in order to provide additional free silver ions (Fig. 11.2(b)). These in turn will eventually be attracted towards the cathode; and so the cycle continues.

This state of affairs is satisfactory only so long as sufficient silver ions exist in the cathode's vicinity and can thus be **captured** or **plated out** on the cathode. The rate at which silver recovery proceeds therefore matches the rate at which fresh silver ions become available.

If, however, the number of silver ions near the cathode falls *or* an attempt is made to plate out silver faster than the rate at which silver ions can be produced by the dissociation of silver complexes, a process known as **sulphiding** can occur. This is the breakdown of thiosulphate itself, a by-product of which is sulphur. When sulphur is released into solution, it reacts with unexposed silver halides to cause film fogging. Fixer which has undergone sulphiding is useless and must be discarded.

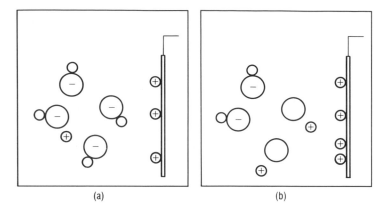

(a)   (b)

Fig. 11.2 The insertion of a negatively charged cathode results in the attraction of the silver ions to its surface. Chemical equilibrium is thus disturbed and in order to restore it silver thiosulphate complexes dissociate. The fresh silver ions are in turn attracted to the cathode and so the cycle continues.

Such disasters can be avoided if the solution is both continually agitated and replenished with 'fresh' used fixer whilst silver recovery is taking place.

Providing that there are adequate silver complexes in solution, agitation helps to bring them within the area of the cathode so that it always has a fresh supply of silver ions for collection.

The electrolytic method of silver recovery used in medical imaging departments in conjunction with automatic processors is known as **high-current-density electrolysis**. An explanation of this term is appropriate before we examine a typical electrolytic silver recovery unit.

Current density This expression refers to the relationship between the current (in amperes) which is used to carry out silver recovery and the surface area (m^2) of the cathode, and is expressed in the following way:

$$\text{Current density} = \frac{\text{Recovery current}}{\text{Area of cathode}}$$

Current density is expressed in A/m^2. A typical value for silver recovery units used in medical imaging departments is $300\,A/m^2$.

Current density affects the *rate* at which silver recovery takes place. The higher the current density, the faster will be the rate at which silver will be plated out on the cathode. The lower the current density, the slower this rate.

The equation above shows us that, for a given surface area, any reduction in plating current will result in a reduction in the rate of silver recovery.

11.3.1.2   High-current-density electrolysis

The description **high current** is used in contradistinction to those silver recovery methods used in the past with manual processing units and which involved the use of very small currents (up to 1 A).

High-current units are used with today's automatic processors and may involve the use of currents up to $\sim 20\,A$.

A typical unit of this type stands about 55 cm high, 33 cm wide, 44 cm deep and is powered by a 240 V mains supply. It is supplied with fixer from the overflow of an automatic processor.

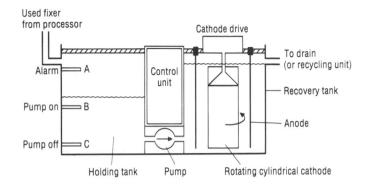

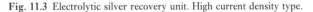

Fig. 11.3 Electrolytic silver recovery unit. High current density type.

Figure 11.3 is a cross-section through a typical recovery unit. It consists of the following sections:

(1) Holding tank.
(2) Recovery tank.
(3) Control unit.

(1) Holding tank
This tank stores the silver-laden used fixer from the automatic processor(s). Silver concentration in solution is typically between 4 and 6 grams of silver per litre.

Contained within the tank are three float-operated switches, A, B and C, controlled by the level of the solution.

In normal use, the level of the fixer in this tank fluctuates between B and C. When the level rises to B, the pump is energized and fixer flows into the recovery vessel via the pump. At the same time, the cathode in the recovery tank rotates and silver plating commences.

Should the level ever fall below the switch C, the pump is automatically stopped. If the level rises above A, either due to pump failure or obstruction, an alarm sounds.

(2) Recovery tank
It is in this tank that electrolytic silver recovery of silver takes place. The tank contains a centrally placed, stainless-steel cylindrical cathode on which the silver is collected. There are four graphite anode rods, one at each corner of the recovery tank. Constant agitation of the solution is achieved by rotating the cathode.

(3) Control unit
This provides a regulated, low-voltage d.c. supply to the electrolytic unit.

A recovery current of between 8 and 15 A is commonly used. The magnitude of this current will depend on the silver content of the fixer. If the concentration of silver is high, the current will need to be increased (current density increased) in order to attract the increased numbers of silver ions in solution. The converse is also true. With older type units it is the operator, e.g. the radiographer, who regularly monitors the incoming fixer solution for silver concentration and adjusts the current according to a recommended table of values supplied with the silver recovery unit. For example: silver concentration 4 g/l, current 8 A; silver concentration 8 g/l, current 12 A.

When the silver concentration falls to 0.5 g/l, the recovery current is switched off automatically.

Some modern units which are microprocessor controlled incorporate a sensor in the recovery tank which monitors the solution for its silver concentration every few minutes and then adjusts the recovery current appropriately.

The complete unit is sealed so as to prevent the escape of fumes and also for security reasons. Fixer from the recovery tank is either discarded via a drain or a proportion of it is recycled for further use (see section 11.3.1.5).

11.3.1.3   Stability of silver content in used fixer solutions

In most medical imaging departments where the type of work and radiographic technique carried out from day to day changes very little, silver concentrations in used fixer will not vary very much. This is because the amount of silver in solution will primarily be determined by the level of replenishment (see section 11.2) and the replenishment rates are governed by the area of film being processed. So, more film processed means more silver in solution, which means more replenishment! Thus, a state of equilibrium is reached whereby, providing the nature of the work or the radiographers' techniques do not change, and the replenishment rates are unaltered, the concentration of silver per litre in the holding tank will remain fairly static.

Once this particular silver concentration level has been determined (using silver estimating papers), the appropriate recovery current can be set and, in practice, seldom needs to be adjusted.

11.3.1.4   Recovering the silver deposit

It is usual when installing a silver recovery unit in a department to negotiate a contract with the supplier whereby the units will be regularly serviced, repaired when necessary and the silver flake removed. The unit should be kept locked, with a senior member of the radiographic staff holding the key.

When silver is due to be collected (e.g. every 2–3 months, depending on a department's workload), the unit should be opened in the presence of a witness (usually a member of the hospital administration department), the silver removed by gently tapping on the cathode with a wooden mallet and then weighed. The cathode must then be cleaned thoroughly before replacement.

A receipt is made out in triplicate, one copy for the medical imaging department, one for the finance department and one to accompany the silver to the refiners.

A service log book should be provided for each recovery vessel and should include sufficient space to enter the following:

(1) Date of contractor's visit.
(2) The weight of silver recovered.
(3) Details of any repairs.
(4) Signature of contractor.
(5) Signature of radiology department manager.
(6) Signature of one other hospital officer.

In due course, the hospital receives payment, less a reduction for the servicing, transport and refining.

The purity of silver obtained by these electrolytic silver recovery units is of the order of 98%.

11.3.1.5   Silver recovery and the recycling of fixer

All silver recovery systems extract silver from solution passed to them via the fixer overflow and silver recovery can be very efficient if monitored regularly. Even so, some silver-laden fixer is nevertheless lost to these systems because of carry-over into the wash tank.

In Fig. 11.4 a silver recovery unit is shown incorporated into the fixer recirculation section of an automatic processor. Used fixer passes from the processor's fixer tank to the silver recovery unit, where the silver content is reduced to around 1 g/l, and from there returned to the processor. In addition, conventional fixer replenishment takes place as described earlier, so that there will be a mix of the two sources of fixer in the processor tank.

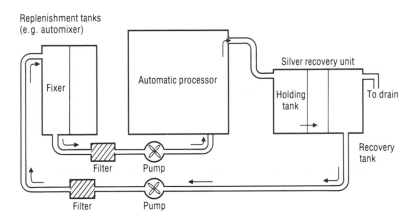

Fig. 11.4 Flow diagram for silver recovery with fixer recycling.

Because the silver content of the processor's fixer is therefore maintained at a very low level, very little will be lost to the drain because of carry-over into the wash tank.

Fixer recycling also means a substantial reduction in the amount of fresh fixer replenishment solution required by the processor. Replenishment rates can be reduced by around 30–50%.

11.3.2   *Silver recovery by metallic replacement*

11.3.2.1   Principle

If base metals such as copper, iron or zinc are placed in a solution containing silver salts, the base metals dissolve into the solution whilst the silver is deposited out of the solution in exchange.

11.3.2.2   Base metal exchange unit

The unit, sometimes called a **silver recovery cartridge** (Fig. 11.5), comprises the following:

(1) A rigid plastic tank (e.g. polyethylene), which is acid resistant and contains inlet and outlet holes;
(2) A **charge** of base metal (e.g. steel wool);

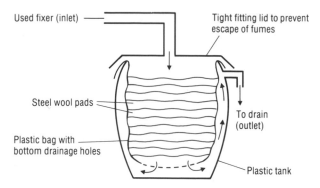

Fig. 11.5 Base metal exchange unit for silver recovery.

(3) A plastic bag or liner to hold the charge;
(4) A tight-fitting lid to prevent the escape of fumes.

The steel-wool charge inside its plastic liner is supported on a base inside the tank, keeping it clear of the floor of the tank.

Silver-laden fixer from the processor enters through the lid and passes down through the steel wool. Metal exchange occurs, the steel wool dissolving to leave a silver precipitate which accumulates in the base of the liner. The silver-free fixer passes through perforations in the liner and leaves the tank via the outlet pipe at the top of the tank. This fixer is unsuitable for recycling.

A single unit will cope with about 25 litres of fixer per day. It is important that the used fixer takes at least 24 h to pass through the recovery vessel. If the processor(s) supplying the recovery unit exceeds the above load, a second unit (known as a **tailing unit**) may be added in series (Fig. 11.6). This additional recovery vessel ensures that all the available silver will have sufficient time in which to be recovered.

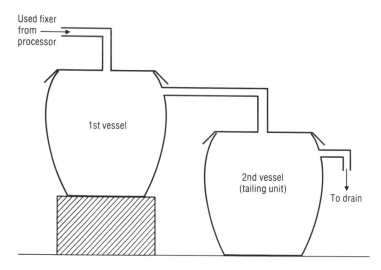

Fig. 11.6 A base metal exchange 'tailing' unit. The tailing unit will recover any silver left by the first recovery unit.

Metal exchange units are periodically checked by the silver refiner, who will collect the exhausted steel-wool charge (i.e. the silver sediment) and at the same time provide a replacement charge.

In order to assess the efficiency of the recovery unit, a sample of the outflow fixer should be collected weekly and tested for its silver content, as described below. The content of the silver effluent should be < 1 g/l if the recovery process is to work efficiently.

11.3.2.3 Monitoring the efficiency of the silver recovery process

The effectiveness, or otherwise, of a silver recovery unit can be checked using silver estimating papers. These are strips of chemically impregnated papers which, when momentarily dipped into the fixer solution and removed, change colour depending on the concentration of silver in solution. The test is usually carried out on the outflow fixer, i.e. the fixer leaving the recovery unit, in order to monitor the efficiency of the recovery process.

The strip is immersed for about 1 s, removed and, after a pause of 30 s, the resultant colour is matched against a colour chart provided with the papers. The concentration of silver (g/l) can thus be ascertained. If the unit is working efficiently, the level of silver in the outflow should be < 1 g/l.

One manufacturer supplies silver estimating papers in the form of plastic strips, with two small squares of paper at one end (Fig. 11.7).

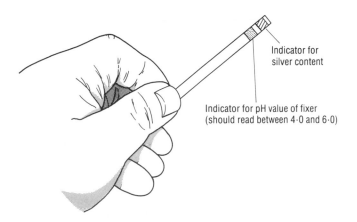

Indicator for
silver content

Indicator for pH value of fixer
(should read between 4·0 and 6·0)

Fig. 11.7 A silver estimating paper which also incorporates a pH indicator. Silver concentrations between 0 and 10 g/l may be measured.

The square at the very end of the strip measures silver concentrations between 0 and 10 g/l using an eight-point colour scale. The second square measures pH values between 4 and 8 using a five-point colour scale. The importance of measuring pH will be seen later.

11.4   Comparison of the two silver recovery methods

11.4.1   Electrolytic method

11.4.1.1   Advantages

(1) Silver yield is of high purity, therefore less costly to refine.
(2) Fixer may be recycled.
(3) Silver easily removed from cathode.
(4) Cleaner method than metal exchange.

11.4.1.2   Disadvantages

(1) Equipment is costly, but can be leased.
(2) Security required when removing silver from cathode.
(3) Efficiency of silver recovery dependent upon regular monitoring.

11.4.2   Metallic replacement

11.4.2.1   Advantages

(1) Equipment relatively inexpensive.
(2) > 98% efficient at silver recovery when charge is new.
(3) Easy to install.
(4) No electrical supply required.
(5) Requires little operator attention.

11.4.2.2   Disadvantages

(1) Fixer cannot be used again.
(2) Assay and refining of silver more involved, and therefore more costly.
(3) The efficiency of the unit falls as the metal charge becomes exhausted.
(4) Smell, if lid not securely fitted.
(5) Not suitable where large volumes of used fixer are being produced.

11.5   Bulk collection of fixer

A department may decide not to carry out its own 'in-house' recovery of silver but, instead, to sell the fixer to a refiner who will carry out the silver recovery on his premises.

This method of recovery does have one advantage in so far as there is no expensive equipment to be purchased. However, it is debatable whether in the long term this is an advantage, since the charges for providing containers, transporting, recovering and refining the bulk fixer are not insignificant and this is of course reflected in the amount of money that the hospitals eventually receive from the sale of the silver.

Other disadvantages

(1) Because the fixer is only sold in bulk, it has to be stored in large tanks on or near the hospital site prior to collection.

(2) It is difficult to measure precisely the volume of fixer being sold.

(3) There is difficulty in accurately assaying the amount of silver in the solution.

11.6   Choice of silver recovery method

The choice of recovery method for a given department is a decision that is best made by the radiology services manager who will have knowledge of the number, siting and output of the departments' processors. In addition, such a person is ideally placed and technically best qualified to be able to evaluate the various methods available and the likely return on investment from one of them. A more involved discussion on the evaluation of silver recovery systems is, however, beyond the scope of this book.

It is important to realize, though, that what may be regarded as the ideal silver recovery method in one imaging department may not necessarily be the most appropriate method for another.

11.7   Silver recovery and pH

The pH of the used fixer is an important factor in silver recovery, the optimum value being around 4. As the pH rises, so recovery slows up and the risk of sulphiding increases. If a test indicates such a rise, a solution of glacial acetic acid can be added to the fixer prior to recovery in order to reduce pH.

11.8   Factors leading to a reduction in the amount of silver recovered

(1) Reduction in the amount of silver in solution.

(2) Too high a flow rate of used fixer through recovery unit.

(3) Current density too low.

(4) Cathode overloaded or metal charge exhausted.

(5) Insufficient agitation.

(6) pH too high.

11.9   Methods of conserving silver

(1) Using films with lower coating weights.

(2) Using the smallest films appropriate to the examination.

(3) Collimating the beam.

(4) Avoiding 'repeat' exposures.

11.10   Recovering silver from scrap film

As we pointed out earlier, some 40% of a film's silver is used in creating the radiographic image, and even this is potentially recoverable once the film has been discarded.

It is a requirement that all films be retained for a certain period. In the UK the recommended time limit is 8 years prior to disposal. At the end of this period, they may be sold along with any scrap or reject films which have accumulated during the previous year.

The procedure adopted by many departments is to collect these annual clear-outs and, along with the scrap or rejected films which have accumulated, sell them to a refiner who has been selected after a careful tendering process.

The availability of film for sale in this way will be different for those departments practising microfilming. In these instances, the film can be disposed of as and when miniaturization of the originals is completed.

11.10.1   *Methods of silver recovery from film*

Chemical

The bulk film is mechanically broken up into small fragments prior to being subjected to a series of chemical washes, the purpose of each being to strip completely all emulsion from the base. The silver-rich solution is then passed through electrolytic recovery cells until all the silver has been recovered.

Burning

This method involves burning the film and recovering the silver from the ash produced. Burning off the unwanted chemical compounds leaves an ash 10–20 times richer in silver than the original material.

In Chapters 10 and 11 we have examined in detail the automatic processor, the chemical automixer and the various methods of silver recovery. In the next chapter we shall take a closer look at the area in which all of these pieces of equipment will be sited.

Chapter 12
The Processing Area

Siting of the processing/viewing/darkroom area
Function of daylight processing area
The viewing area
Darkroom design and construction
Darkroom illumination
Darkroom equipment and its arrangement
Manual processing
Health and safety in processing areas

In the past, the processing area was synonymous with a darkroom/viewing area. However, the advent of daylight processing systems in the 1970s and 1980s, and more recently the electronic imaging systems of the 1990s, has dramatically revolutionized this area. Instead of the solitary 'through-the-wall' processor of the past, many of these rooms will have at least one daylight processing system (see Chapter 13), a laser imager and other equipment associated with the production of hard copy images from digital sources within the department.

The processing area remains, however, a central feature of any imaging department. Many of the principles which were applied both in its design and in its geographic placement are just as relevant in the 1990s. Perhaps the biggest change has been in the provision of darkrooms. They have been mostly dispensed with and the old darkroom/viewing areas have been opened up to create one larger space to accommodate the sort of modern equipment highlighted above. In many cases, the darkroom has only been retained as a very small facility perhaps occupying an unused corner of the department.

The retention of a small darkroom facility may be justified as follows:

- Some daylight systems and laser imagers require their film magazines to be loaded under safelight conditions.
- Some types of films and cassettes are incompatible with daylight systems; e.g. duplicating film, curved cassettes for orthopantomography, etc.
- Dental film processing (although dedicated automatic daylight processors are available for this purpose).

12.1 Siting of the processing/viewing/darkroom area

Processing facilities should be placed in close proximity to where the work of the radiographer is carried out; and moreover, they should serve as many imaging rooms as is geographically possible. This minimizes the number of processors required, as well as being more efficient in terms of radiographers' time and effort spent walking from imaging room to processor.

Figures 12.1 and 12.2 illustrate two different departmental layouts. In Fig. 12.1, a processing area is shown serving three radiographic rooms, whilst in Fig. 12.2 a darkroom provides a similar function. The area should be well ventilated with 12–15 air changes per hour in line with film processor manufacturers' health and safety recommendations (see also section 12.8.3).

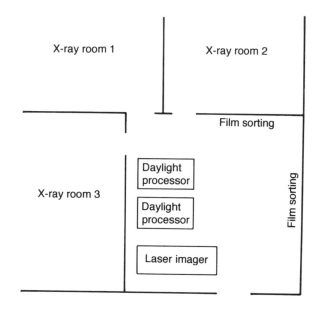

Fig. 12.1 Plan view of a three-room department serviced by one processsing/viewing area.

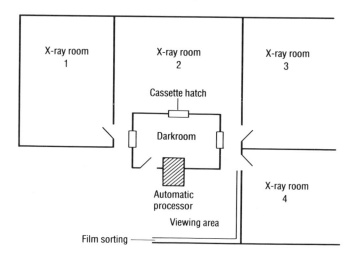
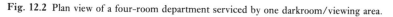

Fig. 12.2 Plan view of a four-room department serviced by one darkroom/viewing area.

12.2 Function of daylight processing areas

(1) Loading/unloading of cassettes by processing equipment.
(2) Care and maintenance of electronic and processing equipment.
(3) Production of hard copy images from digital data.
(4) Storage on unexposed film.
(5) Silver recovery.
(6) Storage area for a small number of replenisher packs.
(7) Site for replenisher tanks or automixer.

A low-level sink unit should be provided for the cleaning of processor racks, and two panels – one controlling the electrical supply and the other the water inlet valves – located near the film processors.

12.3 The viewing area

This should be a room contiguous with the processing area, or even part of the same space if desired. It is the area where the viewing, checking and sorting of films takes place (see Fig. 12.1), and should be out of the sight and sound of patient areas. Furnishings should include:

● Work surfaces;
● Filing compartments or shelving for films or patient categories;
● Cassette storage racks; perhaps vertical compartments under the worktops;
● Viewing boxes and spotlights.

The viewing area is often the site of intense activity and therefore needs to be as large as possible in order to accommodate both the high occupancy and the level of staff movement involved.

12.4 Darkroom design/construction

12.4.1 Location

(1) Centrally sited and serviced by hatches from the adjacent imaging rooms (Figs 12.1 and 12.2).
(2) Sited away from damp or hot areas.
(3) Accessible in terms of power and water supplies.
(4) Adjoining a viewing area/room where processed films can be checked and sorted.

12.4.2 Size

A darkroom which is to be in constant use and where one full-time technician is to be employed requires a minimum floor area of $10\,m^2$ and a ceiling height of around 2.5–3 m. However, where this room is used infrequently and for short periods (e.g. loading film magazines for daylight systems), its size may well be reduced.

12.4.3 Radiation protection

The location of the ideal darkroom will inevitably mean that some walls are shared with adjoining radiodiagnostic rooms and, in the interests of both darkroom staff and film material alike, such walls must be adequately protected from penetration by X-radiation. The same protection standards as detailed in respect to film stores (section 6.1.1.6) apply equally to darkrooms.

If for any reason the adequacy of protection needs to be checked at any time, checks can be carried out using TLDs strategically placed on walls or doors, wherever radiation leakage is suspected. The TLDs should be left in place for at least a week before processing.

12.4.4 *Floors*

A darkroom carrying out solely automatic processing and where the feed tray is the only part of the processor inside the darkroom is sometimes referred to as a **dry** darkroom, since any contact with fluids (cleaning, mixing fresh chemicals, etc.) will take place outside the darkroom. The criteria for darkroom floor material, therefore, need only be for one that is durable and easy to maintain (e.g. plastic tiles).

A light-coloured material will be an advantage to mitigate against the low–light working conditions.

In darkrooms where liquids have to be handled, e.g. where the entire processor is sited inside the darkroom itself, then a non-porous, non-slip flooring material is essential.

12.4.5 *Walls/ceiling*

The walls and ceiling should be:

(1) Light in colour so as to reflect as much light as possible onto working surfaces. A high level of reflected light means that it may be possible to work with fewer safelights and, in addition, the diffuse illumination so created will improve working conditions.
(2) Easy to wipe over and keep clean.

12.4.6 *Ventilation and heating*

These two aspects of darkroom design are important in order to provide for:

(1) Satisfactory working conditions for staff;
(2) Good film handling and storage conditions;
(3) Efficient automatic processor performance.

Where ventilation may be poor and humidity is allowed to rise, heat loss from the processor will be inefficient and a general increase in processor temperature may occur. As a consequence, films may show increased density and fog. An increase in humidity may cause inadequate film drying.

These problems can be prevented by ensuring:

(1) Relative humidity is maintained at around 40–60%.
(2) A minimum of ten air changes per hour.
(3) Room temperatures maintained between 18 and 20°C.

All of these conditions can be achieved by using a good air-conditioning system. Alternatively, fairly satisfactory ventilation can be achieved by using an extractor fan sited higher than and diagonally opposite a second fan, the latter being so placed as to obtain fresh and filtered air from outside. Temperatures may be maintained by ordinary hot-water radiators. Electric fires constitute a fire hazard and should never be used.

12.4.7 Type of entrance

Because of the need to be able to enter and leave a darkroom without admitting white light, the darkroom entrance is necessarily of special design. Four design options are very briefly described.

12.4.7.1 Single-door system

Where access is via a single door, precautions need to be taken in order to ensure that the door is capable of totally excluding light and cannot be opened inadvertently whilst films are being handled. It is customary therefore to link electronically the door-locking mechanism with the lighting circuit, thus preventing the door from being opened if the safelights alone are on.

The single-door system is relatively inexpensive, and economical in terms of space used. However, it is a problem where more than one person is using the darkroom. The locked single door also poses a safety hazard should an accident incapacitate the occupant. Therefore, a means of overriding any safety interlock must be provided.

A type of internal sliding bolt, which is accessible from the outside, could be fitted.

12.4.7.2 Double-door system

Figure 12.3 shows one possible arrangement of the double-door system. Each door should be sturdy in structure and well fitting, in order to exclude all light when closed. Where the doors open in the manner illustrated, the dimensions of the vestibule can be very small, so economizing on space.

If the door nearest the darkroom is a sliding door, then that is an added advantage as far as space is concerned.

An electrical interlock can be fitted in order to prevent either door from being opened unless its fellow is closed.

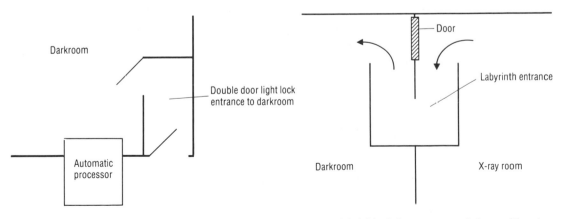

Fig. 12.3 Plan view of a darkroom with a double door light lock entrance.

Fig. 12.4 A labyrinth entrance to a darkroom. Plan view.

12.4.7.3 Labyrinth

A typical labyrinth for a darkroom consists of two parallel passages and a facing wall, as in Fig. 12.4.

The door in the baffle wall provides direct access if moving pieces of equipment in or out, and is useful in the event of an emergency.

The effectiveness of the labyrinth will be greater if:

(1) A matt black paint is used for the interior of the passages, the central baffle and the facing portions of room walls, to help to eliminate internal light reflections;
(2) The vertical height of the entrance is limited to 2 m;
(3) The length of each passage is at least 3 m;
(4) The width of each passage is not more than 700 mm.

Safelights or a white line painted on the labyrinth walls at eye-level are also useful features.

The drawback of the labyrinth design is that it uses a comparatively large amount of space compared to the other systems of entry. It does have the following advantages, however:

(1) Easy and instant access at all times;
(2) Continuous darkroom ventilation.

12.4.7.4 Rotating-door system

One type of design employs a metal cylinder with an opening in its side for entry/exit (Fig. 12.5). To gain entry to the darkroom it is necessary to step into the cylinder and then manually rotate it until the cylinder opening is adjacent to the darkroom. Its one big advantage lies in the fact that it does not require a large floor area for installation.

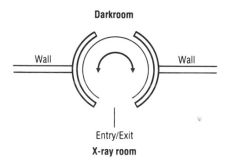

Fig. 12.5 A rotating door entrance for a darkroom.

12.4.8 Fire safety

Ideally, all darkrooms should be provided with an alternative exit, which should be indicated clearly and left unobstructed at all times.

12.5 Darkroom illumination

This may be considered under two headings:

(1) Ordinary white lighting.
(2) Safelighting.

12.5.1   *White lighting*

White lighting is necessary for the following tasks:

(1) Inspection and maintenance of cassettes and screens;
(2) Cleaning of work surfaces and floors;
(3) Servicing of equipment.

White lighting should be:

(1) Sited close to the ceiling to avoid the casting of strong shadows;
(2) Moderate in intensity (e.g. 60 W tungsten, or 30 W fluorescent) in order to make visual accommodation under safelights easier;
(3) Preferably centrally placed, unless the size of the darkroom necessitates additional fixtures, in which case they should be sited over the main working areas.

It may be desirable to have more than one switch if the work surface is remote from the door – one sited near the door, the other at the work area.

If the white light switches are placed higher than the safelight switches, then identification of the respective switches is made easier in the dark and the danger of the wrong light being switched on is minimized.

12.5.2   *Safelighting*

Loading and unloading X-ray cassettes all day in complete darkness would not make for easy or pleasant working conditions!

Whilst all film materials would instantly be fogged if exposed to white light, safelighting, which is the use of dim, coloured lighting, provides sufficient illumination by which one can handle, manipulate and process film. Providing exposure to such lighting is brief, no significant fogging will occur. This last sentence is important, for *there is no totally safe safelighting*! We shall return to this point a little later.

12.5.2.1   How does a safelight work?
When white light is passed through coloured filters, as in Fig. 12.6, certain wavelengths (or colours) are absorbed by the filters, whilst those wavelengths which correspond to the colour of the filters will be transmitted.

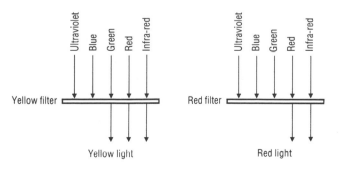

Fig. 12.6 The pigment in the filter selectively attenuates those parts of the spectrum to which the film is most sensitive.

Making the correct selection of safelight filter (or matching the filter to the film, as is sometimes described) means choosing a filter which will transmit a colour to which the film is relatively unresponsive, whilst stopping all light to which the film is most sensitive.

12.5.2.2   Safelight filters

Safelight filters usually consist of a sheet of gelatin dyed to the appropriate colour and sandwiched between two sheets of glass for protection (Fig. 12.7). If used in conjunction with a 25 W lamp and cleaned periodically as recommended, they will give many years of useful life. Gelatin will deteriorate if subjected to extremes of heat and moisture, and so higher-wattage lamps should never be used.

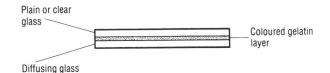

Fig. 12.7 Cross-section through a safelight filter.

12.5.2.3   Spectral transmission graph

Manufacturers produce graphs for their safelights called **spectral transmission** or **filter transmission** graphs (Fig. 12.8). Their purpose is to indicate that part of the visible spectrum which will be transmitted by the filter, and so aid the radiographer in matching the appropriate filter to the type of film in use.

These graphs may appear strange at first because the vertical axis is inverted in comparison to that seen in conventional graphs. In other words, the curve should also be seen as upside down.

On examining the spectral transmission curve illustrated in Fig. 12.8(a), we can see that some of the light which is transmitted by the filter has wavelengths in the region of 550 nm. Such a filter would therefore be inappropriate in a darkroom handling orthochromatic or panchromatic film. It would, however, be suitable for use with monochromatic film materials. A filter which could be used with orthochromatic film is shown in Fig.12.8(b).

Panchromatic film presents special problems, since it will have colour sensitivity extending as far as the red end of the spectrum. It is thus advisable to process such film in complete darkness.

12.5.2.4   How safe is safelighting?

It was mentioned previously that no safelighting is completely safe; all films will become significantly fogged if exposed to safelights for long enough. This is because safelight filters are not perfect absorbers of the undesirable wavelengths and, in truth, *all* films have some sensitivity to *all* wavelengths. Thus, the intensity of illumination and the film-handling time must be kept to a minimum if significant fogging is not to occur.

In practice, the intensity of the undesirable wavelengths transmitted by the filter is small, but their intensity will be increased if the film manufacturer's instructions are ignored by:

(1) Using too small a safelight-to-film distance (intensity increased due to inverse square law);

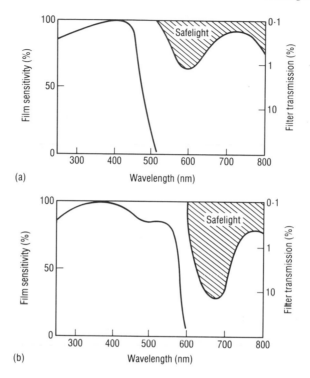

Fig. 12.8 (a) A safelight filter suitable for use with monochromatic film materials. The greatest filter transmission is in the 550 nm wavelength range therefore making it unsuitable for use with orthochromatic film materials. (b) A filter which can be used with orthochromatic film since it transmits light to which the film is insensitive.

(2) Using too high a wattage lamp inside the safelight (a 25 W pearl lamp sited a minimum of 1.2 m from the film is the recommended standard).

12.5.2.5 Sensitivity of exposed/unexposed film

Film which has already been exposed to X-radiation is far more sensitive to safelight fogging than is unexposed material. This is because a small amount of exposure to safelights during handling of a previously *unexposed* film may be insufficient to cause any density increase because its contribution will be less than the threshold level required to trigger such a response (see section 4.5.5.1). However, a film which *has* been previously exposed will already have reached or exceeded the threshold and because all exposures are cumulative, any small additional exposure from safelighting may well result in a noticeable overall increase in density, i.e. the image will be fogged.

Figure 12.9 shows the effect of excessive safelighting on a typical medical X-ray film which has previously had a radiographic exposure (see curve A). Curve B is of an identical film which has been processed correctly without undue exposure to safelights.

Comparing the two curves, it is possible to identify two principal features which occur when film is exposed to safelights for too long (curve A):

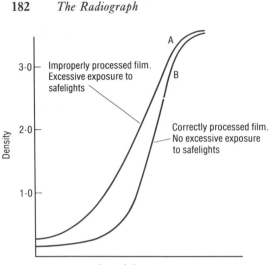

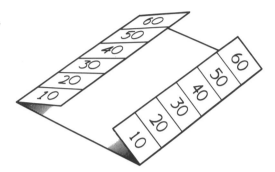

Fig. 12.9 Effect of excessive safelighting exposure on a typical medical X-ray film (film A). The two principal features to be noted are: (1) an increase in gross fog; (2) an overall loss of contrast.

Fig. 12.10 A folded card film holder for carrying out a safe film-handling time test.

(1) An increase in gross fog;
(2) An overall loss of contrast.

12.5.2.6 Safe film-handling time

From the moment an exposed film is taken from its cassette to the instant it disappears inside the processor, it is exposed to safelights. Safe film-handling time is defined as the maximum time for which a film can be exposed to the safelights during the above procedure without causing any appreciable degree of fogging.

How to determine the safe film-handling time
Materials required:

(1) Sheet of 30 × 35 cm card, folded and marked as illustrated in Fig. 12.10. (All markings should be bold enough to be visible under safelight conditions.)
(2) Sheet of 24 × 30 cm card.
(3) A 24 × 30 cm screen-type X-ray film of the fastest variety in use in the department.
(4) A 24 × 30 cm X-ray cassette.
(5) Densitometer (if available).

Method:

(1) Load the cassette with the film in total darkness.
(2) In the X-ray room, mask one-half of the cassette lengthwise with a piece of lead.
(3) Select and make an exposure which will produce, on the exposed portion of film, a uniform density between 0.5 and 1.0 when processed.
(4) In the darkroom, unload the film in total darkness and place in the cardboard holder, with the edges of the holder folded over to cover the long edges of the

film. Place the second sheet of card on top, so as to cover the film and test device.

(5) Position the test device on the workbench at some customary working position.

(6) Switch on the safelight(s) to be tested.

(7) Move the covering card down to the first marked line and expose the uncovered portion of film for 1 min.

(8) The card is moved down to the next line and the uncovered portion of film exposed for 50 s.

(9) Proceed in this way until the entire film has been exposed in accordance with the times marked on the side flaps of the test device.

(10) Turn off the safelights and process the film in total darkness.

The end result is a film with a set of six exposures, as seen in Fig. 12.11, ranging from 10 s to $3\frac{1}{2}$ min.

The film has four distinct portions:

A, which has been pre-exposed to X-radiation but received no safelight exposure during the test;

B, which has been pre-exposed to X-radiation and received safelight exposure;

C, exposed to safelight exposure only;

D, a proportion of the film which has neither been pre-exposed nor received safelight exposure.

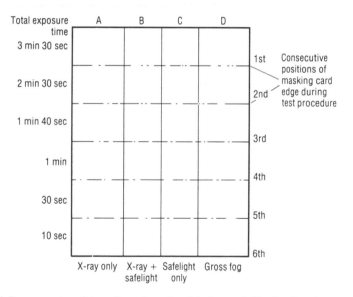

Fig. 12.11 Representation of the radiograph produced during a safe film–handling time assessment.

Inspecting the film Using the densitometer, measure the density at 'D'. This is gross fog. Move next to the bottom of strip 'C' and, working upwards, look for the first density which is 0.05 above gross fog.

As soon as such a density has been found, look to the edge flap on the test card and calculate the total exposure time responsible for this particular density. This time represents the maximum safe film-handling time for unexposed film material.

To discover the safe film-handling time for exposed material, take a densitometer reading of portion 'A' and then, working from the bottom of column 'B', use the densitometer to find the first appearance of a density 0.05 greater than the density at 'A'. Once found, the total time may be calculated from the edge flap. Since the safe film-handling time for exposed material will always be shorter than with unexposed film, it is the former handling time which should be adopted.

It is wise in practice to adopt a somewhat briefer handling time than that estimated at test, in order to provide for a margin of safety.

This test can be carried out without the aid of a densitometer, in which case it will then give a very rough guide to safe film-handling time. The radiographer simply looks for the first visible signs of increased density due to safelight exposure on the portion of film which has been pre-exposed to X-radiation, and reads off the corresponding exposure time.

Typical safe film-handling times average between 20 and 45 s. Excessive safe film-handling times are unnecessary and may indicate too low a level of safelighting.

Remember that the introduction of faster film materials into a department will mean the need for shorter handling times, since such emulsions produce a greater film blackening for a given quantity of light in comparison with slower film emulsions.

12.5.2.7   When should safelight tests be carried out?

(1) Whenever a new darkroom is commissioned.
(2) Where safelights have been changed or additional safelights added.
(3) If faster film material is introduced into a department.
(4) Whenever it is suspected that safelight fogging is occurring.
(5) As part of a quality assurance programme, when the integrity of safelight filters may be checked either annually or biannually.

Should a safelight test indicate that fogging is occurring or that a much shortened film-handling time is required than hitherto in order to prevent film fogging, then one of the following reasons may be suspected:

(1) There is white light leakage, due perhaps to a faulty safelight housing.
(2) A safelight filter is faded, cracked or incorrectly positioned.
(3) The illumination intensity is too great for the particular speed of film material in use. This may be due to:
  (a) Too high a wattage bulb;
  (b) Too many safelights;
  (c) Distance between safelights and film being too small.
(4) The safelight filter is not compatible with the spectral sensitivity of the film being used.

12.5.2.8   Types of safelighting

Direct safelighting
With this form of illumination, light from the safelamp falls directly onto the work surface. A **beehive** safelamp, such as the one illustrated in Fig. 12.12, is an example of direct lighting. Such illumination should be sited a minimum distance of 1.2 m (4 ft) from the working surface, and is the best type of lighting for film loading and unloading areas.

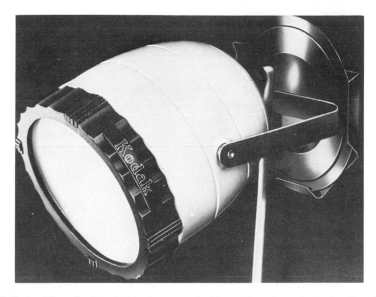

Fig. 12.12 A safelamp for direct lighting known as a beehive safelamp. It may be fixed to the wall or be ceiling suspended. (Courtesy of Kodak Ltd.)

Indirect safelighting
Indirect safelighting is intended to provide general illumination of the darkroom. The safelamp directs the light towards the ceiling, which consequently should be painted in a light colour in order to reflect light back into the room.

Figure 12.13 shows a ceiling-suspended safelamp which includes filters above and below the safelight bulb, thus providing both indirect and direct illumination.

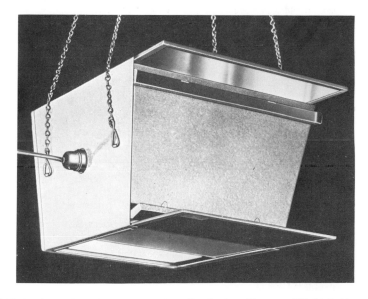

Fig. 12.13 A safelamp for both direct and indirect illumination. (Courtesy of Kodak Ltd.)

These lamps should be suspended at least 2.1 m above floor level in order to prevent head-on collisions with darkroom personnel!

12.6   Darkroom equipment and its arrangement

A well planned automatic processing darkroom will allow an orderly sequence of successive stages of work, with clear 'traffic lanes' so that technicians are not in each others way if there is more than one working in the same room.

Some 'furnishings' necessary for a well-equipped darkroom are listed below:

(1) An automatic processor;
(2) Cassette hatch or hatches;
(3) Film storage hopper(s);
(4) Loading bench/cupboards.

A suitable arrangement for all of these items can be seen in Fig. 12.14.

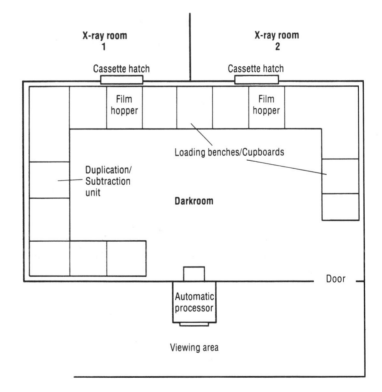

Fig. 12.14 The layout of a typical darkroom well equipped with ample storage and work surfaces.

12.6.1   *Automatic processors*

The main advantage of placing a processor with only the feed tray inside the darkroom (Fig. 12.15) is that processed films may be collected and viewed without any disturbance to darkroom routine. Where a processor is sited inside a darkroom, problems will occur in providing adequate ventilation and in ensuring that heat and fumes are ducted away from the processor.

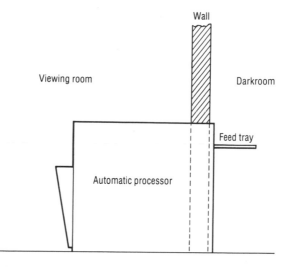

Fig. 12.15 A through-the-wall position for an automatic processor.

For safety, a mains isolator switch serving the processor should be provided both inside as well as outside the darkroom.

12.6.2 *Cassette hatches*

These allow easy transport of film cassettes between radiographic rooms and darkroom.

One door of the hatch is lined with a 2 mm thickness of lead, since it may need to open directly into a radiographic room. The opposite door opens into the darkroom. In addition, the hatch has the following features:

(1) An interlocking device to prevent both doors being opened simultaneously and admitting light into the darkroom;
(2) Partitioning within the hatch to afford two compartments for cassettes, one marked 'exposed' and the other 'unexposed'.

12.6.3 *Film hoppers*

Unexposed films intended for immediate use in reloading cassettes are most conveniently kept in a hopper (Fig. 12.16) under the loading bench. Each compartment accommodates different-sized films.

Besides the obvious requirement that the hopper be light-tight, another safety feature should be considered at the same time as the hopper is installed. This is to link electronically the film hopper microswitch with the white lighting circuit so that the white light goes off if the hopper is inadvertently opened.

12.6.4 *Loading bench/cupboards*

A darkroom loading bench should consist of a workbench and generous cupboard space. Typical units (Fig. 12.17) are supplied in a variety of sizes and configurations to suit most darkrooms.

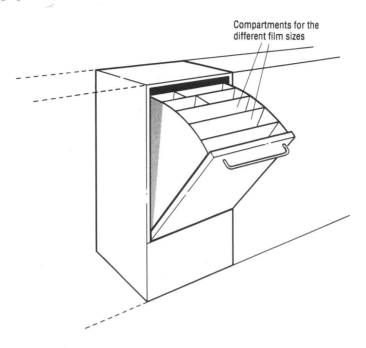

Compartments for the
different film sizes

Fig. 12.16 A film hopper for the darkroom storage of unexposed film materials.

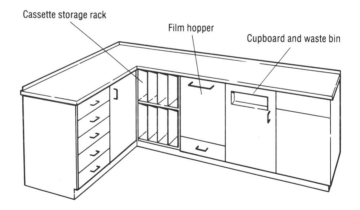

Cassette storage rack

Film hopper

Cupboard and waste bin

Fig. 12.17 A darkroom dry bench system. (Courtesy of Wardray Products Ltd.)

12.7   Manual processing

The modern imaging department, with its accent on automation and daylight processing systems, has been the principal concern of this chapter.

However, since manual processing is not entirely obsolete, this chapter would not be complete without a very brief mention of the special requirements that such a processing procedure demands in terms of darkroom design.

The use of manual processing imposes stricter guidelines on darkroom planning because of the attendant risk of liquid spillage and the proximity of electrical sources to wet areas, etc.

12.7.1 *Floors*

These should be:

(1) Non–slip;
(2) Resistant to staining by chemicals, etc.

12.7.2 *Walls*

Areas in the neighbourhood of sinks and wet processing equipment should be protected to a height of at least 1.3 m with ceramic or plastic tiles.

12.7.3 *Equipment required*

(1) Manual process unit (Fig. 12.18).
(2) Hangers for suspending films when processing.

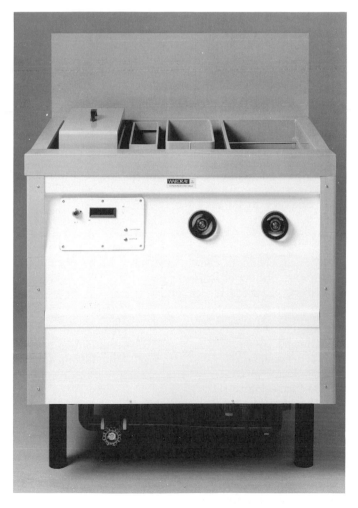

Fig. 12.18 A manual processing unit. (Courtesy of Wardray Products Ltd.)

(3) A drying cabinet.
(4) Wash basin.
(5) Towel dispenser for drying hands.

12.7.4   Electrical safety

Besides the obvious siting of appliances well away from wet areas, staff should always take great care to ensure that their hands are dry before touching any electrical switch or appliance.

12.8   Health and safety in processing areas

12.8.1   Electrical

(1) All electrical equipment to be sited well away from sinks and manual processing equipment.
(2) Electrical appliances to be adequately earthed.
(3) Pull-cord switching for lights.
(4) No trailing cables from appliances.
(5) Pilot lamps incorporated in equipment to indicate when 'on'.
(6) The two mains isolator switches controlling all electrical equipment to be within easy access of all personnel. One sited inside, the other outside the darkroom.

12.8.2   General

(1) The maximum level of safelighting consistent with film sensitivity.
(2) Adequate ventilation.
(3) Second exits for fire safety.

12.8.3   Chemical

Processing chemicals contain many toxic substances and must always be handled with care (Society of Radiographers, 1991). The following are those constituents deserving of particular mention:

Developer	*Fixer*
Acetic acid	Acetic acid
Glutaraldehyde	Ammonium thiosulphate
Hydroquinone	Ammonium sulphate
Diethylene glycol	
Sodium sulphite	
Phenidone (1-phenyl-3-pyrazolidone)	
Potassium hydroxide	

In addition to a well ventilated film processing area (i.e. 12–15 air changes per hour), well maintained automatic film processors and chemical mixers serve to minimize any risks to radiology staff when in the vicinity of, or when handling, such chemicals. Nevertheless, staff should always be aware of the harmful effects of exposure to the chemistry and its fumes through inhalation, ingestion or skin contact.

All staff involved with the handling of film chemistry should be regularly advised to read product labels and mixing instructions before handling solutions. A supply of packs containing safety glasses, face mask, rubber gloves and plastic apron should be available within the processing area for each procedure. The supply should be replenished as and when necessary. However, the **Control of Substances Hazardous to Health (COSHH) Regulations** 1988, which we examine below, make it clear that employers have a responsibility, in so far as is reasonably practicable, to prevent or adequately control exposure to fumes and chemicals using measures other than the personal protective equipment described above. The use of mask, goggles, etc., is still a sensible requirement, but legislation is making it clear that managers cannot abdicate their responsibility for minimising hazards simply by providing safety equipment.

12.8.3.1   COSHH

As one might expect, the COSHH Regulations have significant implications for the diagnostic imaging department; (Photosol, undated, and Society of Radiographers, 1991). The COSHH regulations impose a responsibility upon managers to ensure that the following procedures are carried out in their departments:

(1) Health risk assessments undertaken in order to determine what hazards, if any, exist.
(2) Necessary precautions decided.
(3) Control measures introduced to minimize or eliminate identified risks.
(4) Control measures and working procedures regularly monitored for effectiveness.
(5) If deemed necessary, health surveillance undertaken for early detection of illness due to occupational exposure.
(6) Adequate information, instruction and training afforded to all key staff.

Manufacturers and suppliers of processing chemistry have a statutory obligation under the Health and Safety at Work Act 1974 to provide purchasers with details of the chemical constituents of their processing solutions and any hazards associated with their use. This information is to be found in their **Material Safety Data Sheets** (MSDSs) and is essential reading for radiology managers when carrying out risk assessments.

12.8.3.2   The COSHH assessment (HSE, 1988)

This exercise, which should be carried out in all processing areas, is aimed at identifying:

● The substances being used and their chemical constituents;
● Where and how they are used and handled;
● The hazards associated with each, e.g. the fumes and emissions involved;
● The numbers and type of staff who are likely to be exposed to the hazards;
● The length of time staff are exposed to the hazards;
● The precautions of which staff should be advised.

Ready printed COSHH assessment forms are available from various agencies and enable these procedures to be easily recorded and the findings analysed. Copies should be retained along with manufacturers' MSD sheets, and made freely available for staff to read.

12.8.3.3   Occupational exposure limits (OEL)

Many of the chemicals to be found in film processing areas have a designated exposure limit which can be found in the Health and Safety Executive Document (HSE, 1991) sometimes referred to as **EH40** in the literature. Examples of these are given in Table 12.1. For a more comprehensive list, readers are strongly advised to consult manufacturers' MSD sheets.

Table 12.1 Examples of occupational exposure limit (OEL) set by the Health and Safety Executive for fumes associated with photographic processing. (Source: HSE, 1991.)

Chemical substance	Source	OEL (ppm*)
Acetic acid	Developer and fixer solutions	10
Ammonia	Developer and fixer mixed through spillage	25
Diethylene glycol	Developer	23
Glutaraldehyde	Developer	0.2
Monoethylene glycol	Developer	23
Monopropylene glycol	Developer	150
Hydrogen sulphide	Silver recovery vessels when sulphiding takes place	10
Sulphur dioxide	Fixer	2

* ppm: parts per million.

The advent of more sophisticated daylight processing systems, and increased staff awareness of health and safety issues, has inevitably meant that processing areas are safer places than perhaps they once were.

In the next chapter we will look at some of these automated film–handling or daylight systems in more detail.

Chapter 13
Automated Film-Handling Systems

The attraction of having a system which automatically unloads cassettes, processes films, and reloads cassettes with fresh film, is fairly obvious. There will be less opportunity for film-handling marks and none of the tedium associated with the manual loading and unloading of cassettes under safelights.

Such automatic film-handling systems are commonly called **daylight systems** because all film manipulation is done without the need for a darkroom.

All daylight film-handling systems must perform the following four prime functions if they are to be acceptable:

(1) Load cassettes with unexposed film.
(2) Mark each film with patient's name or number, date, etc.
(3) Unload cassettes.
(4) Process the films.

The two daylight film-handling systems to be described are:

(1) Composite or 'complete' type.
(2) Modular type.

13.1 Cassette load/unload and process system

13.1.1 *Composite type*

The word **composite** means that all of the system's component parts, i.e. film supply magazines or dispensers, film unloading machinery and the processor, are combined in one related unit (Fig. 13.1). Most of these units have a film-loading section which can hold 5–7 film dispensers or magazines.

The precise way in which these systems work varies in mechanical terms, but the principle of operation is common to all of them. For illustration, we shall describe in a very simplified way the operational sequence of the Dupont 'Compact' daylight

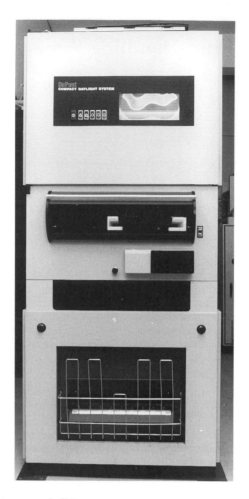

Fig. 13.1 The Dupont compact daylight system.

system (Figs 13.1 and 13.2).

A cassette containing a film for processing is inserted at the front of the unit and the door closed. A bar code (attached to every cassette) is 'read' by the loader microprocessor in order to identify the cassette size.

Inside the unit, the cassette is opened and the film extracted by means of suction cups which move into place over the film. The film is deposited at 'X', the patient's identity and other relevant information is then photographed onto the appropriate corner of the radiograph by means of a prism and lens system, and then transported via a roller and belt system to the rear of the unit where it is fed into the processor.

The film-loading carriage or **sled** moves into position beneath the appropriate film magazine dispenser, a film is then released by the dispenser into the sled and conveyed to the waiting cassette.

After the new film has been transferred from the sled to the cassette, the cassette is closed, the front door to the unit opens and the cassette emerges to be retrieved by the radiographer.

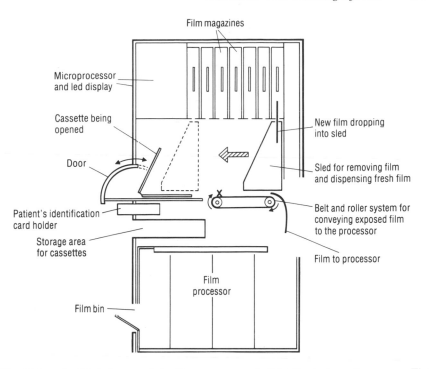

Fig. 13.2 A simplified diagram of the Dupont compact daylight film loader and processor. The sequence of events is as follows once the cassette has been inserted and automatically opened. (1) The sled moves to the appropriate magazine and receives the film. (2) The sled moves to the cassette, extracts the exposed film and dispenses the fresh film into the open cassette. (3) The exposed film is deposited at 'X' and thereby conveyed to the processor. (4) The cassette closed, the door opens and the cassette emerges.

The entire unloading and reloading sequence only takes some 15 s, with each function being communicated to the operator as it happens by means of a multi-language display screen on the front of the unit. The latest version of this daylight system returns the reloaded cassette in 12 seconds.

Other functions that can be carried out by these composite units include:

(1) Unload, process and return empty cassette;
(2) Reload empty cassette and return;
(3) Unload, process and reload CRT and mammography cassettes;
(4) Unload and process AOT or puck film-changer films.

Patient's identification
Films may have the patient's identification photographed onto them using a film identification camera (see section 14.2.2.2) before the cassettes are taken from the imaging room.

Alternatively, identification may be left to the daylight system itself. In the Dupont composite system shown in Figs 13.1 and 13.2, the patient's identification card is placed in a slot at the front of the unit. Antero-posterior or postero-anterior transference of details is then selected, the cassette inserted and, after the film has been extracted from the cassette, the details are photographed onto a corner of the film by means of a prism, lens and mirror system.

Film dispensers

The individual film dispensers supplied with these types of daylight systems are capable of holding at least 100 sheets of unexposed film. (Those in the Agfa Gevaert 'Curix Capacity' system hold up to 135 films.)

The dispensers are usually interchangeable within the loading section, e.g. the 35 × 43 cm dispenser could be placed in any of the film dispenser bays and still be recognizable by the machine as the one containing 35 × 43 cm film.

Cassettes

Manufacturers design their equipment to open a particular type of cassette (usually their own!). Although all the cassettes used with this type of unit are of the standard book-type design, they may vary slightly in some particular locking feature.

It is therefore customary to purchase cassettes from the same manufacturer as the daylight system. These cassettes may be used in the normal way with conventional processing facilities should the need arise.

The processor

The processor may be situated under the loader/unloader section, as, for example, in the Dupont unit described above and the 3M daylight unit. Other manufacturers place their processors in line with the loader (Fig. 13.3(b)).

All of the processors used in the above systems are standard manufacturer's models which can be found in conventional medical imaging darkrooms.

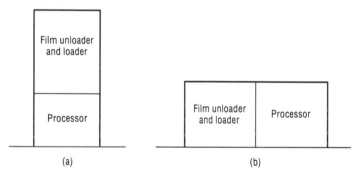

Fig. 13.3 Two types of composite daylight film handling configurations. In (a) the loader/unloader sits above the processor, whilst in (b) the two sections are in line.

13.1.1.1 Microprocessor control of composite daylight systems

The electronic sophistication of these units enables many useful monitoring functions to be carried out. These include:

(1) Monitoring the operating sequence and informing the operator of each step as it happens, by means of a display screen.
(2) Communicating any operator or system error by means of its self-diagnosing system check, and then displaying a fault code which can be identified by the operator so that remedial action may be taken.
(3) Warning the operator when the film supply in a particular magazine is low, and again when it is empty.
(4) Identifying the size and number of films which have been used.

(5) Recording the number and type of equipment faults occurring, so that the data can be called up by the service engineer at any time during his visit.

13.1.2 Modular daylight film-handling system

In this type of daylight system the cassette-loading equipment, i.e. the film dispenser, is separate and can be some distance away from the automatic processor.

Whilst the processor may be centrally located within the department, the film dispensers may be sited in or near the various imaging rooms.

We shall consider the Dupont modular daylight system.

Film dispensers
Separate film dispensers are required for each film size, and they may be wall mounted. In the UK, each dispenser requires a 13 A, 240 V electrical supply.

The film dispenser consists of an upper film storage and dispensing section, and a lower cassette-loading section (Fig. 13.4).

Placing the cassette in the front of the unit and pushing it forwards, actuates the loading cycle mechanism which ensures that the cassette is driven up towards the film storage area. As it does so, two metal pins enter the cassette frame on either side of the film aperture, causing a spring-loaded flap to open. A fresh film is released from the storage compartment and drops into the empty cassette. As the

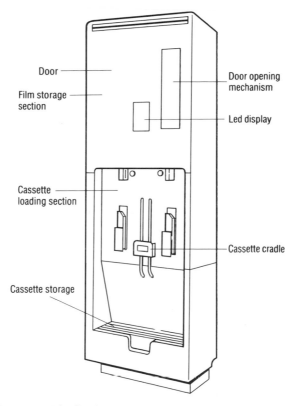

Fig. 13.4 The Dupont modular film dispenser.

cassette is lowered away, so the metal pins disengage and the cassette flap springs shut, safely protecting the film from any light. The returned cassette can then be lifted out of the dispenser.

A display panel on the front of the unit indicates to the operator all of the operation sequences as they take place, as well as indicating the number of supply films remaining.

The films used to restock the dispensers are supplied in special **daylight packs** consisting of 100 sheets of notched film. The film bag containing the films has an extension piece or 'tail' at either end. When loading the empty dispenser with a new supply of film, the bag of film is placed inside the upper section of the dispenser, and the bag top or 'tail' is fed between the two rollers. The bottom 'tail' is cut off by the operator using a special bag-cutter assembly, which swings into position across the bottom of the bag. This piece of bag is then discarded. Next, the door of the dispenser is shut and the following automatic sequence of events occurs. The bag is lifted from the film pack and 'posted' back to the waiting operator through a chute above the door. The film pack is lowered into its correct position within the dispenser and a short high-frequency beep sounds, to inform the operator that the dispenser is ready.

Film cassettes

The cassettes used with the type of modular system described above are not of the conventional hinged or 'book' design, but instead have a flap-sealed slot at one end (Fig. 13.5). This spring-loaded flap can be opened by pressing down on the two springs located on either side of the film aperture. This is automatically carried out by the film dispenser as described above.

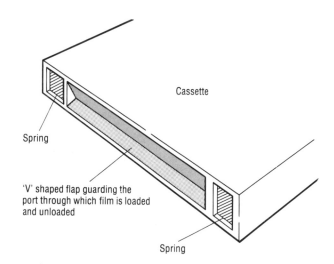

Fig. 13.5 A cassette suitable for use with the modular system seen in Fig. 13.4. The flap is opened by pressure on the two springs. This is automatically carried out by the film dispenser where upon a film drops into the empty cassette.

Some types of cassette have a means of indicating to the operator whether or not the cassette contains a film. This may be a simple mechanism, like a little 'nipple' which is held firmly in the 'out' position when a film is present but which is 'loose' when the cassette is empty (Fig. 13.6).

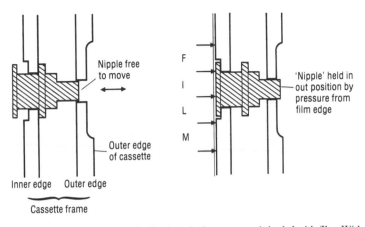

Fig. 13.6 A simple but clever system of indicating whether a cassette is loaded with film. With the film in the cassette the nipple is held firmly in the out position.

Film unloader

The unloader (Fig. 13.7) is used to extract X-ray film automatically from the cassette, apply permanent patient identification data and then feed the film to the processor. It requires an electrical supply similar to the film dispenser described above.

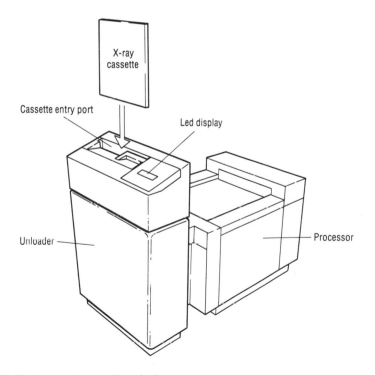

Fig. 13.7 The Dupont daylight film unloader.

Manufacturers naturally match their unloaders to their own particular types of processor, although interfaces are sometimes available to marry the unloader with another manufacturer's automatic processor.

To unload the film, the cassette is inserted into the adjustable entrance port at the top and pushed downwards. The cassette's spring-loaded flap or light gate is automatically opened and screens separate to allow the film to unload. The film drops through the light gate and enters the film chute where the patient's identification is projected onto the film by means of a mirror and lens system, and the film passes into the processor.

A visual display panel on the unloader indicates to the operator each unloading sequence event as it occurs. The date and time are also digitally shown on the panel and can be photographed onto the film at the same time as the patient's identity if required.

The manufacturer Fuji produce a modular daylight system where the film unloader may be used detached from the processor and in a separate location, making the system even more versatile. It automatically unloads cassettes and stores within it up to 25 exposed films of mixed sizes. When required, it can be taken to an automatic processor, attached to the feed side and the films fed automatically to the processor one at a time.

13.2   The choice of system – composite or modular?

The choice is one which the radiology manager makes only after very careful consideration. The many criteria upon which such a decision is based – cost, departmental layout, workload, for example – are unfortunately beyond the scope of this book. However, it is appropriate to look at some of the advantages and disadvantages associated with each type of system.

13.2.1   *The composite system*

13.2.1.1   Advantages

(1) All functions – unloading/loading/processing – are the result of one single action, i.e. placing the cassette into the machine!
(2) In the event of a breakdown, the cassettes can just as easily be handled manually and the film processed through a non-daylight system.
(3) There is no requirement for an extensive darkroom facility. Those systems requiring the loading of dispenser under safelight conditions need only a very small area of the department to be designated as a 'darkroom'.

13.2.1.2   Disadvantages

(1) Because these systems are very often sited in a daylight environment, it means that if one major function fails, e.g. the film loader, then the entire system is out of commission since the processor cannot be used as a separate unit.
(2) In a department with a heavy workload or during periods of intensive activity, congestion may occur in the processing area as several radiographers wait for their cassettes to be reloaded and processed.

13.2.2   *Modular system*

13.2.2.1   Advantages

(1) Greater versatility than the composite system. The film dispensers can be located in or near imaging rooms and the processor in a separate central area. If one particular loader should fail, another of similar size, albeit in a different room location, can be used.
(2) Darkroom facility can be retained so that all types of film, as well as films from the dispensers, can be processed.
(3) Should the processor break down, work can continue, with the films being processed elsewhere.
(4) No hold-up for staff waiting to reload cassettes.

13.2.3   *Summary*

Whichever system is chosen, composite or modular, the advantages of daylight systems over the conventional type of darkroom processing can be summarized as follows:

(1) Faster film handling.
(2) Fewer film-handling marks.
(3) Less space required for the processing function.
(4) Fewer cassettes needed, since they can be reloaded and returned more quickly.
(5) More time can be spent with patient instead of on film-handling activities.
(6) Greater patient throughput because of faster film-handling.
(7) Reduced stress on the radiographer, particularly when working single-handed or on-call.

In this chapter we have studied some of the automatic film-handling systems presently available. In the next chapter we shall look in detail at film presentation and at some of the equipment for viewing the final image.

Chapter 14
Presentation and Viewing of Radiographs

No radiograph is complete unless it has been correctly identified with sufficient patient details imprinted upon it.

The need not only for sufficient, but accurate identification can never be stressed enough. Without it, a radiograph is useless. Besides being dangerous practice, the medicolegal implications which may arise if a poorly or non-identified radiograph is wrongly associated with a particular patient should be a sobering thought for any radiographer.

Providing as much information as possible minimizes the risk of uncertainty over identification, and can help to speed up the sorting process.

It should be the responsibility of the radiographer who takes the film to ensure that the radiograph includes all the necessary information. Careful checking of each radiograph is therefore essential. *There is no exception to this rule.*

All information should be photographically imprinted upon the film by the methods that we describe later, or be put there during radiographic exposure. Adding details by hand after the radiograph has been processed is a sloppy method which only encourages error.

14.1 Types of information

14.1.1 *Identification (essential information)*

(1) Full name.
(2) Date of birth.
(3) Hospital number or code.

(4) Name of hospital.
(5) Date and time of examination.

14.1.2 *Technical*

(1) Right and left markers.
(2) Position of patient or projection, e.g. PA, RAO, ERECT, etc.
(3) Timing of the film in a given sequence, e.g. 5 min, 1 h, etc.
(4) Number of the film in a rapid sequence, e.g. in aortography.
(5) Layer height in tomography.
(6) Tube angulation used.
(7) Whether mobile or ward radiograph.
(8) Stereoradiographs – direction of tube displacement.
(9) Miscellaneous information, e.g. post-micturition, after fatty meal.

14.1.3 *Miscellaneous*

(1) Radiographer's identity.
(2) The particular cassette and screens used. May be identified from letter or numeral on screen surface (see section 8.5). Any faulty screen can be identified quickly from the radiograph and the cassette taken out of circulation.

All information, of whatever type, must be added to the film in such a way that it is:

(1) Legible;
(2) Readable when the radiograph is viewed from the correct aspect (Fig. 14.3);
(3) Not superimposed on any important anatomy;
(4) Included within the collimated area.

14.2 Methods of recording information

(1) Opaque letters and legends.
(2) Actinic marking.
(3) Perforating devices.

14.2.1 *Opaque letters and legends*

A selection of such legends is illustrated in Fig. 14.1. The letters may themselves be radiopaque or radiotransparent on an opaque base. By placing them directly on to the cassette or direct-exposure film, their outline will be exposed onto the radiograph by the subsequent X-ray exposure.

The most common type of marking system is probably the clip-on marker (Fig. 14.2), so called because it can be clipped onto the edge of a cassette. A postero-anterior (PA) and an antero-posterior (AP) form are available.

Selecting the correct type of marker is also important. Clip-on markers are often inappropriate, e.g. when collimating tightly or if using a cone-shaped beam collimating device. Instead, a simple character marker placed on the cassette within the beam area should be used (Fig. 14.3).

(a) (b)

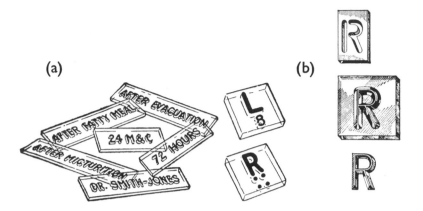

Fig. 14.1 (a) Radiopaque legends and letters for use in marking radiographs. These are engraved on a Perspex base and filled with a radiopaque material. The small character seen under the L and the group of dots under the R are to identify the radiographer. (By courtesy of Cuthbert Andrews.) (b) Markers for radiographs. Upper: The letter is incised in a thin piece of metal. Centre: The letter is lead, mounted in a Perspex plaque. Lower: Single lead character. (By courtesy of Picker International Ltd.)

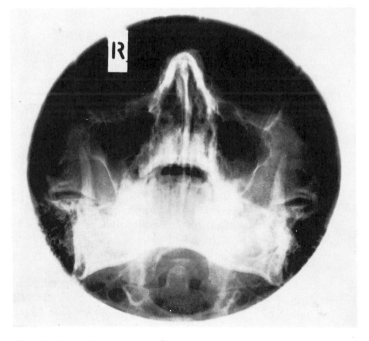

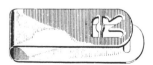

Fig. 14.2 A metal clip-on marker suitable for placing over the edge of a cassette.

Fig. 14.3 A suitable small anatomical marker correctly placed. Occipitomental projection.

14.2.2   *Actinic marking*

Actinic markers are devices which exploit the photographic property of film by using light to print information onto the film.

Such a marking system has *three* advantages:

(1) It provides permanent identification;
(2) It is simple to use;
(3) The information is easy to read.

Whilst there are several types of actinic marker available, they are all, nevertheless, based on either one of two methods:

(1) Contact printing;
(2) Printing using a simple lens system (photographic marker).

Both methods require a small rectangular strip along one edge or corner of the film to have been unexposed to X-radiation. This is achieved by the use of a lead blocker mounted inside the cassette. This unexposed portion of the film is then used for patient identification.

14.2.2.1   **Contact printing**

A unit used for **contact printing** patient information from a typed slip of paper onto a radiograph is illustrated in Fig. 14.4.

Such a unit can be flush mounted with the darkroom bench surface if desired. The typed translucent paper slip is placed over the identification window of the marker unit and held in place by means of a magnetic bar.

Next, the film is removed from the cassette and positioned on top of the paper in

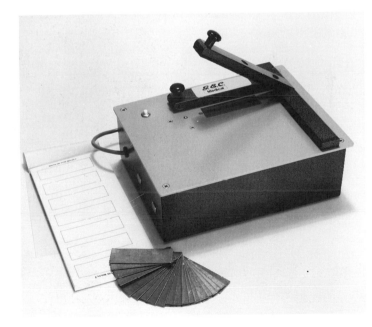

Fig. 14.4 An actinic marker. Also shown are a pad of titling papers, which can be printed with a hospital's name, and a number of lead blockers for fitting to cassettes. (Courtesy of Picker International.)

the angle made by the magnetic bar and the side-positioning stop so that the protected area of the emulsion lies over the window. The hinged spring pressure pad is brought down onto the film, so activating a small flashlamp within the box. The light passes through the slip of paper to the film so that the resultant image will be of white print on a dark background.

In order for film marking to be carried out on films of different speeds, a range of varying light intensities can be selected (e.g. six).

So that the identity slip may be positioned easily on the marker when working under safelight conditions, a neon light is contained within the marker housing to illuminate the marker window. This remains 'on' at all times.

14.2.2.2 Photographic markers

These are perhaps better known as **identification cameras** (Figs. 14.5 and 14.6). They are used extensively in conjunction with daylight film-handling systems. Film marking is done with the film remaining inside the cassette.

Such a method naturally calls for a specially adapted type of cassette, one in which a small rectangular piece of the cassette-back near one corner can be moved aside to provide a 'window' through which patient details may be photographed onto the film. Such a cassette can be seen in Fig. 14.7, with its window half-opened.

The camera is used in the following way.

The patient's details are printed upon a piece of card, which is then placed under the pressure flap of the identification camera with the typed information lying over the glass window.

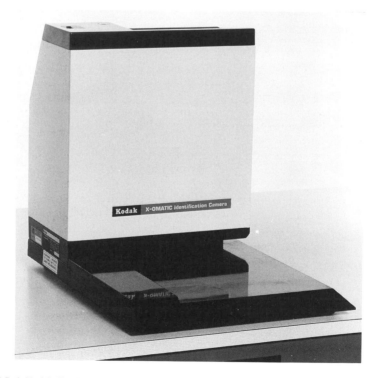

Fig. 14.5 A Kodak film identification camera.

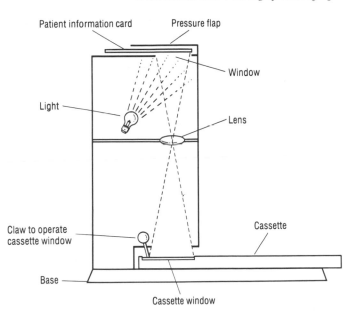

Fig. 14.6 Simplified cross-section through a film identification camera.

When the cassette is inserted at the bottom of the box, a claw automatically moves across the face of the window flap on the cassette, gripping it and sliding it open. Next, a lamp within the marker lights and illuminates the identity card at the top of the unit.

A simple convex lens system focuses the typed information onto the now exposed portion of film. The cassette window is released by the claw and the window shutter, being spring mounted, closes immediately, preventing light entering when the cassette is withdrawn from the camera.

A density control is incorporated within the unit so that the desired film blackening can be obtained as a background for the typed information.

Many of these markers have a 24 h clock, an image of which is photographed onto the film at the same time as the patient's identity (Fig. 14.8).

A significant advantage of the photographic form of marker over the contact printing type is that it may be anywhere in the department. Their placement in radiographic rooms, for example, means that the radiographer responsible for a given examination is able to record the patient details onto the film immediately on completion of a radiographic procedure. Thus, the radiographer carrying out the investigation is made directly responsible for film identification.

Three principal benefits derive from this:

(1) The opportunity for wrong marking is minimized, since no second person (e.g. the darkroom technician) is involved.
(2) The radiographers' responsibility for correct film identification is made easier.
(3) Faster film handling. If the film is to be manually unloaded, then the darkroom technician only has to extract the film and feed it to the processor.

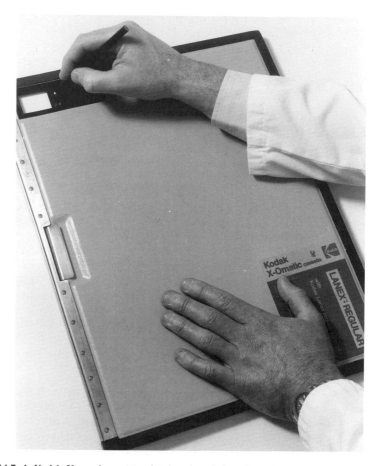

Fig. 14.7 A Kodak X-omatic cassette showing the window through which patient details may be photographed on to the film using the camera illustrated in Fig. 14.5.

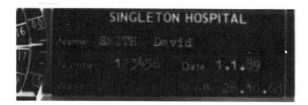
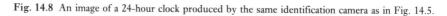

Fig. 14.8 An image of a 24-hour clock produced by the same identification camera as in Fig. 14.5.

14.2.2.3 Specialized photographic markers

These are the type incorporated into most automatic film-handling systems ('daylight' systems), one of which we referred to in section 13.1.1.

14.2.3 Perforating devices

Films and other records may be perforated with letters or figures, as a means of identification, using a perforating machine. More elaborate presses cover a larger range of letters and may be suitable for including the date and the hospital's name.

Compared with the other marking systems that we have looked at, this method is not very useful. It may have an advantage where a large number of radiographs have to be marked with the same legend, but where there is a need to change letters frequently (e.g. patients' names) then it becomes a very slow method of marking.

14.3 Identification of dental films

The size of a dental film precludes it from being individually marked, so the film is made with an embossed dot in one corner. This can be seen on the dental film packet, as well as on the film itself, as a raised dot.

When exposing the film, the convexity of the dot must be towards the X-ray tube, and the film is positioned in the mouth so that the dot is always towards the crowns rather than the apices of the teeth.

Provided that the processed film is then viewed with the dot convexity towards the observer, and the dental formula in Fig. 14.9 is followed, it becomes relatively simple to identify, arrange and mount a set of dental films in the correct anatomical manner.

Note how the radiographs are arranged in such a way that the observer is looking at the images as he would the teeth themselves.

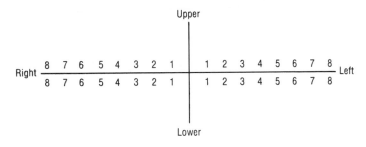

Fig. 14.9 Dental chart formula. When mounting dental films their positioning on the mount should follow the above formula.

14.3.1 Dental mounts

One particular type of mount is made of cellulose acetate, one surface being matt textured and the other glossy. The sheet transmits a diffuse, even illumination when held up to a source of light.

Notches or semicircular incisions, which are used to hold the dental film in place, can be made in the sheet using a special dental mount cutter. The patient's name and other details can be written on the matt surface of the mount.

14.4 Final presentation of the radiograph

All films from a particular examination (e.g. intravenous urography, tomography, etc.) should be arranged in correct sequence before being presented for viewing and possible reporting.

14.5   Viewing equipment

No matter how good the quality of a given film image, all the effort and skill expended in producing it will be wasted unless the conditions under which it is viewed are satisfactory. It is vital, therefore, to place a great deal of importance on providing quality viewing equipment when planning imaging departments.

In Chapter 29 we will look at the relationship between the perception of detail in an image and the conditions under which viewing takes place. For now, we will confine ourselves to examining some of the equipment by which radiographic images, in particular, may be viewed.

The construction of a basic viewing box may be seen in Fig. 14.10. It is approximately 35 cm wide, 55 cm high and 16 cm deep. Power is supplied from the 240 V mains supply.

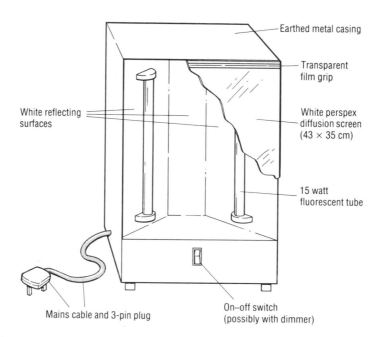

Fig. 14.10 An illuminator for viewing radiographs.

The features of a good illuminator are:

(1) Light of even intensity from edge to edge of the viewing box.
(2) Light should be as 'white' as possible.
(3) Minimal heat given off by the light source.
(4) A facility for varying the brightness.
(5) A high-intensity light (spot or full-screen) incorporated.
(6) Transparent film grips, so that film identification is always visible.

These features are achieved by using two 15 W 18″ fluorescent tubes, a shaped white enamel reflecting surface, and a white perspex screen.

The colour temperature of an X-ray viewing box is 6000 K (see note below).

14.5.1 Colour temperature

The quality of a light source is defined by its **colour temperature**. This is the temperature at which a black-body radiator would emit light of comparable colour. The temperature is expressed in K (kelvin scale).

The definition is best illustrated by the behaviour of a black poker placed into a fire. As the temperature of the poker increases, so its colour changes from black, through a series of different colour reds, and finally to white (if the fire is hot enough, and if the poker hasn't melted!).

Some common types of light source, with their approximate colour temperatures, are given below:

Candle	1930 K
100 W light bulb	2800 K
Electronic flash	5000–6000 K
X-ray viewing box	6000 K
Average daylight	6500 K.

14.5.2 High-intensity light spot

High-intensity light is provided by a 50 W tungsten halogen bulb fitted between the tubes and which produces a *spot* of light at the centre of the screen, the light being operated by a spring-loaded push-switch.

Viewing boxes may be free-standing or wall-mounted, as required, and may be purchased singly or in multiple formats. It is essential when a number of illuminated panels are arranged like this that independent switching for each box is provided, otherwise there will be considerable glare from unused areas when only one or two films are being viewed.

The boxes should also match each other in terms of overall intensity and colour

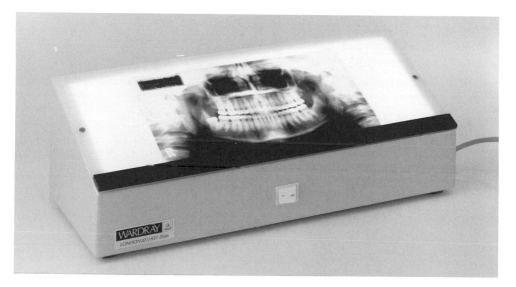

Fig. 14.11 A desk or wall-mounted viewer for 100-mm and dental film. (Courtesy of Wardray Products Ltd.)

of illumination, and within the individual boxes the two or more vertical fluorescent tubes should be identical in light quality and intensity.

It should always be the aim to try to achieve standardization in these regards, not just within the imaging department but throughout the hospital.

14.5.3   Specialized illuminators

14.5.3.1   100 mm Cut film
A typical desk or wall-mounted viewer for 100-mm film can be seen in Fig. 14.11. The viewer is also suitable for dental films.

14.5.3.2   Mammography
One example of a mammography viewer is shown in Fig. 14.12. It incorporates adjustable blinds for masking unused areas of the viewing field, so preventing distracting glare.

14.5.3.3   Teaching viewer
A suitable viewer for the demonstration or conference room can be seen in Fig. 14.13. It has the capacity to hold a large number of films and is motor driven. On the left-hand side are twelve storage frames, each capable of holding eight 35 × 43 cm films. On the right is the illuminated section, mounted on wheels to allow forward and backward movement.

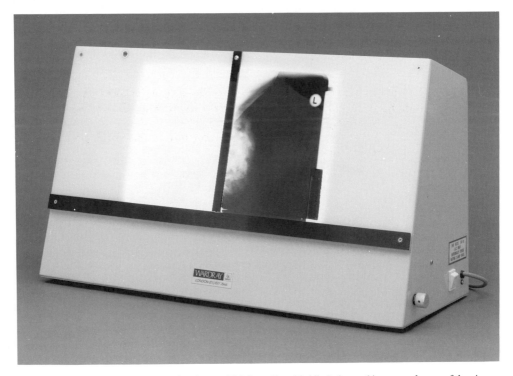

Fig. 14.12 A mammography viewer which has adjustable blinds for masking unused areas of the viewer. (Courtesy of Wardray Products Ltd.)

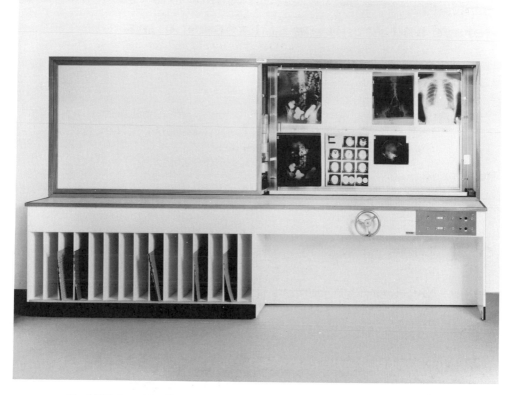

Fig. 14.13 A teaching viewer.

To view a set of films, the selected storage frame is pulled out and the illuminated section moved forward until it is in close proximity with the storage frame.

In the next chapter we discuss how the film images that we have produced are miniaturized and/or stored.

Chapter 15
Storage and Archiving of Exposed Film

Storage
    Shelving
    Other considerations contributing to good store design
Archiving of radiographs
    Miniaturization sizes/options
    The advantages and disadvantages of miniaturization
    Digital archiving

It is a requirement in many parts of the world, including the United Kingdom, that radiographs and other medical images be retained for a specific period by hospitals and clinics.

This advice is based upon two principal considerations:

(1) The need for clinicians to refer to old films in order to observe the course of disease processes;
(2) Health managers have to keep in mind the possibility of litigation and the likely requirement of having to produce films as evidence in any subsequent court case.

15.1 Storage

In the United Kingdom, the recommended minimum time limits for which medical records, including radiographs, should be kept are summarized below:

(1) Ultrasound (obstetric) – 25 years.
(2) Paediatric – until patient's 25th birthday or 8 years after last visit if longer.
(3) All others – 8 years.

The implication in terms of the amount of storage space which may be necessary in order to retain films for such long periods is obvious. To alleviate the problem, many departments carry out miniaturization of their films, thus reducing the amount of storage space required. This is a procedure that we shall consider in detail later.

However, for the foreseeable future, departmental designers will still need to incorporate into their schemes a large-film-format storage area divided into:

(1) **Current store** – for films up to 3 years old.
(2) **Archive store** – for films over 3 years old, which are used less frequently.

The design of such stores will need to take account of features such as adequate lighting and heating, as well as height and spacing of the shelving systems. The various design specifications referred to below are derived from the recommendations set out in the United Kingdom Health Building Regulations (HBN6, 1985) and by Manton *et al.* (1988).

15.1.1 *Shelving*

(1) Fixed shelving racks are preferable to mobile ones. The motor-driven systems are subject to breakdowns, they need regular servicing and are invariably cumbersome.
(2) Shelving should be of metal construction for fire safety and the entire unit subdivided into compartments for easier storage of film packets. Height of shelving should be around 450 mm.
(3) It has been estimated that about 15 m of shelving is required per room per year. So for a store holding films up to 3 years old this means that in a department of six rooms, the shelving space can be calculated thus:

$$6 \times 3 \times 15 = 270 \text{ m of shelving}$$

This could be achieved, for example, by having six ranks of 9 m long shelving, five shelves in height. Other permutations are, of course, possible.
(4) For safety, a maximum height of five or six shelves is advisable.

15.1.2 *Other considerations contributing to good store design*

- Adequate ventilation.
- Satisfactory illumination.
- Dust-free environment.
- Automatic smoke detectors.
- Secure locks, especially if the store is remote from the department.

15.2 Archiving radiographs

The miniaturization of radiographs, i.e. copying a full-sized radiograph onto a small-format film such as 35×35 mm, has long been an attractive option for the imaging department manager seeking to relieve pressure on valuable storage space. More recently, film digitization equipment has become available, allowing departments to digitize their film images and store this data on magnetic or optical disks. In this next section we shall examine these methods in more detail.

15.2.1 *Archiving options*

(1) Miniaturizing to film
    (a) 35×35 mm (sometimes called microfilm or microfiche);
    (b) 100×100 mm.
(2) Digitizing the image to magnetic or optical disk.

15.2.1.1 35×35 mm Miniaturization
The necessary equipment for miniaturization may be purchased by the imaging department and the task carried out on site. Alternatively, the contract for miniaturizing radiographs may be given to a commercial concern who will do the filming either on or off the premises.

Some of the professional 35 mm miniaturizing equipment available nowadays (Fig. 15.1) incorporates an electronic means of ensuring that none of the 'information' recorded on the original radiograph will be lost when transferred to the 35 mm film. Equipment manufacturers have their own names for this technology – Electronic Contrast Modulation (ECM) from Johnsons and LogEtronics (Log E) from MAB Film Services are but two examples.

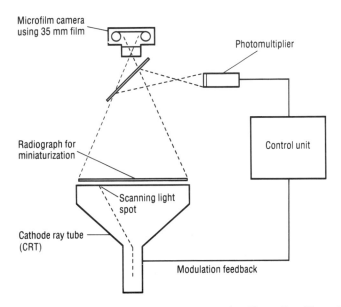

Fig. 15.1 The Johnson 'Scanatron' miniaturization system using 35 mm film. The radiograph for miniaturization is pre-scanned with the CRT light spot. The light passes through the film and is 'sampled' by the photomultiplier. Areas of high density on the radiograph result in a low-intensity light beam reaching the photomultiplier, which can then direct the control unit to modulate the initial light spot intensity so increasing its intensity. Areas of low radiographic density will result in the opposite effect with the CRT light spot intensity being decreased. In this way all of the radiographic densities can be modulated in order to fit the characteristic curve of 35 mm film.

The advantages of such systems may be understood by considering the difference between the sensitometric characteristics of a duplitized emulsion for use with intensifying screens, and those of a typical single emulsion 35 mm photographic film (Fig. 15.2).

Whilst the density range of the former can extend to 3.0 or more due to the combined effect of the two emulsions, the latter film can only produce a maximum density of around half of this. So how can it be possible to accommodate such a large range of densities on a miniature-type film with such a short density range?

The answer lies in the way in which these electronic systems examine each of the densities present in the original radiograph and then change or **modulate** them so that they will 'fit' the shorter straight-line portion of the 35 mm H and D curve. In this way, none of the information represented by the various density values in the original will be lost in the copying. The densities present on the original will all be represented on the 35 mm film.

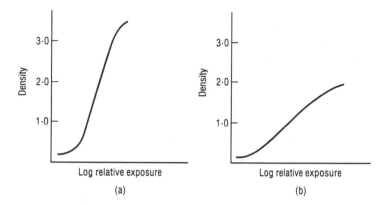

Fig. 15.2 Typical characteristic curves for (a) screen type duplitized film and (b) 35-mm single emulsion black and white film. Such a disparity makes it difficult to accommodate all of the densities of the original radiograph when making a copy on 35 mm film.

How is contrast modulation carried out?

The modulation of the different densities on the original is carried out by pre-scanning the original with a CRT light spot, the light which has passed through the film being 'sampled' by a photomultiplier tube.

Where the intensity of this light is great (corresponding to an area of low density on the radiograph), the scanning light spot intensity will be decreased during the copying cycle. Where the intensity of the transmitted light is small (corresponding to a dense region on the original), then the light spot intensity will be increased when making the copy.

Once the radiograph has been pre-scanned and beam modulations electronically assessed, the film is rescanned, this time with the 35 mm film being simultaneously exposed.

Thus, all the densities on the original will have been modulated in order to fit the characteristic curve of the miniature film.

The 35 mm film

A wide-latitude black and white film is used. The operator may opt for a negative-type film, so producing a 'black' bone image, or a reversal (slide)-type film, in which case the bones will appear 'white'.

Following processing, the film may be left as a roll, coded and filed or it may be cut into strips according to patient and mounted in clear plastic envelopes.

Microfiche/microfilm

The process of copying images onto 35 mm film is sometimes referred to as **microfilming**, with the 35 mm film described as **microfilm**.

A series of images relating to any one patient is commonly called a **microfiche**.

Film readers

Microfiches can be inserted into a special film reader, which will project onto a screen an image similar in size to the original radiograph.

If the 35 mm copies are kept on the roll, then a subsequent search for a particular patient's films will require that a projector with a reel-to-reel facility be made available. This is possibly a more time consuming exercise but experience has shown that requests by clinicians to see 'old' films, especially those over 3 years old, are rarely met with in practice.

NB It is possible to produce large copies (e.g. 35 × 43 cm) from the miniature films, if required, by using special film enlargers.

Storage of 35 × 35 mm miniature film
Storage cabinets are available which have a capacity for storing up to 35 000 microfiche.

15.2.1.2   100 × 100 mm Miniaturization

A copying/miniaturization system using 100 mm sheet film is available (Fig. 15.3). The equipment incorporates:

- Ultraviolet light source (situated inside the lid);
- A glass-copying surface to take the large films;'
- 100 mm film supply cassette;
- 100 mm take-up cassette;
- A 'reducing' lens system (see section 20.24).

The copy is made by placing the radiograph on the glass-copying surface and closing the lid. Lid closure initiates exposure, the duration of which can be pre-selected. The exposed film is then automatically transferred to the take-up cassette,

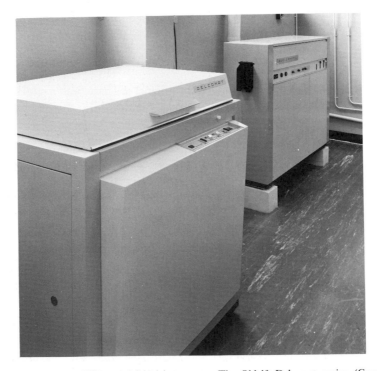

Fig. 15.3 A 100 mm × 100 mm miniaturizing system. The Oldelft Delcomat copier. (Courtesy of Oldelft England Ltd.)

whilst a fresh film is supplied automatically to the exposure area by the supply magazine.

The take-up cassette can hold up to 50 sheets of exposed film, and when full is withdrawn from the copying unit and attached to a dedicated processing unit. The processor automatically unloads the magazine, film by film. Thus, with this sort of equipment configuration, copying and processing can be carried out in the same room or area with no safelighting requirement.

100 × 100 mm film

The film used is of the reversal type thus producing a negative image just like the original, i.e. a 'white' bone image.

15.2.1.3   The advantages and disadvantages of miniaturization

Advantages

(1) Huge saving in valuable storage space.
(2) Versatility. Films are small enough to be filed in cabinets or with patient's notes.
(3) The original large films can be released for silver recovery purposes.
(4) No expensive large film bags are required if miniaturization is done immediately following reporting. The plastic storage envelopes used with miniature film are relatively cheap.
(5) Miniature-format film has a guaranteed archival permanence of 25 years.
(6) Films can be filed easily in an automatic film-retrieval system.

Disadvantages

(1) Large initial cost of providing miniaturizing equipment.
(2) Need to provide film readers, particularly for the 35 mm format, which is too small to view satisfactorily with the naked eye.
(3) Reluctance on the part of some clinicians to accept change.

15.2.1.4   Digital archiving

Film digitization is a process by which the analogue optical densities present in a radiographic image are converted into discrete picture elements (pixels), each of which will have a digital value whose magnitude depends on the original film density at the point sampled. The original hard copy image is consequently converted to a digital matrix, and the information stored on magnetic or optical disk. The film digitizer illustrated in Fig. 15.4 performs this function and in this instance is combined with a workstation, allowing the operator to view retrieved archived images on the monitor if required. Having the original radiograph in digital format thus enables the radiographer or radiologist to manipulate the image in just the same way as with a CT, MRI or other digital system image. The digitization of radiographs is an essential requirement in a filmless radiology department because of the need to digitize any films brought into the department from other hospitals. It also plays an important part in the preparation prior to a department converting to filmless operation, when a programme of selective digitization of some of the department's existing radiographs is being implemented (Strickland, 1994).

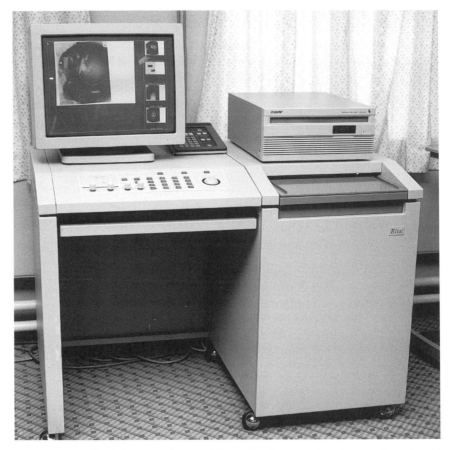

Fig. 15.4 Vision Ten VT4000 Rita! combined X-ray film digitizer and workstation. (Reproduced by courtesy of Laser Lines Ltd.)

The digitization process
NB *The reader is referred to section 22.4.2 for details of the principles of digitization.*

A schematic drawing of a film digitizer is shown in Fig. 15.5. The leading edge of the film is presented to the entry rollers which take over the automatic transport of the radiograph. Inside the digitizer, the film passes beneath a stabilized strip light source which creates a fine line of light on the film. This thin strip of light passes through the radiographic image to a **bending** or **folding mirror** whose function is to reflect the light beam in the direction of a focusing lens and thence to a linear **charge coupled device (CCD)**.

The CCD chip itself comprises 6000 elements, although only the central 3384 elements are used when scanning the film. On the chip, the varying light intensities within the beam will be converted into corresponding amounts of electrical charge which are assigned numerical values. The process is performed by an **analogue to digital converter (ADC)**. Each CCD element represents one pixel. For a 35 × 43 cm radiograph, the fine strip of light previously mentioned is responsible for producing a maximum of 3384 pixels across the width of the film for each line

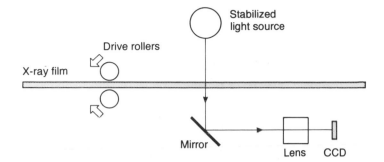

Fig. 15.5 A charge coupled device (CCD) film digitizer. (Courtesy of Laser Lines Ltd.)

scanned by the beam. During the film digitization process, a total of 4096 lines may be scanned along the length of the film. Depending on whether 8-bit or 12-bit sampling is used, 256 or 4096 grey scale levels can be stored by each pixel. Matrix size is also variable. For the highest possible resolution with pixel size at 105 μm, a 4k matrix, giving 3384 pixels per line and 4096 lines can be used. A 35 × 43 cm chest radiograph digitized at such a resolution and with an 8-bit system would require 13.5 megabytes (Mb) of memory. Using the same 8-bit technology, but a 1k matrix (846 pixels per line, 1024 lines), the chest radiograph would require about 1 Mb of memory.

Storage of digital images

The methods available for storing digital image data may be categorized into short-term (on-line) storage and long-term (off-line or archival) storage:

Short-term data storage Short-term (on-line) storage, for use as an **image buffer**, is provided by a **hard disk drive**. Large capacity storage can be achieved with a stack of rotating rigid disks sometimes known as **RAID** (redundant array of independent disks), six to eight in number, each carrying a ferromagnetic coating similar to that used on magnetic videotape (see section 23.1). As the disks spin, write heads, positioned a few micrometres from the surface of each disk, transfer or *write* the digital signals into their magnetic coating in the form of patterns of magnetisation. The data can be retrieved by using the same heads in their *read* mode. These actions correspond closely to the record and playback functions of a videotape recorder. The hard disk drive is totally enclosed in a sealed housing to exclude dust, and is located inside the casing of the computer. The read and write functions are extremely rapid, e.g. enabling a 35 × 43 cm chest radiograph on a 1k matrix (demanding 1 Mb of disk space) to be saved to disk in a few seconds, and retrieved from disk even more quickly. These times increase slightly if loss-less **data compression** techniques are used, but the images then require less than a third of the disk space. The hard disks used in digital imaging have capacities ranging from around 500 Mb to one or two gigabytes (1000–2000 Mb). Unfortunately, since the data stored on hard disks can be corrupted by the influence of external magnetic fields, hard disks are not a suitable medium for archival storage of data.

Long-term data storage The most common method of archival storage of digital data is the **optical disk**. This consists of a rigid glass disk, housed in a protective cartridge and coated on both sides with a thin film of metal alloy. Digital data are written onto the disk by means of a modulated laser beam which burns into the coating of the disk as it rotates, changing its reflecting properties. The data is read by scanning the rotating disk surface with a laser beam and monitoring the light reflected from its surface. Unlike magnetic disks, most optical disks can be written onto only once, although they can be read any number of times. This property gives rise to the term **WORM** disks (write once, read many) which is used to describe this technology. WORM disks are ideal for archival storage because the data they contain cannot be erased: they are non-corruptible.

Saving dating to, and retrieving data from WORM disks is a slower process than for hard disks. For example, the 35×43 cm chest image would take under a minute to save and less again to retrieve. The storage capacity of WORM disks depends partly on their size. The most popular size is $5\frac{1}{4}''$ diameter, having a capacity of 940 Mb to 1.3 Gb (equivalent to 1100–1500 1k matrix chest images). Less popular are $12''$ disks with 6–10 Gb capacity.

WORM disks may be stored in a 'Jukebox', an auto-loading disk system which can swap disks in 10–12 seconds and is capable of handling some 50 disks at a time.

Picture archiving and communication systems (PACS)

One of the most significant benefits of working with digitized images is the opportunity to transmit the images over short or long distances using **local area networks** *(LANs)* or telephone lines (**teleradiography**), so that they can be displayed on remote diagnostic workstations. Any electronic network set up to receive, archive and transmit digital images to another area is known as a picture archiving and communications system, or **PACS**. Systems can range from a single departmental configuration where digital image output from, say, CT, MR, DSI or CR (see Chapter 28) is fed to a central archive, stored and thereby made available for transmitting to viewing consoles in radiologists' offices or to a laser imager if a hard copy image is required. More sophisticated systems may involve linking other departments and other hospitals.

Benefits of PACS The principal gains to be achieved are in the improved patient management through more rapid access to information (e.g. patients' films and reports) throughout the department and hospital. Part of this stems from improved efficiency and clinical performance on the part of the clinician (Todd-Prokropek, 1994). The opportunity for radiologists to use high resolution computer screens to view and compare images from a range of different imaging modalities is one example. An additional advantage of a PACS environment is the reduction in the need for film filing areas and the consequent greater ease and efficiency in retrieving images.

Many of these advantages are only attainable if the PAC system in use allows speedy access to multimedia data stored in different medical information systems such as the Hospital (**HIS**), and Radiology (**RIS**) Information Systems. These systems therefore need to be fully integrated with PACS for maximum benefit.

So far we have studied the way in which film images are produced, presented and stored. In the next chapter we shall take a closer look at the technical aspects of the film image.

Chapter 16
The Radiographic Image

We have now completed our study of the methods used to produce, display and observe a radiograph. For a number of reasons the radiographic image is never a perfect reproduction of the anatomical structures that it aims to portray. It is the purpose of this chapter to examine critically the technical aspects of the image recorded on the radiograph, to describe its limitations and to attempt to identify their causes. Such an analytical approach is an essential skill, which we practise as radiographers whenever we check a radiograph.

It is beyond the scope of this book to consider the anatomical and pathological significance of the radiographic image, so we will limit our considerations to those features of the image which are associated with defects in the image-forming process. If we can identify the origin of such image defects, we can attempt to rectify them and so improve the standard of the images we produce.

We shall describe the image defects under seven main headings:

1 Unsharpness.
2 Over- or underpenetration.
3 Poor contrast.
4 Graininess.
5 Image artefacts.
6 Distortion.
7 Double images.

16.1 The unsharp image

For reasons we described in Chapters 3, 5 and 7, a radiographic image is never perfectly sharp. However, when we check the quality of a radiograph we assess whether there is any *noticeable* blurring, and if so, whether it reduces the diagnostic

223

value of the radiograph. Radiographic unsharpness is caused by geometric, photographic and movement factors.

16.1.1   *Geometric unsharpness*

This is due to the finite size of the X-ray source (Eastman Kodak, undated). There should be no appreciable geometric unsharpness in images of the extremities and other areas where the body part under investigation can be positioned very close to the film or film–screen system. Where this is not possible, modifications to radiographic technique can be made to minimize geometric unsharpness, e.g. increasing the focus–film distance or selecting a finer focal spot (see section 3.1.2.3).

Macroradiographs may exhibit geometric unsharpness due to the large object–film distance essential to this magnification technique (see Chapter 26). However, the magnification factor should be chosen to ensure that for the available focal spot, geometric unsharpness is not intrusive.

A radiograph of a thick body part may demonstrate some structures more sharply than others. For example, on a fronto-occipital projection of the skull, anterior structures may not be shown as clearly as posterior structures because they suffer greater geometric unsharpness. In some situations, this may improve the visualization of structures close to the film by selectively blurring out those over-lying structures whose superimposed outlines might confuse the image.

16.1.2   *Photographic (intrinsic) unsharpness*

This is due to limitations in the film–screen system. Blurring due to the cross–over effect and light scatter within the intensifying screens was discussed in section 7.2. Such effects tend to become more noticeable in situations where high-speed, low-dose techniques are required. Photographic unsharpness can be reduced if it is feasible to use a slower, high-resolution, single-screen or non-screen system.

Unsharpness due to the poor film–screen contact associated with badly designed or damaged cassettes should not be tolerated.

16.1.3   *Motional (kinetic) unsharpness*

This is due to relative movement during the exposure between the invisible X-ray image and the film or film–screen system.

The amount of motional unsharpness depends on the extent of relative move-ment occurring during the exposure. It therefore depends on:

(1) **Speed of movement** (fast movement produces the greatest blurring);
(2) **Direction of movement** (movement *across* the direction of the X-ray beam produces the greatest blurring);
(3) **Duration of exposure** (long exposure times produce the greatest blurring).

Relative motion may be caused by movement of the patient, the film or the X-ray tube, but in the majority of cases patient movement is the culprit.

Patient movement Patients often experience difficulty in keeping still during a radiographic exposure. This may be due to their age or physical and mental state, or because the position they have been asked to adopt is uncomfortable, painful or unstable. Reassuring the patient to reduce anxiety and tension and the use of positioning aids and immobilizing devices will usually ease the problem. The effect of involuntary motion of internal organs, such as the heart or abdominal viscera, is more difficult to control. In all cases, the extent of movement during the exposure, and therefore the amount of motional unsharpness, may be reduced by employing the shortest possible exposure time

Film movement This source of blurring is normally eliminated by ensuring that the film cassette is securely fixed in the bucky tray or cassette-holder. But it is possible for badly designed bucky trays to vibrate slightly when the moving grid mechanism is operating. Occasionally, the clamps which immobilize the cassette in its tray may work loose, allowing the cassette to move. Unsharpness due to such problems is rare. However, blurring may arise if the cassette is inadequately supported (e.g. during ward radiography) or is held by the patient when some degree of movement is to be expected if a stable position is not adopted.

X-ray tube movement Blurring due to this cause is suggestive of poor equipment design or failure to activate the tube suspension locks. In rare cases, the whole tube assembly may oscillate or drift during the exposure and possibly cause motional unsharpness.

16.1.4 Total image unsharpness

The total unsharpness (U_T) of an image is a combined effect due to geometric (U_G), photographic (U_P) and motional (U_M) factors, linked approximately by the relationship:

$$U_T = \sqrt{(U_G{}^2 + U_P{}^2 + U_M{}^2)} \quad \text{(Hay, 1982)}$$

It is unfortunately true that in attempting to reduce one source of unsharpness the radiographer may inadvertently increase another to a point where the overall effect is an image which is *less* sharp. For example, when selecting an ultrafast film–screen combination in order to shorten exposure time, the resulting improvement in motional unsharpness may be outweighed by an increase in photographic unsharpness associated with the high-speed screens. The result is then the opposite of what was intended. It is the task of the radiographer to balance the various factors causing unsharpness in order to arrive at an optimum overall result, i.e. minimum total unsharpness.

16.1.5 Identifying the sources of unsharpness

We have reviewed the main causes of unsharpness in the radiographic image. The experienced radiographer maintains control over these factors and produces radiographs which do not exhibit noticeable unsharpness. Nevertheless, there are times when difficulties arise during a radiographic examination and an unsharp radiograph is the result. How can the radiographer identify the cause of such unsharpness when the radiograph is examined?

Probably the easiest form of blurring to identify is that due to movement. Motional unsharpness tends to produce a characteristic linear streaking effect in the image due to the directional nature of the movement, e.g. the vertical blurring of the diaphragm on a chest radiograph due to failure to arrest respiratory activity.

Geometric and most forms of photographic unsharpness are difficult to differentiate with any certainty on a radiograph because they tend to pervade the whole area of the image. An exception is blurring due to poor film–screen contact (section 7.2), which exhibits a characteristic diffuse effect over a limited area of the image. However, careful consideration of the conditions under which a radiograph was produced often suggests to the radiographer the most likely reason for a blurred image.

16.2   The over- or underpenetrated radiograph

One of the most common reasons for having to repeat a radiograph is that the image is too dark or too light. There are a number of causes of over- or underpenetrated radiographs but they may be grouped into one of three broad categories: radiographer errors, equipment failure and processing errors.

Radiographer errors, such as:

(1) Poor choice of exposure factors due to misjudgement of the patient's tissue thickness or tissue type.
(2) Failure to match exposure factors to the film–screen system.
(3) Use of non-standard focus–film distance.
(4) Lack of familiarity with automatic exposure devices (selection of wrong measuring field, overenthusiastic collimation, etc.).
(5) Grid cut-off, e.g. due to angulation across the grid, off-centring of the beam, or using the wrong focus–film distance. **Grid cut-off** or **edge cut-off** produces a loss of image density which may be more noticeable near the edges of the film.

Equipment failure, such as:

(1) Reduced X-ray tube output, e.g. when the tube is near the end of its working life.
(2) Premature termination of exposure, e.g. due to a faulty exposure timing mechanism.
(3) Inadequate mains electrical supply, especially during ward radiography with a mains-dependent mobile unit.

Processing errors Over- or underdevelopment (leading to excessive or reduced density) due to causes such as abnormal developer temperatures or inappropriate developer replenishment rates.

16.2.1   *Identifying the causes of abnormal density*

Processing errors can often be identified as the cause of abnormal density because not only is the radiographic image of the wrong density, but so too is the identification panel on the film, produced by the actinic film marker. Additionally, processing faults tend to affect a whole series of films produced by different radiographers in different X-ray rooms.

Equipment failure may be diagnosed by monitoring the displays on the X-ray unit control console before and after each exposure; the mAs reading is particularly informative.

Radiographer errors may be diagnosed by the process of eliminating other factors. The reject analyses undertaken as part of quality assurance programmes generally show that radiographer error is the most likely cause of over- or underexposed films.

16.3   Poor contrast and fogging

Lack of contrast or, less commonly, excessive contrast reduces the information which can be gleaned from a radiographic image.

We saw in Chapter 3 that the **subject contrast** generated by differential attenuation as the X-ray beam passes through the patient is affected by factors such as the inherent differences in the patient's tissues, the presence of contrast agent, the X-ray tube kilovoltage and the X-ray beam filtration. Subject contrast is reduced by the presence of secondary radiation, particularly that due to scatter. In Chapters 5 and 7 we described the way in which subject contrast is amplified during the process of recording the image by the **film contrast** and **screen contrast** of X-ray films and intensifying screens. In Chapter 9 we noted the effects on film contrast of processing conditions. We described the way **fogging** of the image is produced by safelighting (Chapter 12) and film storage conditions (Chapter 6).

The combined effects of subject contrast, film and screen contrast and fogging determine the **radiographic contrast** in the final radiograph, i.e.:

Radiographic contrast = Subject contrast + Screen contrast − Fogging

Thus if radiographic contrast is too low (or too high) the radiographer can trace the cause to one or more of the individual contributory factors identified briefly above and discussed in more detail in the chapters indicated.

How is it possible to identify which of the many possible factors is the cause of poor contrast in a radiograph? Let us firstly consider the case of *low* radiographic contrast.

16.3.1   *Identifying the cause(s) of low contrast*

Low contrast may be a feature of the subject area under investigation, e.g. it is an inherent characteristic of conventional mammographic images because the tissue differences being imaged are minimal. In other words, low-contrast images must be expected when such areas are being examined.

Selection of an inappropriately high tube kilovoltage will result in a low–contrast radiograph. This must be placed high on the list of possible causes of low contrast. Consideration of the kVp employed, in relation to the subject of the radiograph, should enable the radiographer to determine whether the kVp chosen was appropriate.

X-ray beam filtration and kilovoltage waveform are fixed parameters in the case of most X-ray units and are therefore unlikely to be the cause of occasional loss of image contrast.

Similarly, the film emulsions used in radiography do not differ greatly and the film or intensifying screen characteristics cannot be responsible for the radiograph displaying unexpectedly low contrast.

However, film processing conditions may well suffer rapid changes, which could lead to a sudden deterioration in radiographic contrast. This would affect *all* radiographs fed through the ailing processor, enabling the cause of the problem to be confirmed.

Fogging is a common cause of loss of radiographic contrast and is one of the easiest to identify. Low contrast may be due to safelight fogging or X-radiation fogging. The effects of fogging are discussed below.

16.3.1.1 Fogging
Image fogging may be due to:

X-radiation, e.g. due to scatter generated when the radiograph was exposed, or to background radiation due to poor storage of the unexposed film. X-radiation fogging usually produces a general increase in image density. Radiation fogging which occurred before the film was loaded into its cassette affects the entire area of the radiograph, including the patient identification 'window'. Radiation fogging of the film through the back of its cassette may produce superimposed images of constructional features of the cassette, such as the clasps which hold it closed. Fogging due to scatter passing through the cassette front during exposure does not affect the patient identification area of the film, since the cassette is designed specifically to protect this part of the film from radiation passing through the cassette front. Such cases of fogging due to scatter are a consequence of inadequate beam collimation, failure to employ a grid or air gap, patient obesity or high kilovoltage techniques.

Safelighting The appearance of safelight fog is similar to that of X-radiation fog except that the patient identification area of the film is affected no less than the rest of the film. Occasionally, part of the film may have been protected from safelight fogging, e.g. by another film lying on top of it on the darkroom bench. Safelighting may be confirmed as the cause of low contrast by carrying out the simple test described in section 12.2.5.6.

White light Exposure of the film to white light, whether from daylight or artificial sources, in most cases produces total blackening of the affected area. Such an effect can scarcely be described as 'low contrast' since contrast is completely absent. Leakage of white light into a cassette, usually at its edge due to incomplete closure, produces a characteristic blacking of the film along the affected edge, and a larger patch of fog penetrating inwards towards the centre of the film (Fig. 16.1).

Fig. 16.1 White light fogging. In this case the light has leaked into the cassette along its bottom edge and produced a large patch of dense fog.

16.3.2 *Identifying the cause(s) of high contrast*

Excessive overall contrast on a radiograph may result in localized regions of the image suffering from an absence of contrast because they are black (or white). A radiograph of a barium-filled stomach illustrates this problem. In most cases the excessive radiographic contrast is generated by high inherent tissue contrast due to the gross differences in tissue thickness or tissue type which are characteristic of steep-range radiography. The use of high-kilovoltage techniques helps to nullify these effects by moderating subject contrast.

Raised contrast *could* be a consequence of the film–screen system being used. If so, it is indicative of the failure of the radiographer to select an exposure technique appropriate to the contrast characteristics of the system.

16.4 Graininess

An intrusive grainy appearance on a radiograph can be traced to a number of causes (Pizzutiello & Cullinan, 1993).

Structure mottle

As we saw in Chapter 4, the images on radiographs are formed from particles of metallic silver, but under normal viewing conditions the granular nature of the image is too fine to be visible. Under abnormal conditions, such as excessive processing temperatures, the silver grains may clump together to form particles which may be coarse enough to give the image a grainy appearance.

The phosphor grains in the fluorescent layer of an intensifying screen may also produce graininess, but in most cases this effect is suppressed by the inherent unsharpness of film–screen systems.

Quantum mottle

The use of a high-speed, rare-earth intensifying screen combined with low mAs exposure may result in the appearance of quantum mottle on the radiograph (section 7.11). The effect is enhanced if the film–screen system has high-contrast characteristics.

16.5 Image artefacts

A radiograph is sometimes marred by the presence of sundry marks or **artefacts** on its surface or superimposed on its image. We provide below details of some of the more common causes of image artefacts but readers should note that the list is by no means exhaustive.

16.5.1 *Screen marks*

Any deposit on the surface of an intensifying screen in a cassette is likely to interrupt light in its passage from the screen phosphor to the film emulsion, resulting in a sharply defined image artefact which appears white on the radiograph. Screen marks may be caused by dust particles, fluff, hair or other foreign matter inside the cassette, or by surface scratches or other damage to the intensifying screen supercoat. The identity of the offending cassette should be noted so that its condition can be checked.

16.5.2   *Pressure marks*

The application of undue pressure or stress to film emulsion before or during development may result in pressure marks appearing on the radiographic image.

Careless handling of film in the darkroom is a major cause of pressure marks, the most common example being the small, crescent-shaped **crimp mark** which may appear either dark (on a light background) or light (on a dark background); see Fig. 16.2. It is widely believed amongst radiographers that crimp marks are caused by fingernail pressure but this is rarely the case. Crimp marks occur during handling if a film becomes kinked or creased when it droops under its own weight if supported only near its edge (Fig. 16.3).

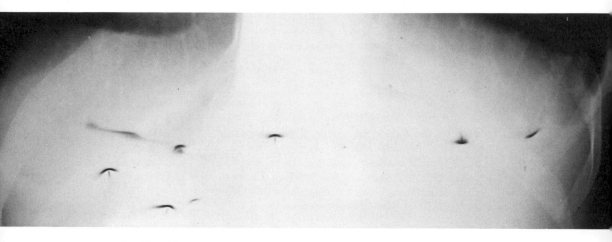

Fig. 16.2 Crimp marks. This section of a P-A chest radiograph shows several dark crescent shaped pressure marks caused by poor darkroom handling technique.

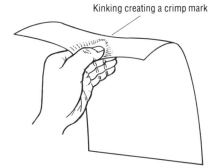

Kinking creating a crimp mark

Fig. 16.3 Creation of a crimp mark due to faulty film handling.

Automatic 'daylight' film-handling systems eliminate those image faults which are associated with the handling of film by the human operator. However, they have been replaced by a small number of different artefacts which occur during the mechanized handling of film (see *Static marks* below).

Storage. Larger, usually white pressure marks may be produced by poor film-storage conditions; e.g. by stacking boxes of film horizontally on top of one another rather than on edge.

Manufacture. Rarely, pressure marks occur due to stresses suffered by the emulsion during the film manufacturing process. Such marks are unpredictable in appearance and are likely to affect a number of films from the same batch. It is thus the repeated incidence of pressure marks of similar appearance on films from the same box which characterizes this form of artefact.

It is often claimed that if pressure damage to film emulsion (especially crimping) occurs *before* the film is radiographically exposed, the pressure mark produced is white, while if the damage occurs *after* exposure the mark is black (e.g. Fuji, 1983). If true, this simple rule would be helpful in tracing the origin of a particular pressure artefact. However, it is doubtful whether the statement is universally valid. Experiment shows that the *magnitude* of pressure is just as likely to determine the appearance of the pressure mark as the time it occurred in relation to exposure. The reader may wish to carry out tests to investigate this problem further.

16.5.3 Static marks

In the dry atmosphere of hospitals, it is common for static electrical charges to accumulate as a result of friction. The handling of film, whether by machine or the human operator, may generate static which could discharge onto or from the film. Such electrical discharge triggers chemical changes in the emulsion which mimic exposure and result in characteristic black **static marks** on the radiographic image. Most static marks are easy to identify and can usually be traced to the film transport systems of rapid film changers, the feed mechanism of film processors, or cassette loading and unloading activities. Certain synthetic clothing materials, such as nylon, are notorious for generating static charges. If static marks are prevalent when cassettes are loaded and unloaded by a particular individual, clothing should be considered as a possible cause.

The most spectacular static marks, which pervade almost the entire area of the radiograph, are produced during film manufacture (Fig. 16.4).

Depending on their appearance, static marks may be described as:

- Tree static;
- Crown static;
- Pin static;
- Crow's feet.

16.5.4 Finger marks

Handling the surface of a film with the fingers before it has been processed may lead to the formation of artefacts. Moisture transferred to the film surface from the skin modifies the action of developer during processing and may produce finger-print marks on the radiograph. Hands previously contaminated by contact with chemicals or metals are more likely to cause such marking of the image. Films processed by hand are even more at risk if great care is not taken, because of the possibility of spotting or splashing the film surface with developer, fixer or even water. Automated film-handling eliminates these problems.

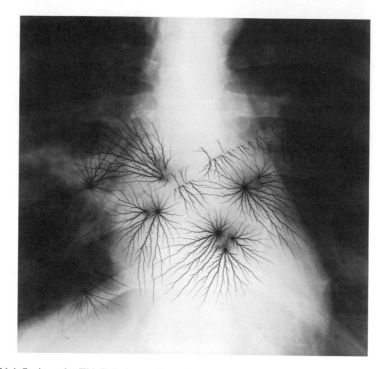

Fig. 16.4 Static marks. This P-A chest radiograph was ruined by the presence of multiple static marks caused by electrical discharge onto the film prior to processing.

16.5.5   *Chemical staining*

Inadequate fixing or washing during film processing leads to eventual yellow or brown staining of the image due to the presence in the emulsion of unstable sulphur compounds. These stains are not immediately apparent but form gradually over the weeks, months or even years of storage of the radiograph.

16.5.6   *Surface damage*

Film emulsion is particularly delicate and prone to damage during processing. A badly adjusted processor film transport system may cause abrasions to the emulsion surface, which remain as visible marks on the finished radiograph. For example, so-called **pi marks** spaced regularly across a film are suggestive of damage produced by one of the transport rollers in the film processor.

Surface damage is best detected by viewing the radiograph carefully under *reflected* light, as well as by transmitted light, and its surface should be examined gently with the fingertips to locate any roughness. Often the damage can then be seen to affect only one side of the radiograph.

Under adverse processing conditions the emulsion may partially detach from its base, causing **reticulation** or **frilling**. It may even detach completely, exposing the glossy surface of the base material.

16.5.7   *Radiopaque artefacts*

The presence of radiopaque artefacts in the path of the X-ray beam produces annoying image opacities which may obscure or confuse vital anatomical detail. Radiographs spoilt by the presence on the patient of items such as hairgrips, safety pins, hearing aids, dentures, wristwatches or jewellery are perhaps more common than one would wish. It is the presence of an unexpected artefact giving rise to an ambiguous appearance which probably has the most serious consequence. For example, a damaged secondary radiation grid may produce a linear marking which could be mistaken for a fracture line. A trace of barium sulphate contrast agent on a patient's gown could be identified mistakenly as a chest lesion.

The range of possible image artefacts is enormous and it is the radiographer's task, as far as possible, to prevent such artefacts from appearing on the radiograph. In spite of such efforts, artefacts may still occur and every radiograph must be checked with this in mind. The examination of a radiograph for image artefacts is a skill which requires practice to perfect. Having detected an artefact, it must be identified positively and the appropriate action taken. Careful study of the appearance of an image artefact and a knowledge of the exposure and processing conditions, together with the pool of experience available in the radiography department, should enable the origin of most artefacts to be identified successfully.

16.6   The distorted image

Distortion is present if the proportions of an image differ from those of the structure that it represents (Pizzutiello & Cullinan, 1993). A distorted image gives a misleading view of the object.

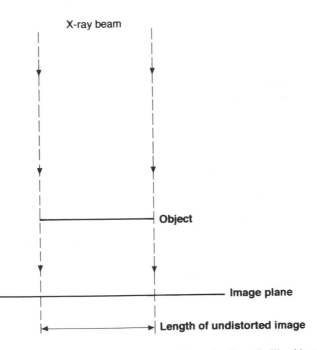

Fig. 16.5 The ideal conditions for the production of an undistorted radiograph. The object is parallel to the image plane, and both are perpendicular to the X-ray beam.

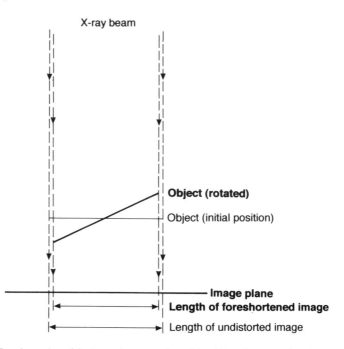

Fig. 16.6 Foreshortening of the image due to rotation of the object plane away from its initial position.

16.6.1   *Distortion due to the object plane–image plane relationship*

Distortion is due largely to the relationship between the directions of the object plane and the image plane. Distortion is not normally apparent as long as the object plane is parallel to the image plane, regardless of the X-ray beam direction. In practice however, the most common arrangement is for the beam to be directed at right angles to both the object and image planes (Fig. 16.5). We shall therefore adopt this as the initial condition for the purposes of the discussion which follows.

Radiographic image distortion appears either in the form of **foreshortening** or **elongation**.

16.6.1.1   **Foreshortening**
Assuming the image plane remains at right angles to the beam, any rotation of the object plane away from its initial position produces foreshortening along one axis of the image (see Fig. 16.6). For example, failure to position the feet in internal rotation causes foreshortening of the femoral necks on an antero-posterior projection of the pelvis. Internal rotation sets the neck of femur horizontally, i.e. parallel to the film (see Fig. 16.7).

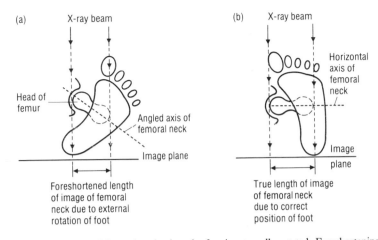

Fig. 16.7 (a) Orientation of femoral neck when the foot is externally rotated. Foreshortening occurs because axis of the femoral neck is not parallel to the image plane. (b) Femoral neck in the correct position due to slight *internal* rotation of the foot. The image of the femoral neck is therefore undistorted.

16.6.1.2 Elongation

Assuming the object plane remains at right angles to the beam, any rotation of the image plane away from its initial position produces elongation along one axis of the image (see Fig. 16.8). For example, the characteristic elongated egg-shaped appearance of the cranium on a 30° fronto-occipital (Townes or half-axial) projection

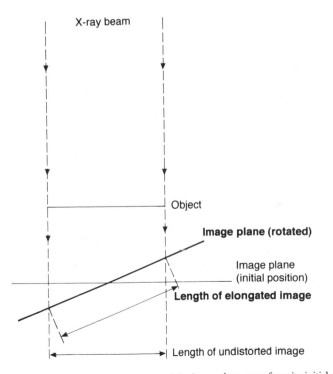

Fig. 16.8 Elongation of the image due to rotation of the image plane away from its initial position.

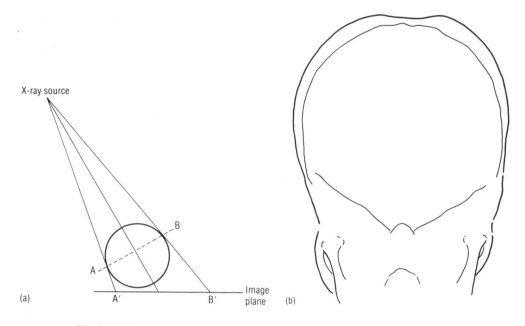

Fig. 16.9 (a) Elongated image A′ B′ of skull section AB due to the 30° angle between the object plane and the film at the image plane. This diagram reproduces the exposure conditions under which a Townes (half axial) projection is produced on a Lysholm type of skull unit. (b) A tracing of a radiograph showing the elongated cranial outline in the Townes projection produced under the conditions shown in (a).

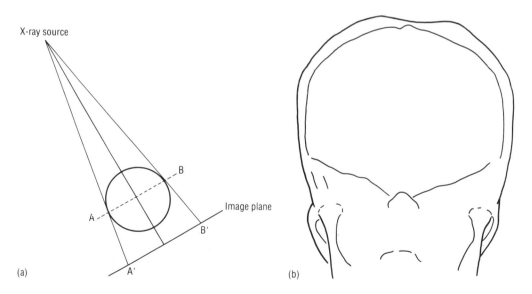

Fig. 16.10 (a) Image A′ B′ of skull section AB is undistorted because the image plane is parallel to the object plane. This reproduces the conditions under which a Townes projection is produced on an isocentric skull unit. (b) A tracing of a radiograph showing the relatively undistorted cranial outline in the Townes projection produced under the conditions shown in (a).

of the skull when taken on a Lysholm type of skull unit such as the Siemens CRT-4, is due to the 30° angle between the object plane and the film (Fig. 16.9). The equivalent projection produced on an isocentric skull unit gives a relatively undistorted image because the object plane and film are parallel (Fig. 16.10).

16.6.1.3   Avoidance of distortion

Rotation of both the object plane and image plane by the same angle and in the *same* direction, such that they remain mutually parallel, eliminates distortion of structures in the object plane (Fig. 16.11). But note that structures lying outside the object plane *are* subject to distortion.

Rotation of the object plane and image plane by the same angle in *opposite* directions also produces an undistorted image (see Fig. 16.12), because under these conditions, foreshortening created by the object plane rotation is exactly counterbalanced by elongation resulting from the image plane rotation. This is the origin of the strategy adopted to avoid image distortion during intra-oral radiography of the teeth (Fig. 16.13).

16.6.2   *Distortion due to X-ray beam divergence*

For the sake of simplicity, our discussion of image distortion has thus far ignored any effects caused by the divergent nature of the X-ray beam. Indeed, if the object plane and image plane are parallel to each other, beam divergence causes magni-

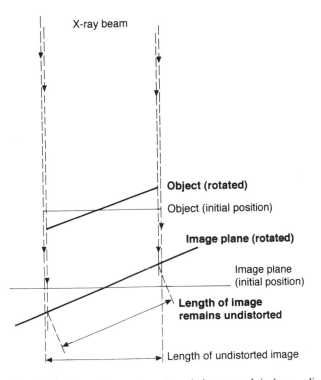

Fig. 16.11 Rotation of both object and image planes through the *same* angle in the *same* direction results in an undistorted image of structures within the object plane.

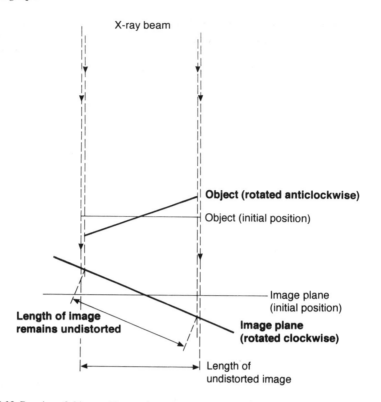

Fig. 16.12 Rotation of object and image planes through the *same* angle in *opposite* directions results in an undistorted image of structures within the object plane.

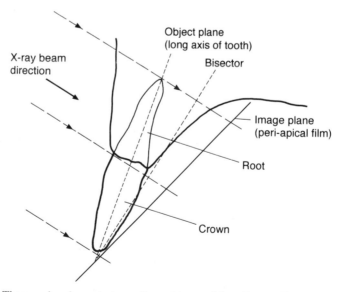

Fig. 16.13 The procedure for producing undistorted intra-oral dental images. The classical method is to direct the X-ray beam at right angles to the bisector of the angle between the planes of the tooth and the film. This ensures that the object and image planes are rotated by the same angle, but in opposite directions.

fication but not distortion. However, if these two planes are *not* parallel, beam divergence produces a third form of distortion in addition to foreshortening and elongation. **Differential magnification** occurs, where different parts of the object plane are recorded with different degrees of magnification (e.g. Fig. 16.14).

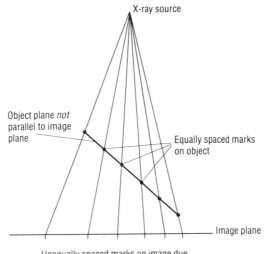

Fig. 16.14 Differential magnification. Different parts of the object are imaged with different degrees of magnification because the beam is divergent and the object plane is not parallel to the image plane.

As a general rule, radiographic positioning minimizes differential magnification by bringing the principal plane of the structure under examination parallel to the film. Additionally, if object–film distance is small relative to focus–film distance, image magnification is minimal and differential magnification is not significant.

We should remind ourselves that any attempt to represent a three-dimensional structure in a planar two-dimensional image is bound to result in some form of distortion. One advantage of defining standard, widely accepted radiographic projections is that the distortion present on such images is expected and understood. If we deviate from these standards, the projections that we produce may exhibit unfamiliar distortions, which the observer has difficulty in interpreting.

16.7 Double images

It is not unusual for a radiograph to be produced which carries two images superimposed on top of each other. This may occur, for example, if a previously exposed cassette is re-exposed before the original film has been removed for processing. The two images are generally quite distinct and it is easy to identify what has happened.

Another possibility is that the radiographer operating the X-ray unit exposure button inadvertently produced a double exposure. In this case, the two near-identical images are almost perfectly superimposed and very close inspection of

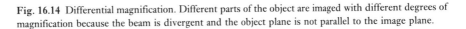

the radiograph may be required to confirm that a double exposure has occurred.

Duplitized X-ray film carries two identical images, one on each side of its base. In theory, careful examination should distinguish the existence of two images, especially if the radiograph is viewed obliquely. Although widely quoted (e.g. Kodak, 1982), this **parallax** effect is not detectable under normal viewing conditions.

The technical analysis and checking of radiographs is a wide-ranging and fascinating subject in which every radiographer must become proficient. In this chapter we have only been able to provide a limited treatment of what is essentially a practical skill. Illustrations in books are poor substitutes for actual radiographs. To complement this account, we therefore recommend that the reader devotes time to examining in detail and at leisure a random selection of rejected radiographs with the help of an experienced radiographer.

In the next chapter we direct our attention to the influence of exposure factors on the radiographic image, and the ways in which exposure factors may be manipulated to optimize image quality.

Chapter 17
The Influence of Exposure Factors

In this chapter we identify the controlling factors which affect the density and contrast of a radiographic image. We shall concern ourselves solely with those factors over which the radiographer has an important influence and we shall examine the ways in which such factors can be manipulated to suit the conditions ruling at the time the exposure is made.

Whether a radiographic image is produced by the action on film emulsion of X-rays directly or of fluorescent light from intensifying screens, the resulting change in optical density is a consequence of the absorption of energy by the emulsion. This absorption of energy is influenced by a number of variables which must be assessed by the radiographer in the selection of radiographic techniques. Two broad categories may be defined, into which these variables fall.

Exposure factors, i.e. those factors which affect the quantity and distribution of radiation energy to which the image receptor (film or film-screen system) is exposed.

Film–screen factors, i.e. those factors which affect the way in which the energy received by the image receptor is absorbed and translated into image density and contrast.

Note that the term **exposure factors** is often used as a blanket term, in which no discrimination is made between the two categories defined above. Thus, the film-

241

screen system may be included as one of the exposure factors. However, in this chapter we shall retain the distinction between exposure factors and film–screen factors.

17.1 Exposure factors

There are many factors which affect the quantity and distribution of radiation energy reaching the image receptor and over which the radiographer has some control. We shall describe these factors firstly by examining the generation of X-rays in the X-ray tube and then by following the path of the X-ray beam from the tube focus to the image receptor.

The radiographer controls the quantity and quality of X-rays generated, primarily by choice of the electrical factors supplied to the X-ray tube, i.e. tube kilovoltage and milliamperseconds.

17.1.1 Kilovoltage (kVp)

Altering tube kilovoltage affects two characteristics of the X-ray beam emitted from the tube target: its quality and its intensity (Ball & Moore, 1986).

17.1.1.1 Quality

The quality of a beam is an expression of the effective photon energy of the beam. Its significance in radiographic imaging is threefold:

(1) It influences the ability of the X-ray beam to penetrate matter: an increase in tube kVp produces an increase in penetrating power. Thus, in general, a higher tube kVp is required for thick or dense patient tissues.
(2) It influences radiographic contrast. As we saw in Chapter 3, tube kVp has an important effect on differential attenuation of the beam and therefore on subject contrast. Reduction of kVp leads to an increase in radiographic contrast.
(3) It influences radiation dose to the patient. There is no simple rule to follow here but it is generally true to say that the radiation dose to structures within the limits of the primary beam can be reduced if kVp is increased.

Note that the kilovoltage waveform, whether pulsating, rippling, constant or decaying exponentially, also influences beam quality. Although waveform is not under the control of the radiographer at the time of the exposure, it may well be a factor taken into account when choosing an X-ray generator.

17.1.1.2 Intensity

The intensity of the beam emitted from the X-ray tube target is an expression of the rate of flow of radiation energy per unit area of cross-section of that beam. Raising the tube kilovoltage increases both the intensity of radiation emitted from the tube target and the intensity of radiation reaching the film, and thus leads to an increase in image density.

We learn from physics (Wilks, 1987) that the intensity (I) of an X-ray beam increases approximately as the square of the peak tube kilovoltage:

$$I \propto (kVp)^2$$

However, since this relationship does not hold true for the intensity of the X-ray beam reaching the film cassette, it is of little practical value to the radiographer.

17.1.2   Milliampereseconds (mAs)

Altering the mAs affects the total X-ray beam energy produced by the X-ray tube during the exposure; it does not affect the quality of the beam (Ball & Moore, 1986). The X-ray output of the tube and the energy delivered to the image receptor during the exposure both vary directly with the mAs, e.g. if mAs is doubled then the film–screen system receives twice the energy. Thus, in the time-scale method of sensitometry described in section 4.5.4.1, we were justified in assuming that exposure to the film–screen system was directly proportional to mAs.

While it is common for radiographers to treat mAs as a single factor, it is the product of *two* quantities:

(1) The current (mA) flowing from the cathode to the anode of the X-ray tube during the exposure;
(2) The duration of the exposure in seconds.

Thus, whatever the individual values of mA and exposure time, if their product is constant, the energy incident upon the image receptor is the same, e.g.:

```
 20 mA for 1 s
 40 mA for 0.5 s
 80 mA for 0.25 s
200 mA for 0.1 s
500 mA for 0.04 s
```

All these combinations produce 20 mAs and all result in the same level of radiation energy reaching the film (assuming that no other factors have been altered). We shall see later, however, that the photographic effect of these exposures is not necessarily identical (section 17.2.2.3).

As a general rule, radiographers prefer to use an mA and exposure time combination in which time is as short as possible to minimize movement unsharpness. For a given selected mAs value, most modern X-ray control systems automatically provide maximum mA and minimum time combinations, unless the radiographer specifically requests otherwise. Automatic exposure devices (AEDs), such as the Siemens' Iontomat, also provide maximum mA and minimum time exposures (Carter, 1994).

Occasionally, the radiographer may wish to depart from a maximum mA and minimum time combination. The selection of an exposure time of several seconds is essential for the technique of autotomography, where selective blurring of some anatomical structures is deliberately encouraged, e.g. in the 'moving jaw' technique for the antero-posterior projection of the cervical spine.

17.1.3   Focal spot

Closely allied to the selection of mAs is the choice of size of the tube focus. Most X-ray tubes offer two possible effective focal spot sizes, known as fine and broad focus. The size combinations differ in different X-ray tubes, but common focal spot pairings available are: 0.6 and 1.2 mm, 0.3 and 1.2 mm, and 0.4 and 0.8 mm.

Fine focus should be selected when geometric factors are likely to limit image quality, e.g. when object–film distance is large. An ultrafine focus (0.3 mm or less) is needed for macroradiography (see section 26.2.1).

Broad focus should be chosen when geometric factors are more favourable and when no visible advantage would be gained by using the fine focus. Broad focus permits higher tube loading and enables maximum mA to be used; thus, broad focus is necessary when a high mAs and minimum exposure time are required.

It is an unfortunate feature of the control systems used on many modern X-ray units that the radiographer does not have to make a conscious selection of focal spot size and may therefore be unaware of which focus is in use.

17.1.4   Filtration

As the X-ray beam emerges from the tube, it is modified by the effects of inherent and added filtration. However, only in a few special cases, such as mammography, is filtration adjustable and directly under the radiographer's control. In these instances, increasing beam filtration produces both an increase in the quality and a reduction in the intensity of the beam leaving the X-ray tube. Only the *intensity* of the beam reaching the image receptor is significantly affected by a change in filtration unless other factors, such as kVp, having a more direct effect on transmitted beam quality, are altered.

17.1.5   Focus–film distance

The natural divergence of the primary X-ray beam causes its intensity to reduce with increasing distance. Its energy is spread over an increasing area as distance from the source increases. Under specified conditions, an inverse square relationship may exist between beam intensity (I) and distance (d) from the X-ray source:

$$I \; \alpha \; \frac{1}{d^2}$$

The qualifying conditions are that the X-ray source is infinitely small (a point source) and that there is no attenuating medium in the path of the beam. These theoretical conditions are very different from those experienced by an X-ray beam which exposes a radiograph, and one would not expect the inverse square law to be of any practical value. Surprisingly, in spite of this, the inverse square law seems to work reasonably well in practice and can be applied with some confidence to exposure manipulations involving changes of focus–film distance (FFD). Thus, if FFD is doubled, say from 90 to 180 cm, the energy received by the image receptor is reduced to approximately one-quarter (see section 17.3.2).

Changing the FFD is usually accomplished by moving the X-ray tube nearer to or further from the patient. In such cases only the *intensity* of the beam reaching the film is affected. But if, exceptionally, the FFD is altered by changing the patient–film distance, beam *quality* is also affected due to modification of the air-gap between patient and film (see section 3.1.1.2).

17.1.6   Collimation

The radiation energy received by the image receptor during an exposure is from two sources: primary and scattered radiation. Tighter collimation of the beam has the effect of reducing the area covered by the primary beam and therefore the volume of patient tissue irradiated. This in turn reduces the amount of scattered radiation reaching the film and thus the total energy it receives. Consequently, as the X-ray field size is reduced by collimation, not only is subject contrast improved, but also the intensity of the beam reaching the film is reduced and a compensatory increase in the kVp or mAs may be necessary. Unfortunately, when producing a localized projection of (say) a single vertebra, there is no simple relationship between the reduction in field size from the scout view and the exposure adjustment needed to maintain image density: the radiographer must judge on past experience what modification is required.

17.1.7 *Table-top attenuation*

Various materials and thicknesses are used in the construction of the radiolucent top of the X-ray couch that supports the weight of the patient. Since different designs vary in the amount of attenuation they impose on the X-ray beam, radiographing a patient through different couch tops introduces an additional exposure variable which the radiographer may wish to consider. Current thinking favours the use of carbon-fibre technology, which reduces beam attenuation and helps to minimize the radiation dose to the patient (Hufton & Russell, 1986).

17.1.8 *Grid*

Secondary-radiation grids modify the amount of radiation energy reaching the image receptor. The reader is referred to Carter (1994) for details of the construction and mode of operation of secondary-radiation grids and to Aichinger *et al.* (1992) for an assessment of their performance. By design, the radiopaque slats of the grids attenuate scattered radiation and therefore reduce the total energy received by the film. But **primary** radiation is also attenuated, as it penetrates through the protective grid cover and either the relatively radiolucent interspaces or as it strikes a radiopaque slat (Fig. 17.1). The effect of a grid in reducing the intensity of radiation reaching the film is expressed as a **grid factor**. The grid factor depends on the quality of radiation concerned (and therefore on tube kilo-

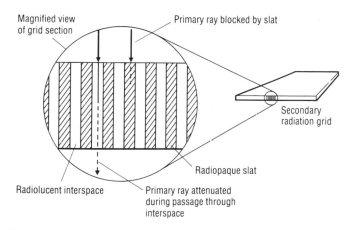

Fig. 17.1 Attenuation of primary radiation by a secondary radiation grid. Some rays are attenuated as they pass through the relatively radiolucent interspaces. Others are totally blocked by the radiopaque slats. Note that the grid illustrated is unfocused (parallel) and has a grid ratio of 8:1. Note also that the 'rays' referred to represent *streams* of X-ray photons rather than single, individual photons.

voltage), as well as on the design characteristics of the grid. In general, high-ratio grids attenuate the X-ray beam more than those of medium ratio, while fine-line grids may attenuate more than coarse grids. In recent years, the use of carbon fibre as a grid cover material has improved the transmission properties of grids.

The one critical factor that we have not included here is the patient. As we described in section 3.1.1.1, the attenuating properties of the body part being imaged have a major influence on the X-ray beam before it reaches the image receptor. The patient is not generally thought of as being one of the exposure factors, but the radiographer's assessment of tissue type and tissue thickness is clearly crucial in determining what exposure factors should be selected.

It should be emphasized that of the eight factors affecting exposure described above, only the first two (kVp and mAs) are used by the radiographer to control directly the density of the radiographic image, and only kVp, collimation and grids are used to control its contrast. The remaining factors are varied for other reasons and their effects on density and contrast, though important, are incidental.

17.2　Film–screen factors

We have previously defined film–screen factors as being those factors which affect the way that the energy received by an image receptor (direct-exposure X-ray film or film–screen system) is absorbed and transformed into image density and contrast. There are fundamental differences between the conditions of exposure for direct-exposure film and film–screen systems, so we will describe the relevant factors separately.

17.2.1　*Direct-exposure film*

We explained in section 4.4 that the photographic effect which takes place in direct-exposure film (non-screen film) is produced solely by the direct action of X-radiation on the film emulsion.

Direct-exposure film is individually packed ('double-wrapped') in strong, light-proof, paper envelopes which are almost perfectly radiolucent. Thus, there is no significant attenuation of the X-ray beam as it penetrates through the envelope. The major criterion to be considered for exposure selection is the speed of the film.

17.2.1.1　Relative film speed

It is essential that as high a proportion as possible of the X-ray energy incident on the film is absorbed within the emulsion layers of the film. This characteristic is sometimes known as the quantum detection efficiency or absorption efficiency of the film.

Having absorbed X-ray energy, the photographic effect, together with chemical development, must convert this energy into adequate image density. Conversion efficiency is a term applied to this characteristic of the film.

The effects of quantum detection efficiency and conversion efficiency are combined in the expression of the **speed** of the film. The speed of *photographic* film is commonly quoted as an **ISO number** (e.g. ISO 200/24°, ISO 400/27°, etc.), a system which has largely replaced the older ASA (American Standards Association) and DIN (Deutsche Industrie-Norm) systems. The ISO (International Standards Organisation) number indicates the response of a film to exposure to light under precisely controlled conditions but unfortunately, the ISO system is not a suitable method for expressing the response of a film to *X-ray* exposure. In fact, there is no widely accepted method for expressing X-ray film speed in absolute terms but we noted in Chapter 4 that *relative* speed can be useful when considering radiographic exposure requirements, e.g. if film A is twice the speed of film B it requires only half the exposure to give an image of the same average density. Relative speed tends to vary in value at different tube kilovoltages, but even so it is a factor which can be employed successfully in exposure calculations.

17.2.1.2   Reciprocity

The photographic response to X-rays of direct-exposure film depends on the total energy received during the exposure. It depends directly on the selected mAs. The response is the same whether the energy arrives at low intensity over a long period, or at high intensity over a very short period. Thus, as long as all other exposure factors remain constant, any combination of mA and exposure time that gives the same mAs value produces the same image density: 25 mA for 3 s (75 mAs), 75 mA for 1 s (75 mAs) and 750 mA for 0.1 s (75 mAs) produce exactly the same image density. The response is said to obey the **reciprocity law** (Pizzutiello & Cullinan, 1993).

17.2.2   Film–screen systems

The film–screen system consists of a screen-type X-ray film used in conjunction with single or twin intensifying screens. The photographic effect on film emulsion is produced almost wholly by exposure to light from the screen(s) rather than to X-radiation (see section 4.4.1.4). The film–screen combination is always contained within a cassette specially designed to maintain intimate contact between the film and intensifying screen, and to exclude light. The cassette forms such an integral part of the image receptor that we will include it in our considerations.

17.2.2.1   Cassette attenuation

The incident X-ray beam must penetrate through the cassette front in order to reach and activate the intensifying screens inside. We saw in section 8.1.4 that a range of materials having differing attenuating properties may be used in the construction of the front of a cassette. Thus, a radiographer using a cassette with an aluminium alloy front may need to give a greater exposure than would be necessary with a carbon-fibre cassette, even though the two cassettes contain identical film–screen combinations. A convenient way of comparing the attenuating properties of cassettes is to quote their **aluminium equivalents** at a specified tube kilovoltage, e.g. 1 mm Al at 60 kVp.

The exposure adjustments required to compensate for different cassette designs are generally determined empirically, so it is undesirable for there to be too many different cassette designs in use in a single X-ray department.

17.2.2.2   Screen speed

The speed of an intensifying screen is a measure of the luminance that results from a specified exposure to X-rays. It depends on the screen's absorption efficiency for X-rays photons (quantum detection efficiency) and on its conversion efficiency. An indication of the speeds of different screens is provided by the quantity known as the **intensification factor**.

Intensification factor (see section 7.10)
This is defined as the ratio of the X-ray exposure required to produce a given density on screen-type film alone to that required to produce the same density on the same type of film when used with intensifying screens. Since screen-type films should not be used without intensifying screens, the basis on which the intensification factor is defined is rather academic. However, it can be of value in comparing the speeds of different screens. For example, if screen A has twice the intensification factor of screen B, it is twice as fast and requires only half the exposure to produce the same density when used with the same type of film. If the two screens are used with *different* films, comparisons between their intensification factors are no longer valid.

17.2.2.3 Film speed

The speed of a screen-type film is a measure of the visible light exposure required to produce a specified image density. It depends on the emulsion's ability to absorb light and on the efficiency with which image density is produced by the photographic process.

Reciprocity failure
The response of a film to exposure to visible light does not always adhere to the reciprocity law. Thus, an exposure of 25 mA for 3 s may not produce the same image density as 750 mA for 0.1 s, even though they both equate to the same mAs. At both the upper and lower extremes of exposure time, the photographic response is less than that for intermediate values, i.e. film speed varies over a range of exposure times, being at its maximum for mid-range values. In practice it is rare for reciprocity failure to be the cause of a wrongly exposed radiograph, because exposure manipulations do not normally range over such extremes of exposure time and the effects of reciprocity failure can thus be ignored.

17.2.2.4 System speed

The concept of relative *film* speed is of doubtful value in comparing the speeds of screen-type films because it fails to take into account the possible differences in matching between the films and their intensifying screens.

In practice, screens and films are used *together* rather than in isolation from one another, and it is the speed of the combined film–screen system that should be considered. In this context, the matching of screen and film characteristics has a vital influence on system speed (section 7.5). The most satisfactory and useful method of expressing the speed of film–screen combinations is to compare the relative speeds of the systems *as a whole*, including the effect of cassette attenuation. The relative speed of system A to system B is then defined as the reciprocal of the ratio of the respective X-ray exposures required to produce the same density under the same exposure conditions:

$$\text{Speed of A relative to B} = \frac{\text{Exposure (mAs) to B}}{\text{Exposure (mAs) to A}}$$

to give the same density at the same kVp.

Note that the value of relative speed is likely to vary with changing tube kilovoltage.

Speed class

In recent years, it has become common to express the relative speeds of different film–screen combinations in terms of a **speed class**. The system is based on assigning the value 100 to the speed class of a traditional 'regular' or 'par speed' system (calcium tungstate screens with monochromatic film). The speeds of other film–screen systems are then expressed by comparison with this reference value. For example, an ultra-fast rare-earth system might be described as of speed class 800, indicating that it requires only one eighth of the exposure of the reference system to produce the same density. The radiographer should treat such claims with caution, especially when using speed class to draw comparisons between the products of different manufacturers.

17.2.2.5 Contrast

Film–screen systems exhibit a markedly higher contrast response than direct-exposure film. Manufacturers market a wide choice of film–screen combinations from which the radiology manager or superintendent radiographer can select a system with contrast and latitude appropriate to the department's needs, but for the radiographer working within the department the choice is more limited. There may be only two systems from which to choose for general radiography, e.g. a 'fast' system and a slower 'high-resolution' system. Speed and resolution rather than contrast are likely to be the criteria on which the individual radiographer makes a decision. Radiographic contrast then becomes a factor which can be influenced only through control of subject contrast. In special cases, such as mammography, the contrast characteristics of the film or film–screen system may be given higher priority.

We have examined the various factors which influence the density and contrast of the radiographic image. We shall next investigate how the factors under the radiographer's control can be manipulated in order to ensure a satisfactory result.

17.3 Manipulation of exposure factors

Consideration of the infinite variety of shapes, sizes and types of patient who present themselves for X-ray makes it inconceivable that a radiographer could remember all the possible combinations of exposure factors required to produce correctly exposed radiographs. In practice, the task is made easier by limiting the choices available, e.g. only two or three film–screen systems may be available, the FFD is standardized at 90 or 180 cm, only one type of grid may be in use, etc. The radiographer can thus remember representative exposure factor combinations for a limited range of techniques, applicable to an 'average patient'. Some departments provide charts, in each X-ray room, giving suggested exposure factors for a range of examinations and projections. Alternatively, the exposure factors may have been previously keyed into the memory of the X-ray unit, ready to be recalled at the touch of a button on the control panel. In either case, each new patient is assessed by reference to the average, so that adjustments to exposure can be estimated. The skill required to assess the patient develops with experience, although some radiographers seem to be endowed with more natural ability than others in this respect.

The need to manipulate exposure factors arises when conditions vary from the typical, e.g.:

(1) The patient may be unable to keep still during the exposure: the radiographer must then modify the factors to minimize exposure time.
(2) The patient may be badly injured: thus, a gridded cassette may have to be used instead of a Potter–Bucky.
(3) A supine antero–posterior chest radiograph may have to be produced at an FFD rather less than the standard 180 cm.

In each of these cases, the radiographer has two options:

Either (1) try to memorize a different set of exposure factors for each new set of circumstances;
Or   (2) learn how to adapt familiar exposure techniques by altering them to suit the new circumstances.

In most cases, modifications are made to the selected mAs and/or kVp to ensure that the correct radiation dose is received by the image receptor. We shall now work through some examples of this type.

17.3.1 *Modifying exposure time*

There are two possibilities. The radiographer wishes to:

(1) *Reduce* exposure time from the 'standard' exposure in order to eliminate movement unsharpness;
(2) *Increase* exposure time in order to use autotomographic techniques.

Example 1 Suppose that the standard exposure required for an anteroposterior radiograph of the pelvis on a male patient of average build is 65 kVp, 200 mA, 0.2 s at 90 cm FFD. However, the patient to be examined is restless and cannot be immobilized properly. How can the exposure factors be modified to allow the radiographer to reduce the exposure time to 0.05 s in order to minimize the possibility of the radiograph suffering from movement unsharpness?

17.3.1.1 mA correction

The simplest solution is to increase tube current (mA) while maintaining the same mAs and kVp, since this will result in an image of the same density and contrast as would have been produced by the standard exposure.

$$mAs = mA \times time$$

$$Standard\ mAs = 200\ mA \times 0.2\ s$$

$$= 40\ mAs$$

The new mA setting required is then given by:

$$New\ mA = \frac{mAs}{New\ time}$$

$$= \frac{40}{0.05}$$

$$= 800\ mA$$

Probably a more sensible method would be to realize that the required time (0.05 s) is one-fourth of the original time (0.2 s), thus the mA must be increased four times (i.e. from 200 to 800 mA) in order to maintain the same mAs.

17.3.1.2   kVp correction

A solution requiring more thought would be to increase the tube kilovoltage (kVp) rather than the mA. This method, if applied correctly, can still result in an image of the same average density, although radiographic contrast would be reduced.

10 kV rule

The relationship between kVp and mAs is complex. Many radiographers use a simple rule-of-thumb known as the '10 kV rule', which works surprisingly well in practice. The rule states that increasing (or decreasing) the tube kilovoltage by 10 kV has approximately the same effect on image density as doubling (or halving) the mAs. Thus, if mAs is cut by half, raising the tube kilovoltage by ten restores the image to its original density.

It is important to realize that the 10 kV relationship *is* only an approximation to the truth and is most accurate in the midrange of diagnostic kilovoltages, say between 50 and 75 kV. Let us try applying the 10 kV rule to our current problem.

We wish to reduce the exposure time by a factor of four, i.e. we wish to halve it, and halve it again. The effect on image density of halving the exposure time (and therefore halving the mAs) can be corrected by increasing the kVp by ten. Thus, 65 kVp, 200 mA and 0.2 s can be modified to 75 kVp, 200 mA and 0.1 s while image density remains the same.

Let us halve the time and add 10 kV again: 75 kVp, 200 mA and 0.1 s then becomes 85 kVp, 200 mA, 0.05 s. This *could* give a satisfactory result but we may be expecting rather too much of the 10 kV rule if we apply it at 85 kVp. Image contrast is also likely to have deteriorated as a result of our increase of kilovoltage. Even so, the 10 kV rule remains a most useful weapon in the radiographer's armoury.

An alternative but rather less practical method of estimating the kilovoltage adjustment required to compensate for a given change in mAs is to use the relationship below:

$$\frac{(\text{New kVp})^4}{(\text{Old kVp})^4} = \frac{\text{Old mAs}}{\text{New mAs}} = \frac{\text{Old exposure time}}{\text{New exposure time}}$$

where the 'old' exposure factors refer to the original or standard factors.

NB *The above relationship applies only to film–screen systems. For direct exposure, non-screen techniques the $(kVp)^4$ factors are replaced by $(kVp)^2$.*

Applying the relationship to our current problem we recall that:

Old exposure time = 0.2 s	Old kVp = 65 kV
New exposure time = 0.05 s	New kVp = ?

Then

$$\frac{(\text{New kVp})^4}{(65)^4} = \frac{0.2}{0.05}$$

$$(\text{New kVp})^4 = \frac{0.2}{0.05} \times (65)^4$$

$$(\text{New kVp})^4 = 4 \times (65)^4$$

New kVp $\simeq 1.4 \times 65$

$\simeq 92$ kVp

Thus, an exposure of about 92 kVp, 200 mA, 0.05 s is required. Note that there is a discrepancy of 7 kVp between this result and the one produced by the 10 kV rule, indicating that at least one of the two results is in error. In fact *neither* result is correct because the relationship involving the fourth powers of kilovoltage is also an approximation. Radiographers should therefore not be deceived into believing that the results of their mathematical computations (e.g. the eight digit display on an electronic calculator) are accurate to several decimal places!

17.3.1.3   Combined mA and kVp correction

It is possible, and often advisable, to increase both mA *and* kVp if exposure time is to be greatly reduced. In our example, the reduction of time by a factor of four can be achieved by doubling the mA while also increasing kVp by ten, i.e. instead of 65 kVp, 200 mA, 0.2 s we could select 75 kVp, 400 mA, 0.05 s. By limiting the kilovoltage rise, we ensure minimal loss of contrast; by limiting the current, we avoid excessive wear on the tube filament.

We shall now apply the same principles to an example where the radiographer wishes to *increase* exposure time.

Example 2 Suppose the standard exposure for an antero-posterior projection of the cervical spine is 60 kVp, 100 mA, 0.2 s and the radiographer wishes to modify this to provide an exposure time of 3 s so that the moving jaw technique can be employed. What adjustments could be made to kVp and mA to maintain the correct image density?

The exposure time needs to be multiplied by a factor of 15 to increase it from 0.2 to 3.0 s. This *could* be achieved by merely reducing mA by the same factor, i.e. $100 \div 15 \simeq 7$ mA. The chosen factors are then 60 kVp, 7 mA and 3 s.

Alternatively, we could incorporate a reduction in kilovoltage as well as a drop in mA, e.g. reduce the kilovoltage from 60 to 50 kVp. The 10 kV rule predicts that this will have the same effect on image density as halving the mA, so the mA now only needs to be reduced by a factor of 7.5 instead of 15, i.e. $100 \div 7.5 \simeq 13$ mA. Thus, the chosen factors are now 50 kVp, 13 mA and 3 s.

17.3.2   *Modifying focus–film distance (FFD)*

Most radiography is carried out with the X-ray focus at a standard distance from the film, e.g. 180, 100 or 90 cm. Occasionally, the radiographer may have to produce a radiograph at a non-standard FFD. The exposure factors which are appropriate at the standard distance then need to be modified in order to produce an image of correct density.

Example 1 Using a mobile X-ray unit, a supine antero-posterior chest radiograph was produced of a bed-ridden patient on the orthopaedic ward. The factors used were 55 kVp and 4 mAs at 120 cm FFD. A follow-up chest radiograph was requested the next day, but because of traction bars attached to the bed the radiographer was forced to employ a shorter FFD of 100 cm. What modification to the mAs should the radiographer make to produce a radiograph of comparable density?

At the shorter distance, the X-ray beam reaching the film will be of increased intensity, and without modification to mAs the image density will be too great. Thus, the selected mAs must be reduced.

We can use the inverse square law to derive an approximate relationship between required mAs and FFD:

$$\frac{\text{New mAs}}{\text{Old mAs}} = \frac{(\text{New FFD})^2}{(\text{Old FFD})^2}$$

In our current example:

Old FFD = 120 cm	New FFD = 100 cm
Old mAs = 4 mAs	New mAs = ?

and

$$\frac{\text{New mAs}}{4} = \frac{100 \times 100}{120 \times 120}$$

$$\therefore \text{New mAs} = \frac{100}{144} \times 4$$

$$\simeq 3 \text{ mAs}$$

The radiographer must therefore select 55 kVp and 3 mAs at 100 cm FFD to give the required result.

Note that confusion can easily occur in applying this 'square law' relationship, and the radiographer should always check that the computed answer is sensible before making the X-ray exposure. A common error is to invert the ratio of FFDs. The calculated value for new mAs is then *greater* than the original value (it would be 5.76 mAs in the example above) while common sense tells us that a *reduction* of exposure is required.

Application of the FFD relationship can produce surprising results. It is not always appreciated, for example, that a 10% increase in FFD requires *more* than a 10% increase in mAs to maintain constant image density (in fact the mAs should be increased by > 20%). Radiographers often underestimate the effect on the image of FFD errors introduced through failure to adhere to a standard FFD.

17.3.3 Changing the film–screen system

Exposure factors appropriate to one film–screen combination can easily be converted to apply to another. Such a conversation may be necessary when a new film–screen system is introduced into a department. It is necessary to determine the relative speed of the two systems but once this has been done the exposure conversion is straightforward.

Example 1 A department changes over from a traditional fast tungstate screen – monochromatic film system to a rare-earth screen – orthochromatic film system. At 75 kVp, the new system is found to be 2.5 times faster than the old. The previous exposure factors used for the lateral projection of a typical lumbar spine were 75 kVp and 200 mAs at 90 cm FFD. How could these factors be modified to enable them to be used with the new film–screen system?

Since the new system is 2.5 times faster, it requires 2.5 times less exposure to produce the same image density. Thus, the new mAs is given by:

$$\frac{\text{New mAs}}{\text{Old mAs}} = \frac{1}{2.5}$$

In our example, Old mAs = 200 mAs, so:

$$\frac{\text{New mAs}}{200} = \frac{1}{2.5}$$

$$\therefore \text{New mAs} = \frac{1}{2.5} \times 200$$

$$= 80 \text{ mAs}$$

The exposure factors required are therefore 75 kVp and 80 mAs at 90 cm FFD. Note that if an exposure conversion is required at kilovoltages other than 75 kVp, the relative speed of the two systems should be reassessed. In practice, assessments done at (say) 15 kVp intervals over the diagnostic range should be sufficient to enable reasonable exposure conversions to be made.

Example 2 A department acquires some new high–resolution screens to complement the high–speed screens currently in use. The same film is to be used with both systems. The high–speed screens have an intensification factor (IF) of 90, while the high–resolution screens have an IF of 40. The IF values were assessed at 50 kVp using the same film.

Using the high–speed screens, a lateral projection of the facial bones requires 50 kVp and 20 mAs at 90 cm FFD. By what factor should the mAs be modified to render it suitable for use with the high–resolution screen system?

The relative speed of the two systems can be deduced from the values of the intensification factor provided, since the relative speed of new screens compared to old is given by:

$$\text{Relative speed} = \frac{\text{New IF}}{\text{Old IF}}$$

In our example, Old IF = 90 and New IF = 40, so:

$$\text{Relative speed} = \frac{40}{90}$$

$$\simeq 0.4$$

Thus, the high–resolution system is 0.4 times slower than the high–speed system and the New mAs that it requires is therefore greater than the Old mAs:

$$\frac{\text{New mAs}}{\text{Old mAs}} = \frac{1}{0.4}$$

$$\therefore \text{New mAs} = \frac{1}{0.4} \times 20$$

$$= 50 \text{ mAs}$$

The exposure required on the new screens is therefore 50 kVp, 50 mAs with an unchanged FFD. Since intensification factors may vary with tube kilovoltage, the exposure conversation factor calculated above may only be valid at the specified kVp.

Example 3 Because of industrial action, an X-ray department can no longer obtain supplies of its usual film and has to switch over to an alternative brand. At 65 kVp, the speed of the new brand is found to be 1.4 times greater than the original film when used with the same intensifying screens. If typical exposure factors for a lateral skull radiograph using the original film were 65 kVp and 60 mAs at 90 cm FFD, what exposure should be selected with the new film to give an image of similar density?

Since we know the relative speeds of the two films at the specified kVp, the problem is simple. The new film is 1.4 times faster, so the mAs required is 1.4 times less, i.e.:

$$\text{New mAs} = \frac{\text{Old mAs}}{1.4}$$

$$= \frac{60}{1.4}$$

$$\simeq 43 \text{ mAs}$$

The exposure should be corrected to 65 kVp, 43 mAs at the same FFD.

17.3.4   Changing the grid

Secondary-radiation grids have different beam transmission characteristics determined by the materials used in their construction and by the details of their design. Thus, a radiographer may need to modify exposure factors, e.g. when changing from a Potter-Bucky technique to one using a gridded cassette, or when switching from a grid to a no-grid technique.

17.3.4.1   Grid factor

In section 17.1.8 we stated that the grid factor expresses the amount by which radiation is attenuated as it passes through a secondary-radiation grid. The grid factor is defined (Carter, 1994) as the ratio of exposure (mAs) required to produce a given image density when using a grid to that required to produce the same density with the same film–screen system when no grid is used, i.e.:

$$\text{Grid factor} = \frac{\text{Exposure (mAs) with grid}}{\text{Exposure (mAs) without grid}}$$

All other factors, including kVp, must remain constant.

Example 1 A radiographer produces an antero-posterior radiograph of the shoulder using 55 kVp, 10 mAs at an FFD of 90 cm using a high-resolution film–screen system. The image is of the correct average density but the radiographer feels that the image contrast would be improved by the use of a grid. If the grid factor at 55 kVp is 3:1, what mAs should the radiographer employ?

By definition, a grid with a grid factor of 3:1 requires the mAs to be tripled to maintain the same image density. Thus, New mAs is given by:

$$\text{New mAs (with grid)} = \text{Old mAs (no grid)} \times \text{Grid factor}$$
$$= 10 \times 3$$
$$= 30 \text{ mAs}$$

So the required exposure is 55 kVp, 30 mAs with the other factors unchanged.

Example 2 The gridded cassettes in an X-ray department are to be replaced. The grid factor was 4:1 for the old grids at a tube voltage of 60 kVp while for the new grids it is 3:1. What modification to exposure will the radiographers need to make?

Grid factors can be used to compare the performance of different grids by using the relationship:

$$\frac{\text{mAs with new grid}}{\text{mAs with old grid}} = \frac{\text{New grid factor}}{\text{Old grid factor}}$$

$$\therefore \text{New mAs} = \frac{\text{New grid factor}}{\text{Old grid factor}} \times \text{Old mAs}$$

$$= \frac{3}{4} \times \text{Old mAs}$$

So the radiographers need give only three-quarters of the previous mAs. It is important always to double-check that the calculated answer is reasonable, remembering that the required mAs should increase as the grid factor increases. In this example, the grid factor was reduced, resulting (as expected) in a decrease in the required mAs.

17.3.4.2 Moving grids

It is often stated that a moving grid technique (as in a Potter-Bucky mechanism) requires a greater exposure than a stationary grid technique. This statement is misleading, since it implies that the motion of a grid *per se* increases the grid factor. This is *not* the case. However, a different exposure may well be required for a radiograph produced using a Potter-Bucky and one produced with a *separate* stationary grid, e.g. in a gridded cassette. The differences here may be due to:

(1) The different characteristics of grids used in Potter-Bucky tables compared with those used as stationary grids;
(2) Attenuation in the table-top which is present when a Potter-Bucky mechanism is employed;
(3) Grid cut-off (see section 16.2) caused by the lateral displacement of the grid as it oscillates in the Potter-Bucky. Aichinger *et al.* (1992) have shown that transmission of the primary beam may be reduced by up to 11% due to the off-centring associated with grid movement.

17.3.5 *Multiple exposure changes*

Occasionally, the radiographer may wish to modify *several* aspects of exposure rather than just a single factor. The combined effect of the changes can be calculated by working through the effect of each change separately, step by step, using the methods that we have described.

Example A chest radiograph is produced using 55 kVp, 6 mAs at 180 cm FFD with the cassette in a chest stand; no secondary radiation grid is used. What exposure should be selected if the same chest is radiographed using an upright bucky (grid factor 4:1) at an FFD of 100 cm?

Step 1
Consider the effect on exposure of using a bucky. A grid factor of 4:1 indicates that

the mAs must be increased by a factor of four to maintain the same image density, i.e. $4 \times 6 = 24$ mAs. Thus, if this was the only change, an exposure of 55 kVp, 24 mAs would be required.

Step 2
Consider now the effect of the change of FFD. We use the relationship:

$$\frac{\text{New mAs}}{\text{Old mAs}} = \frac{(\text{New FFD})^2}{(\text{Old FFD})^2}$$

We use the 24 mAs just obtained as the value of Old mAs in this part of the calculation. Thus:

$$\frac{\text{New mAs}}{24} = \frac{(100)^2}{(180)^2}$$

$$\text{New mAs} = \frac{100 \times 100}{180 \times 180} \times 24$$

$$\simeq 7 \text{ mAs}$$

The exposure factors required under the new conditions are therefore 55 kVp and 7 mAs at 100 cm FFD using the upright bucky.

When solving problems of this type, it is advisable to deal first with the simplest exposure manipulations and leave the most complicated part of the calculation (e.g. FFD or kVp changes) until the final step.

17.4   Programmed exposure factors

The accurate selection of exposure factors by the radiographer requires great skill and judgement. When errors are made, image quality suffers and repeat radiographs may be necessary, thus increasing the radiation dose received by the patient. In recent years, attempts have been made to eliminate exposure errors by programming into the memory of the X-ray unit various combinations of exposure factors appropriate to the different radiographic projections of a wide range of anatomical regions of the body. Anatomically programmed radiography (APR) systems largely remove the need for radiographers to memorize vast numbers of exposure factors. Moreover, even without APR, it is now less common for radiographers to select both X-ray tube mA and exposure time as separate entities. Instead, the radiographer selects mAs and kVp as part of a 'two-knob' control system. Such systems are tending to make some of the exposure calculations described in this chapter of academic rather than practical interest.

Automatic exposure devices (AEDs) such as the Siemens Iontomat, greatly simplify exposure selection, requiring only the kVp to be chosen ('one-knob' control). APR systems, used in conjunction with automatic exposure devices, simplify the selection of exposure factors even further and should lead to a reduced incidence of repeat radiographs. However, there is a risk that the undoubted benefits of programmed exposures and AEDs are achieved at the expense of a loss of flexibility in exposure selection.

In the next chapter we study how the quality of radiographic images can be maintained at an optimum standard by systematic testing of imaging materials and processes as part of an organized quality assurance programme.

Chapter 18
Image Quality Control

This chapter deals with some of the methods used by radiographers to ensure that radiographs of optimum quality are consistently being produced.

Because the medical imaging department is a very costly hospital department to run, any programme of monitoring which encompasses imaging as well as processing equipment is an invaluable aid to ensuring that top-quality images are being produced in the most cost-effective way. Such a monitoring programme is often referred to as a **quality assurance** or **quality control** programme.

The benefits of such close control are:

(1) A reduction in the number of 'repeat' radiographs.
(2) A reduction in the radiation dose to the public.
(3) Improvement in the rate of flow of patients through the department.
(4) Good quality radiographs, consistently produced.
(5) Standardization of radiographic results from one processor to the next.
(6) Automatic processor and imaging equipment reliability, with efficiency maintained.
(7) A more informed selection of future equipment can be made because of accurate knowledge of the reliability of existing apparatus.

18.1 Elements of imaging which need to be monitored

Any radiographic quality assurance programme that is intended to be comprehensive will need to monitor the following:

(1) Imaging equipment (X-ray tubes, generators, etc.).

259

(2) Recording system (cassettes, screens and films).
(3) Processing equipment (automatic processors; safelights, etc.).
(4) Reject radiographs.

An analysis of item (4) will often indicate problems with items (1), (2) and (3); we shall examine a reject film analysis programme, as it is called, later in this chapter.

A discussion on the monitoring of imaging equipment is, we believe, better understood when dealt with in the context of an equipment textbook and so we have intentionally omitted this element. We shall therefore start with the recording system.

18.2   Monitoring the recording system

Under this heading, the main tasks that a radiographer will need to carry out, besides the regular cleaning of screens and cassettes, include:

(1) Investigating suspected poor screen–film contact in an X-ray cassette;
(2) Checking a cassette for suspected light leakage;
(3) Comparing the relative speeds of two different film materials;
(4) Comparing the relative speeds of two different types of intensifying screen;
(5) Comparing the relative speeds of two different film–screen systems.

18.2.1   Checking a cassette for poor film–screen contact

The test is carried out by radiographing a specially made test object. This is a sheet of zinc or copper about 1 mm thick and continuously perforated with holes of 2.5 mm diameter about 4 mm apart. There should be about 3 or 4 holes per centimetre.

At the centre of the sheet is a 13 mm diameter hole, the purpose of which is to produce on the film an exposed area large enough for image density to be measured easily. The sheet should be large enough to cover completely the cassette to be tested. To carry out the test, the suspect cassette is loaded with film, placed on the X-ray table and the test sheet laid on top of the cassette.

The exposure is made at an FFD of 1.5 m using a focal spot of 1.0–1.5 mm. The tube should be centred to the middle of the sheet. The filtration of the X-ray beam should not be more than 2 mm Al equivalent. The exposure factors should be 40–50 kVp (to avoid penetrating the metal of the test sheet) and about 4–5 mAs. The combined exposure should be such as to produce a density of 2–3 (measured on the film at the central 13 mm 'hole').

The film should be viewed on a conventional viewing box at a minimum distance of 4 m. Where there is lack of contact in the cassette between the film and the intensifying screens, dark areas appear on the radiograph (Fig. 18.2). If film–screen contact is good, the test sheet image will be uniform in density (Fig. 18.1).

The dark patches in Fig. 18.2 result from the scattering of light from the screens over areas of the film which should not have been exposed, since they underlie the metal of the test object.

Poor film–screen contact usually arises as a result of damage to a cassette, the front or back surface being dented or distorted, for example. Such damage is usually irreparable and the cassette should be discarded.

It is a good idea to carry out the screen contact test on all new cassettes prior to their entering service and of course whenever a cassette is under suspicion.

Fig. 18.1 The test radiograph of a perforated metal sheet obtained from a cassette in which screen contact is good. The central cut-out area facilitates the measurement of density. (Courtesy of G.M. Ardran.)

18.2.2 *Testing a cassette for light leakage*

Broken fastenings or hinges, buckled corners or loose fronts are the usual causes of light leakage in an X-ray cassette. A test which involves exposing a loaded cassette to intense light is carried out in the following manner.

The cassette is loaded with film and closed. Each side and edge of the cassette is subjected in turn to light from a 100 W tungsten lamp for a period of 15 min at a distance of 1.22 m from the cassette (i.e. six 15 min periods).

The film is then processed and viewed. Any edge darkening of < 3.2 mm in width should be considered to be insignificant.

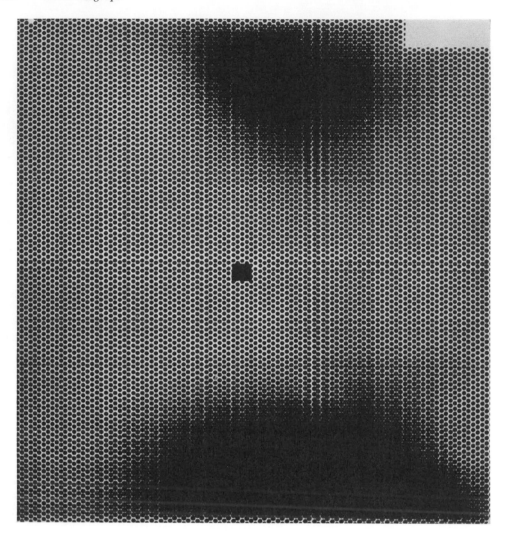

Fig. 18.2 The test radiograph obtained from a cassette in which screen contact is poor. (Courtesy of G.M. Ardran.)

18.3 Relative speed tests

Before any new film or intensifying screen can be assimilated properly into an imaging department, it will be necessary to know the speed of that material in comparison with the old one. Is it slower or faster? And by how much? The answers to these questions are important in order for old exposure factors to be modified.

Whilst film and screen manufacturers will endeavour to supply the answers, the most reliable and accurate method of obtaining this information is to carry out your own relative speed tests.

The three relative speed tests that we shall consider will be on the following subjects:

(1) Film.
(2) Screens.
(3) Film–screen combinations.

18.3.1 *Comparing the relative speed of two films*

Before introducing new film material into a department it is necessary to ascertain the relative speed of the new film in relation to the old one. Is it faster? How much faster? The radiographer could use time-scale sensitometry (section 4.5.4.1) and construct characteristic curves for both old and new material and then compare them in the manner described in Chapter 4.

The method that we describe below is also based on time-scale sensitometry, but avoids the need to draw characteristic curves.

(1) Select two 24 × 30 cm cassettes identical in design and containing identical intensifying screens.
(2) Load one cassette with the old film material (A), and the other with the new film material (B). Take the cassettes to the X-ray room.
(3) Place the two cassettes on the X-ray table with their long edges together.
(4) Protect a small area of each cassette (e.g. a corner) with a piece of lead. These areas will be used to assess which of the two films has the higher base-plus-fog density.
(5) Collimate the beam to produce a narrow rectangular exposed area on both cassettes as shown in Fig. 18.3.

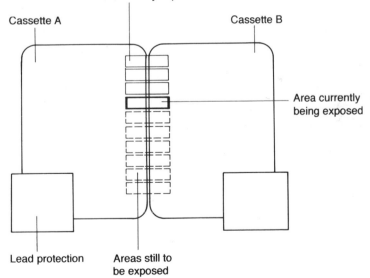

Fig. 18.3 The arrangement of cassettes for assessing the relative speed of two films.

(6) Being careful to avoid overlaps, make a series of radiographic exposures proceeding down the length of the cassettes, increasing the exposure time for each exposure by a constant factor (e.g. 2). The series of exposures might be as shown in Table 18.1.

Table 18.1 A possible series of radiographic exposures.

Steps on film	Exposure (mAs)
1	1
2	2
3	4
4	8
5	16
6	32
7	64
8	128
9	256

(7) As you proceed, cover with lead the areas you have previously exposed and the areas yet to be exposed. This will avoid these areas being fogged by scattered radiation.

(8) Process both films in the same processor, preferably alongside each other.

NB The duration of the exposure must be the *only* variable. All other conditions – X-ray tube, mA, kVp, FFD, focal spot size, beam collimation, cassette, intensifying screens, processor – must remain constant.

(9) Using a densitometer, find two steps (one on each film) which match in density. Try to find a density which is in the middle part of the useful density range (between 1.0 and 1.5). Let us suppose that you have found the matched densities in the two areas identified in Fig. 18.4 (step 4 on Film A and Step 6 on Film B).

(10) Check the table of exposures to find the two mAs values which produced the two densities. In our example 32 mAs for film B and 8 mAs for film A. The

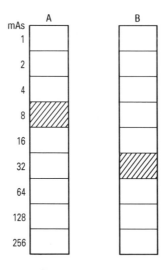

Fig. 18.4 Using test strips to compare film speed. The two matched densities correspond to step 4 (8 mAs) on strip A and step 6 (32 mAs) on film strip B. The ratio of these exposures is 32/8 = 4 so film A is four times faster than film B.

ratio of these exposures is $32/8 = 4$. So film A is four times faster than film B and requires only 25 per cent of the exposure necessary for film B.

The above method has the drawback that there may be no densities within the useful density range which exactly match between the two films. It would then be necessary to select the two densities which showed the least difference.

In some circumstances, the procedure we have described may need to be modified due to limitations in the exposure selection system of the X-ray unit. For example it may not be possible for the radiographer:

(1) To select mAs values which follow precisely the geometric progression sequence suggested;
(2) To set a constant mA value and control mAs by varying the exposure time alone.

However, it may be possible to circumvent both of these problems by repeating the exposure a number of times over the same area of the cassettes; e.g.:

- A single exposure on the first area (say 2 mAs);
- Two exposures of 2 mAs on the next area (equivalent to 4 mAs);
- Four exposures of 2 mAs on the next area (equivalent to 8 mAs).

and so on. . . .

Even allowing for these possible complications, the time-scale method is none-theless a simple, straightforward and generally accurate means of determining relative film speeds.

18.3.2   Comparing the relative speed of two screens

The test is similar to that described above for assessing the relative speed of film. Providing that the new screens have the same colour light emission as the ones they are being compared with, then an identical type of film may be used between each pair and time-scale sensitometry can be used to ascertain their relative speeds.

18.3.3   Determining the relative speed of two film-intensifying screen combinations

It is far more likely that instead of having to assess the relative speed of two different films or two screens of similar phosphor, you will be required at some stage to assess the relative speed of two different film–screen combinations. In other words, not only will the screens be of different phosphors but the films may also be different in order to match the light emission from the particular screen.

A time-scale intensity test such as the one that we have just described could be used. However, a second and more accurate method of determining relative speed is one that depends on the use of a calibrated step-wedge (section 4.5.5.5).

Let us examine its use in this instance.

18.3.3.1   Equipment

(1) Two similar cassettes fitted with different screens and each loaded with an appropriate film for the screens under test. The two screen–film systems will be identified as 'A' and 'B'.
(2) A calibrated step-wedge about 75 mm wide and consisting preferably of between 12 and 16 steps.
(3) A densitometer.

(4) Identification markers, e.g. 'A' and 'B'.
(5) X-ray equipment.

18.3.3.2 Method

We shall assume that the step-wedge to be used is the same as the one that we calibrated in section 4.5.5.5.

(1) The two cassettes 'A' and 'B' are placed edge to edge on the X-ray table, with the step-wedge positioned on top as shown in Fig. 18.5.

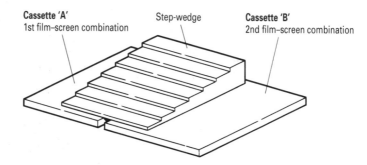

Cassette 'A'
1st film–screen combination   Step-wedge   **Cassette 'B'**
2nd film–screen combination

Fig. 18.5 Determining the relative speed of two different film–screen combinations.

(2) Centre the X-ray beam to the middle of the step-wedge and collimate to the borders of the wedge.
(3) Place identification markers on each cassette.
(4) Make an exposure using the same kV as was used to calibrate the step-wedge, e.g. 70 kVp.
(5) Process both films.
(6) Put both films side by side on the viewing box, adjusting them until two densities of ~ 1.0 are adjacent to each other (Fig. 18.6). Let us assume that steps 7 and 4 are the matching densities.
(7) On film A there are six exposure changes between steps 1 and 7, whilst the other film has three exposure changes. This is where the calibrated step-wedge now becomes useful. We know that the log relative exposure per step at 70 kVp was 0.12 (section 4.5.5.5), so the log exposure value of step 7 on film A is $6 \times 0.12 = 0.72$. The log exposure value of step 4 on film B is $3 \times 0.12 = 0.36$.
(8) The relative speed of system B is found by subtracting the two log relative exposures and finding the antilog of the answer. So:

$$0.72 - 0.36 = 0.36$$
$$\text{antilog } 0.36 = 2.29$$

The relative speed of system B is expressed as follows:

system A : system B = 1:2.29

In other words, system B is ~ 2.3 times faster than system A when used at 70 kVp.

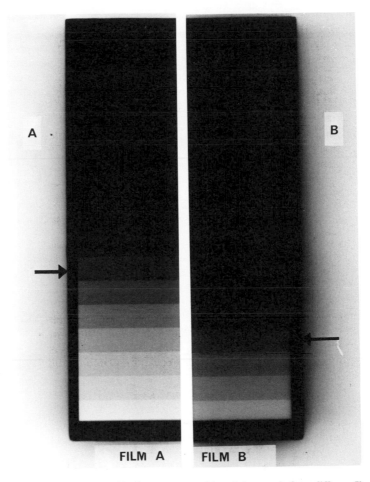

Fig. 18.6 Step-wedge images used in the assessment of the relative speed of two different film–screen combinations. Step 7 on film A and step 4 on film B are the matching densities approximating to $D = 1.0$.

18.4   Monitoring the automatic processor

In a department of medical imaging, consistency in the quality of the films and radiographs produced is essential. This is only possible, however, when automatic processors function to a set standard with maintained uniformity. In departments with more than one processor and where each is handling similar types of film, it is advisable to ensure that processor performance is standardized. In other words, a particular film–screen combination exposed to a given exposure should produce a similar image whichever automatic processor is used to process it.

18.4.1   Principles of processor monitoring

In Chapter 10, when we explained the film development aspect of automatic processing, we pointed out the ways in which various processing parameters like developer temperature and activity affect the density of the processed image. When these change for any reason, so will film density.

Processor monitoring therefore depends upon regularly processing sensitometric strips (Fig. 18.7) and analysing them with the aid of a densitometer in order to identify subtle changes in density values from one day to the next. Any changes from one strip to another are charted to see whether there is a trend. If there is, then the cause must be identified and corrective action taken.

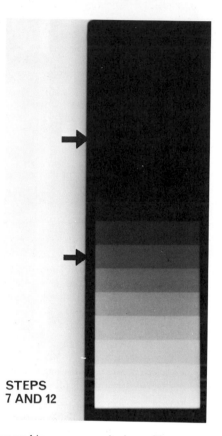

STEPS
7 AND 12

Fig. 18.7 Step-wedge image used in processor monitoring and known as a sensitometric strip. Step 7 will be used on a day-to-day basis to assess speed, whilst the difference between steps 12 and 7 will be used to measure contrast.

As we shall discover, monitoring in this way is so sensitive that it is possible to identify processing faults long before their effect becomes visible to the naked eye.

18.4.1.1   Sensitometric film strips and their production

Such a film strip has a series of increasing densities or stepped exposures (e.g. 16) ranging from ~ 0.2 to 3.0. The strip's use was explained in section 4.5.4, when we described the construction of a film's characteristic curve.

Sensitometric strips for processor monitoring are best obtained by using an intensity-scale method. Time-scale methods are more time consuming and, because several exposures are necessary to produce the film strip, the possibility of error is compounded.

One of the drawbacks with any method of producing sensitometric strips is the need for absolute consistency on the part of the radiographer. The strip must be produced in the same way, using the same step-wedge, cassette, X-ray tube and identical exposure factors, etc.

Another problem is that any failure, no matter how small, on the part of the equipment to produce a consistent kV or mA from one day to the next will also lead to the erroneous impression that it is the processor which is the cause of the inconsistency in the stepped densities so produced.

The use of a sensitometer (section 4.5.4.1) to obtain such a strip does have the advantage of eliminating many of the variables mentioned above. However, it is perfectly feasible to use an ordinary step-wedge and produce consistent sensitometric strips from day to day, providing that the following factors remain the same:

● X-ray set;
● Exposure factors;
● Film–focus distance (FFD);
● Step-wedge;
● Cassette;
● Type of film (a box should be set aside for this task).

It is possible to purchase boxes of 'ready made', unprocessed sensitometric film strips. However, these films are far less sensitive to variations in processor performance than freshly produced ones, and for that reason it is better to produce sensitometric strips as and when they are required.

The ideal film strip should comprise a set of densities ranging from ~0.2 to 3.0 (Fig. 18.7) and a small portion of the film should be shielded so that it does not receive any exposure. This area will be used subsequently to determine density due to base plus fog.

18.4.1.2 Evaluation of the processed film strips

Throughout this section we have stressed the importance of being able to duplicate, from one day to the next, the conditions of strip production so that any measured changes in the step-wedge densities can be attributed correctly to processor developer variations rather than careless preparation of the test strips.

Deviations from the normal development conditions of the processor are revealed by checking three important parameters. These are:

(1) Speed.
(2) Contrast.
(3) Density of the base plus fog (gross fog).

Reference to a typical film characteristic curve reminds us of the fact that the most important part of the curve is the so-called straight-line portion, and it is this portion which is most sensitive to changes in developer activity.

Consequently, when setting up a processor monitoring programme, the sensitometric test strip is examined carefully with the aid of a densitometer to identify two densities which represent the lower and upper parts of the straight-line portion. These are usually near 1.0 and 2.0, respectively. These two densities will become the reference values. The wedge steps corresponding to these values are recorded, because the same two steps will be used for evaluating processor performance on a day-to-day basis. Let us assume that those two steps are numbers 7 and 12 (Fig. 18.7).

Film speed

Film speed is a very sensitive indicator of changes in developer activity. Any increase in developer activity (e.g. due to an increase in temperature) will result in an increase in all of the strip densities. In other words, there will have been an increase in speed, since for the same X-ray exposure a greater response has been elicited from the film emulsion.

The step that we shall use for assessing speed will be number 7.

Contrast

Contrast is stated to be the difference in density. Using our sensitometric strip, we can determine the contrast by measuring the densities on our selected steps (numbers 7 and 12) and subtracting the lower density from the higher one.

To make sure of a difference in density that is adequate for measurement, it is worthwhile selecting two steps which are not immediately adjacent. This point should be borne in mind at the beginning of a monitoring programme, when two steps are being selected.

Gross fog

The third parameter examined in a processor monitoring programme is gross fog, defined as the density of the film base plus any fog density contributed by the development of unexposed silver halide.

This is checked easily by using the densitometer on a part of the film that has been protected carefully from exposure during the production of the step-wedge image.

An increase in the density of base plug fog is not a sensitive indicator of processor performance. Speed and contrast are affected at a much earlier stage should developer activity vary.

Speed, contrast and gross fog are plotted separately on a processor control chart, as described below.

18.4.2 Processor monitoring in practice

A box of films and a specific cassette should be set aside for the monitoring programme. A large number of test strips, e.g. 6–10, are produced and processed over the period of one day.

The first sensitometric strip is examined and upper and lower reference values are decided upon as described earlier. The identical number of steps on the remaining strips are also measured with a densitometer and an average value for each of the two steps is calculated. These become the reference values, and the two particular steps on the wedge which produced these readings will be the ones examined on each subsequent day of the monitoring programme.

Producing a processor control chart

Let us assume that the reference values obtained from averaging the readings from several test strips are as follows:

Speed (step 7 on the wedge)	0.90
Contrast (step 12 minus step 7)	1.10
Base plus fog	0.20

These values establish the reference or baselines for the three sections of the control chart (Fig. 18.8). Subsequent measurements, known as the **speed index, contrast index** and **fog index**, are charted in the same way.

The following data should be recorded on the chart:

- Identity of the processor being monitored;
- Developer temperature;
- Developer replenishment rate;
- Specific gravity of the developer;
- Fixer replenishment rate;
- Date on which test strip was processed.

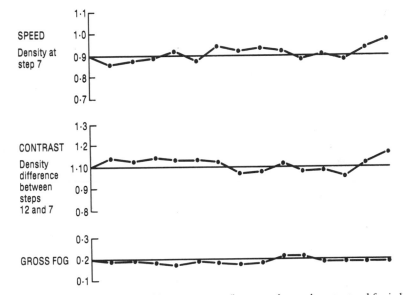

Fig. 18.8 A processor control chart with measurements (known as the speed, contrast and fog indices) recorded daily.

Establishing tolerance limits

Limits must be set for the speed, contrast and fog indices, so that should these levels be exceeded remedial action can be taken.

What limits are acceptable will depend on the requirements of individual departments, but they are usually set in the range 15–20% of the reference values.

All processors undergo fluctuations in performance, as any processor control chart will demonstrate. This is to be expected. The importance of processor control charts, however, is not the individual reading, which may be at variance with previous ones and upon which no action need be taken, but those readings which, taken together, demonstrate a trend. Trends of change are significant and need to be acted upon *before* the changes become visually apparent in the radiographs. Table 18.2 shows possible causes of three of the more common trends found on processor control charts.

Interpretation of control chart findings

If a daily reading is markedly at variance with previous measurements, the densitometer should be checked to ensure that it has been correctly zeroed, and the

Table 18.2 Problems of processor monitoring.

Problem	Likely causes
Speed and contrast increasing	(1) Developer temperature too high (2) Developer over-replenishment (3) Film transport speed reduced
Speed and contrast falling	(1) Developer temperature too low (2) Developer under-replenishment (3) Film transport speed increased (4) Poor developer recirculation
Speed and fog increasing; contrast falling	(1) Developer contamination (2) Faulty safelighting (3) Test strip fogged. New box of films needed?

reading taken again. If the variation is maintained, a fresh sensitometric strip should be produced and processed.

Should all remedial action fail to bring the processor under control, all the developer, along with its replenisher, should be drained off and fresh solutions made up.

A new monitoring programme should then be implemented within a day or so, in order to establish reference values for the new developer.

Frequency of testing

The testing should be done whenever a new machine is installed and thereafter on at least three days per week, e.g. Monday, Wednesday and Friday. The test strips should be processed mid to late morning after the processor has had time to warm up and become stable.

Following processor servicing and on any other occasion when all chemistry has been changed, it is advisable to allow the processor to settle down over a period of a couple of days before implementing a fresh monitoring programme following the procedure outlined earlier.

18.4.2.1 Testing the adequacy of fixer replenishment

In the modern automatic processor, the volume of fixer replenishment is matched to the surface area of film processed. The greater the number of films processed, the more fixer replenisher used. So, providing the type of work does not change and the rate of replenishment per square metre of film remains constant, a state of equilibrium is reached whereby the silver content of the fixer should remain fairly constant.

This useful fact makes it easy for the radiographer to assess the best fixer replenishment rate, simply by estimating the level of silver in solution with silver-estimating papers.

A fixer replenishment rate that is too low will be indicated by an increase in the quantity of silver in solution. Too high a replenishment rate means that the silver-estimating papers would show a low silver content.

Once a department has decided upon an acceptable level of silver in solution, e.g. 5 g/l, this level can easily be checked by silver-estimating papers on a weekly basis and the replenishment rates adjusted up or down if necessary in order to maintain this standard.

Over-replenishment is wasteful, whilst under-replenishment can lead to inefficient fixation and thereby loss of archival permanence.

18.4.2.2 Testing the efficiency of the washing process

Unless films are adequately washed, thiosulphate from the fixing process will
remain in the emulsion and, in time (perhaps after several years), cause staining.

To ensure image permanence, a weekly check may be made on a processed
radiograph for evidence of residual thiosulphate.

Method

A couple of drops of chemical reagent, such as Thiodet, is dropped onto a clear
(unexposed) area of the radiograph and left for 2 min. The reagent is then blotted
off and the colour of the resultant stain compared to a set of tints on a comparator
chart provided with the reagent. The inspection should be made immediately,
because the stain will gradually darken with exposure to light and produce a reading
which would be misleadingly high.

A thiosulphate level of $< 3\ \mu g/cm^2$ is recommended for archival permanence.

If the result of the test shows the washing to be inefficient, the fault may lie with
one of the following:

- Water flow rate inadequate;
- Water circulation pump malfunctioning;
- Wash-water too cold.

We shall now turn our attention to the final element in the quality assurance
programme that we outlined at the beginning of this chapter: reject film analysis.

18.5 Reject film analysis

Reject film analysis is a method of determining, from the analysis of a department's
reject films, just how cost effective and consistent both staff and equipment are in
producing good quality images (radiographs).

The objectives of a reject film analysis programme may be summarized as
follows:

(1) To ensure that high standards of radiographic technique and film handling are
    maintained throughout the department.
(2) To ensure that radiographic equipment is consistently operating to a high
    standard.
(3) To ensure that film materials are used in the most cost-effective way.

18.5.1 Method

There are several versions of reject analysis programmes. The one that we shall
describe is a fairly comprehensive one, involving a great deal of data collection. The
end result, however, is that a reject rate can be determined for each imaging room
and each type of examination, in addition to one for the department as a whole.

Before commencing any programme of this type, it is important to determine:

- The period for which you want the analysis to run (e.g. 4 weeks);
- The number of people who are to supervise the programme. (For example, 2 or

3 basic-grade radiographers supervised by a senior radiographer is ideal. Results can be discussed with the quality manager.)

Immediately before the survey commences, record:

(1) The number of unexposed films in the processing areas (including those in cassettes).
(2) Any unexposed films in each imaging room.

Determine the number of reject categories to be used. The following are suggested:

- Overexposure;
- Underexposure;
- Positioning;
- Motion;
- Processing;
- Equipment;
- Miscellaneous (unidentified faults, etc.).

In addition to identifying the reason for rejection, films should also be sorted by the analysis team into examination categories, e.g. chest, abdomen, cervical spine, etc.

Once the programme is under way, the following steps are taken:

(3) Each room keeps a record of the number of examinations by type, and the number of films taken. In addition, all of the room's reject films are retained for collection.
(4) The analysis team make a weekly collection from each room, as well as assimilating the room data that have been recorded. The reject films are then sorted into the appropriate rejection categories, as well as being identified by examination type.

18.5.2 *Evaluation of results*

On completion of the survey period, the following data should be available for analysis:

- Total amount of film used during survey (A).
- Total number of reject radiographs (B).
- Total film usage for each room.
- Total rejects per room.
- Total films for each type of examination.
- Total reject films for each type of examination.
- Total films in each reject category.

$$\text{The overall percentage reject rate} = \frac{B}{A} \times 100\%$$

Anecdotal evidence appears to indicate that the reject rate in those imaging departments using a reject analysis programme averages between 10 and 15%. The greatest number of repeats is due to exposure error.

It is impossible to be precise as to what is an acceptable reject rate, since standards can vary from one department to the next. What may be regarded as a film fit only for rejection in one department may be accepted in another.

Nevertheless, reject analysis does have a valuable place, not in comparing one hospital imaging department with another but in assessing whether the standards set in a particular department are being maintained.

A higher-then-average rejection rate should always be investigated to identify problem areas. If a comprehensive reject analysis programme such as the one that we have outlined is followed, then it will be possible to identify very precisely the types of examination technique which may be giving rise to particular problems.

18.5.3 Conclusion

Running a reject film analysis programme is a time-consuming procedure. It demands the active participation of every member of staff if it is to produce worthwhile results. It is not something that can be done in isolation, but should form part of an all-embracing quality assurance programme which includes both processor monitoring and equipment testing.

We have now completed our study of the radiographic image. In the next chapter we shall turn our attention to the fluoroscopic image and, in particular, the role of the image intensifier.

Part 4
The Fluoroscopic Image

Chapter 19
The Image Intensifier

In the next series of chapters we describe the imaging systems which are used to display and record the fluorescent, dynamic images generated by image intensifiers and fluoroscopic screens.

19.1 Direct fluoroscopy

It is possible to view directly, with the naked eye, the fluorescent image produced by a simple phosphor-coated screen. Such **direct fluoroscopy** is fraught with difficulties, primarily because the brightness and contrast of the image are unacceptably low (Hay, 1982). However, until the 1960s this was the only technique widely available for demonstrating, in real time, the movements of dynamic processes of the body, such as peristalsis.

Modern fluoroscopy depends on the electronic amplification of image brightness using a vacuum device known as an **image intensifier**. It is this device which is the subject of discussion in this chapter.

19.2 Image intensification

Image intensification is a process by which the brightness (and contrast) of an image is increased. It is sometimes known as **image amplification**.

Image intensification is most commonly achieved by using an **electrostatic image intensifier tube**. This is a vacuum device which converts a low-intensity, full-sized image into a high-intensity, miniaturized image. It is exposed to the X-ray beam that has been transmitted through the patient and is used in one of two configurations, as shown in Fig. 19.1. The traditional arrangement is to use an undercouch X-ray tube and to attach the intensifier tube to a serial cassette changer located immediately above the patient. The alternative, more recent arrangement is to use an overcouch X-ray tube and to position the image intensifier underneath the table top. The second method is usually associated with a remote-control facility. Discussion of the pros and cons of these designs is beyond the scope of this book and the reader is referred to textbooks on diagnostic X-ray equipment for such information (e.g. Carter, 1994).

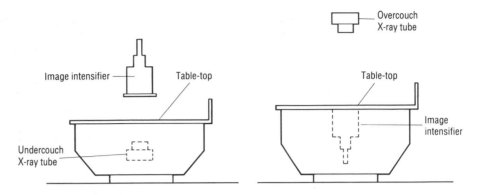

Fig. 19.1 Image intensifier–X-ray tube configurations. The overcouch tube, undercouch intensifier is the more recent development.

It is usual to employ a closed-circuit television (CCTV) system to permit instantaneous (real time) viewing of the intensified image, in which case the image is displayed on the screen of a television monitor (see section 22.1.1.3). Additionally, the image may be recorded photographically on fluorographic film as a miniature static image, which is examined using a magnifying viewing system.

19.2.1 *Principles of operation*

Figure 19.2 illustrates the principal components of an image intensifier tube. The circular **input phosphor** at the end of the tube nearest to the patient is 25–57 cm in diameter and uses sodium-activated **caesium iodide** as its phosphor material. Exposure of the input phosphor to the X-ray beam that has been transmitted through the patient causes it to emit light. The brightness of light emitted is proportional to the intensity of the incident X-rays. Thus, a fluorescent image is formed, but this image is of very low intensity.

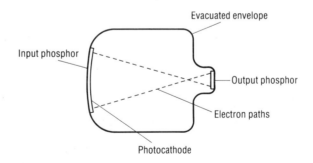

Fig. 19.2 The electrostatic image intensifier. Electrons released from the photocathode, under the action of light from the input phosphor, are accelerated and focused onto the output phosphor. Note that the accelerating, and focusing electrodes are omitted from this diagram.

Coated onto the input phosphor is a **photocathode** layer which releases electrons from its surface in numbers related to the intensity of the light to which it is exposed. The number of electrons emitted from a given point on the photocathode is therefore dependent on the X-ray intensity at the corresponding point on the input phosphor, e.g. where X-ray intensity is high, light emission and ultimately electron emission is high. There is thus a pattern of electron emission from the photocathode which mimics the pattern of intensities in the transmitted X-ray beam: an **electron image** is produced.

In the body of the image intensifier tube the electrons are accelerated through a potential difference of 25–35 kV, and focused electrostatically onto a circular **output phosphor** 2.5– 3.5 cm in diameter. This has a coating of zinc–cadmium sulphide, which fluoresces when bombarded with electrons. The light image so produced may be up to 9000 times brighter than the input phosphor image. There are two reasons for the gain in brightness.

Electron acceleration Electronics emitted from the photocathode gain kinetic energy from the electric field inside the intensifier tube. This energy is converted into light at the output phosphor.

Reduction in image size The area of the output phosphor image is about one-hundredth that of the input phosphor. This, in itself, increases the image brightness one-hundred times.

19.2.2 Output phosphor image quality

We have explained that the image produced by an image intensifier may be up to 9000 times brighter than would be the case if a simple fluorescent screen were used. Image contrast is also increased. These represent very worthwhile improvements in image quality but, as with any imaging system, the resulting image is not perfect. As we discussed in Chapter 3, there are deficiencies already present in the invisible image in the X-ray beam transmitted through the patient. The image intensifier introduces further losses, although these are generally far outweighed by the gains in image brightness and contrast. Let us examine some aspects of the quality of the intensified image.

19.2.2.1 Unsharpness
Geometric unsharpness may be minimized by positioning the intensifier input phosphor as close as possible to the patient, but other forms of image unsharpness may arise *during* the intensification process.

Input phosphor The finite thickness of the caesium iodide layer means that light produced in the layer may spread and be scattered before it reaches the photocathode. (Note that this effect was described in section 7.2 in relation to intensifying screens.) A point source of light in the phosphor results in the photocathode being exposed to a small **disc** of light, and the electrons are emitted from a finite area rather than from a point. The spreading of light within the input phosphor is minimized by using needle-shaped caesium iodide microcrystals. When the fluorescent layer is formed, the crystals are deposited in such a way that the long axis of each crystal is perpendicular to the plane of the input phosphor (see Fig. 19.3). The principle of the **light-pipe** used in fibre-optic technology then operates (see section 20.1.1.2). Light emitted within each crystal is internally reflected within the crystal and exits only at its end (Fig. 19.4). Thus, the spreading of light is limited and the consequent image unsharpness is minimized.

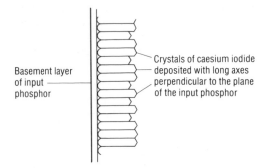

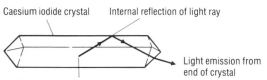

Fig. 19.3 Alignment of caesium iodide crystals on the input phosphor.

Fig. 19.4 The light-pipe principle operating in a caesium iodide crystal. Lateral spread of light is minimized by total internal reflection within the crystal, thus improving image sharpness.

Electron focusing Electrons emitted from the photocathode are focused onto the output phosphor. Electrons arising from a point on the photocathode should hit the output phosphor at a point. In fact, limitations in the electrostatic focusing system result in a slight divergence and the electrons hit the output phosphor over a finite area rather than a point (Fig. 19.5). It is difficult to design a focusing system which is equally effective over the entire image field. Most systems provide optimum sharpness in the central regions of the image, with reduced sharpness at the periphery.

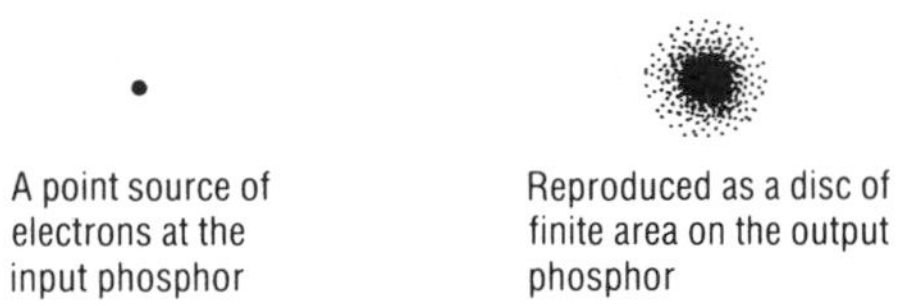

Fig. 19.5 Imperfect electron focusing in an image intensifier. Focusing tends to deteriorate towards the edges of the image field.

Output phosphor As with the input phosphor, problems are created by the spreading and scattering of light within the fluorescent layer of the output phosphor. These effects are minimized by adopting methods similar to those referred to in section 7.3.3 in relation to intensifying screens.

19.2.2.2 Noise

Quantum noise A consequence of the gain in image brightness produced by the image intensifier is that the X-ray intensity required to provide a satisfactory image is very low. In such situations there is a danger that the quantum nature of the X-ray beam will become visible and the image will suffer quantum noise. Loss of image quality due to quantum effects is minimized by ensuring that the input phosphor has a high **quantum detection efficiency**, i.e. the caesium iodide layer absorbs a high proportion of the X-ray quanta incident upon it. Note, however, that quantum noise on the output phosphor image is not necessarily created within the image intensifier but is a result of the reduced X-ray exposures associated with the use of image intensifiers.

Structure mottle The input phosphor, photocathode and output phosphor display a graininess in their structure due to the finite size of the microcrystals which they contain. This could produce an intrusive grainy appearance on the output phosphor image, known as **structure mottle**. In practice, this effect is masked by the more significant **quantum noise**.

19.2.2.3 Resolution

The output phosphor image is only 2.5–3.5 cm in diameter and must be magnified before it is displayed to the observer. It is therefore vital that the miniature image is of the highest possible resolution. The loss of image sharpness and the effect of noise described above influence the maximum resolution achievable with an image intensifier. The limiting resolution of the intensified image is typically between 5 and 7 line-pairs/mm at the centre of the image field, but rather less than this at the periphery (e.g. STD, 1987). It is also the case that brightness may reduce towards the edges of the image, producing an effect known as **vignetting**.

19.2.2.4 Distortion

The electron image or pattern created as electrons are emitted from the photocathode of an image intensifier should be duplicated in miniature when the electrons bombard the output phosphor. Any deviation from this pattern results in **distortion** of the intensified image which, if present, is likely to be more noticeable towards the edges of the image field. Distortion at this stage may indicate a design fault in the image intensifier itself, or maladjustment of the electron optical system which focuses the electron stream. The effect of stray magnetic fields in the X-ray room, perhaps due to the rolled steel joists (RSJs) used in the building construction, may cause a characteristic 'S' distortion (Fig. 19.6(a)). Many image intensifiers exhibit 'pin-cushion' distortion (Fig. 19.6(b)) due to the fact that the input phosphor is curved whilst the output phosphor is flat (MDD, 1994). Note, however, that distortion in the *final* image may well be caused by limitations in the optical lens system (section 20.2.6.2) employed as part of the fluorographic camera or in the television system rather than in the image intensifier tube.

19.2.2.5 Spectral emission

Manufacturers specify the spectral emission characteristics of a phosphor by means of a numerical code. The zinc–cadmium sulphide output screen phosphor of an image intensifier is usually quoted as a **P20** type, which fluoresces predominantly in the yellow–green part of the visible light spectrum (500–650 nm), with maximum intensity occurring at 560 nm (Fig. 19.7). The photographic film which records the intensified image must have its spectral sensitivity matched to the wavelengths of light emitted by the output phosphor.

19.2.2.6 Gas spots

Image intensifier tubes sometimes suffer from the presence of traces of gas inside the vacuum. When the tube is operated, the gas becomes ionized and a stream of ions is drawn onto the output phosphor, producing an irregular patch or bright spot on the image. Gas spots tend to appear if the image intensifier has not been used for a while. An intensifier in regular use should not suffer from this image defect.

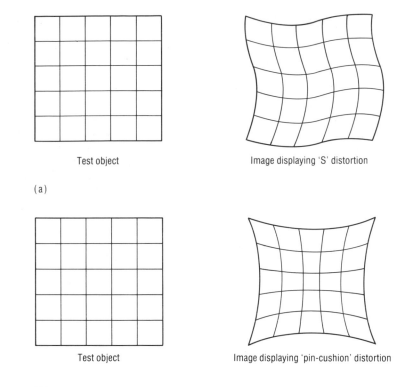

Test object   Image displaying 'S' distortion

(a)

Test object   Image displaying 'pin-cushion' distortion

(b)

Fig. 19.6 (a) 'S' distortion in image intensifiers. Straight lines in the subject are reproduced as stretched 'S' shapes in the image. The effect is produced by stray magnetic fields. The illustration exaggerates the effect for purposes of demonstration. (b) 'Pin cushion' distortion in image intensifiers. Image magnification increases towards the edges of the image field. The effect is exaggerated in the diagram.

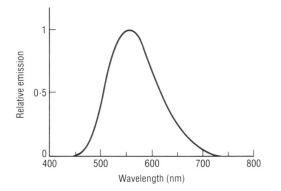

Fig. 19.7 Spectral emission of a P20 type image intensifier output phosphor. Peak emission occurs at 560 nm (yellow–green).

19.2.3 Multifield image intensifiers

It is common for image intensifiers to offer a facility where the electron optical system can be switched between two modes such that either the entire input phosphor image or just the central part of the image is transferred to the output phosphor. Such a system is described as a **dual-field** image intensifier. For example, it may provide a choice between 27 or 17 cm input image fields (a '27/17' system). Whichever input field is selected, the output image field remains the same. Thus, switching to the smaller input field produces an output image which appears magnified relative to that given by the larger input field (see Fig. 19.8). Image intensifiers are currently available with a triple-field option, giving a choice of three input field sizes. There may be some loss of image quality when used in the magnification mode compared with the full-field image.

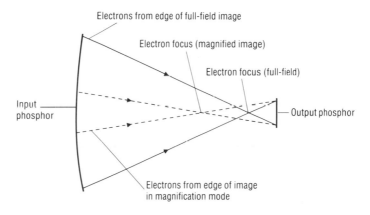

Fig. 19.8 The dual-field image intensifer. By altering the position of the electron focus the image on a small central section of the input phosphor can be made to occupy the whole area of the output phosphor, giving the effect of a magnified image.

It should be noted that a reduction in the input field size is accompanied by a reduction in the amount by which image brightness is amplified. Thus, to maintain the brightness of the output phosphor image at a constant level, the X-ray beam is increased in intensity by raising X-ray tube kilovoltage (kVp) or current (mA). There is normally an **automatic brightness control** (ABC) system incorporated to maintain constant output image brightness, whichever magnification mode is employed. The ABC system also compensates for the effect of different tissue thicknesses due to various patient body types and radiographic projections (Carter, 1994).

In this chapter we have outlined the method by which image amplification is achieved in an electrostatic image intensifier and we have described some of the characteristics of the image that it produces on its output phosphor. In the next chapter, we describe how light from the output phosphor is distributed and focused onto the various image receptors available.

Chapter 20
Lens Systems and Image Distributors

The image on the output phosphor of an image intensifier is not viewed directly. Rather, it is focused onto the pick-up tube of a television system for instant viewing or onto fluorographic film to be photographically recorded. In this chapter we shall examine the behaviour of the lens system used to focus the intensified image, and the distribution system which diverts the image to the fluorographic or television camera.

Before describing the lens focusing system, it is necessary that we first study some of the basic principles of optics: the science of the formation of optical images.

20.1 Optics

20.1.1 Wave properties of light

As we saw in Chapter 4, light is a form of electromagnetic radiation and many aspects of its behaviour can be explained by reference to the wave nature of light. Because light is a wave, it exhibits the phenomena of refraction and reflection, on which the formation of light images with lenses and mirrors depends (England *et al.*, 1990).

20.1.1.1 Refraction
In general, when a light ray passes from one transparent medium into another, it changes direction at the interface between the media (Fig. 20.1). When passing from a rare medium (e.g. air) into a denser medium (e.g. glass), the light ray is bent *towards* the normal (the **normal** is a line drawn perpendicular to the interface).

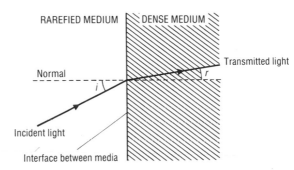

Fig. 20.1 Refraction of light at an interface between two media. The diagram shows the angles of incidence (*i*) and refraction (*r*).

When passing from a dense to rare medium, the ray deviates *away* from the normal. Only if it meets the interface at right angles is it transmitted without deviation. This phenomenon of bending of light is known as **refraction**.

Snell's law

The angle between the incident ray and the normal is known as the **angle of incidence** (*i*). The angle between the refracted ray and the normal is called the **angle of refraction** (*r*); see Fig. 20.1. For a given interface, a mathematical relationship known as Snell's law exists between these angles:

$$\frac{\sin i}{\sin r} = n$$

where *n* is a constant known as the **refractive index**. An interface with a high refractive index produces more refraction than one with a low refractive index. Note that if $n = 1$, no refraction takes place. Some examples of the refractive indices of various materials when interfaced with a vacuum are quoted in Table 20.1.

Table 20.1 Example of values of refractive indices. In each case the value quoted is for a vacuum–material interface, which in practice is the same as for an air–material interface.

Material	Refractive index
Air	1.00028
Water	1.33
Eye	
Aqueous humour	1.33
Vitreous humour	1.34
Cornea	1.38
Crystalline Lens	1.4
Glass	1.5–1.6
Diamond	2.42

The effect of colour

The values of refractive index vary slightly for different wavelengths of light. Thus, different colours of light are refracted by different amounts, as demonstrated in Fig. 20.2 which shows white light being split into a spectrum of colours as it is refracted

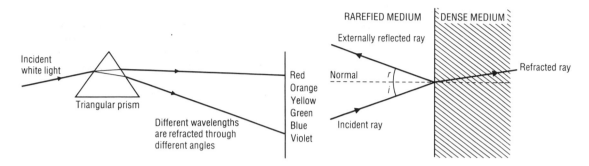

Fig. 20.2 Production of the visible light spectrum by passing white light through a triangular glass prism.

Fig. 20.3 Reflection of light at an interface. The angles of incidence (i) and reflection (r) are equal. The diagram illustrates partial external reflection, the remaining light being transmitted and refracted through the interface.

by a triangular prism. Note that short-wavelength light (e.g. blue–violet) is refracted more than long-wavelength light (e.g. red). These differences can cause complications in the design of lens systems (see section 20.2.6.3).

20.1.1.2   Reflection

Light may be **reflected** as well as refracted at an interface. An interface may reflect light **directly** (e.g. from an optically smooth surface) or *diffusely* (e.g. by scattering from an optically roughened surface). We shall consider only direct reflection since it is of greater importance in optics (Fig. 20.3). In this case, the angle between the reflected ray and the normal (the *angle of reflection*) is always *equal* to the angle of incidence. All wavelengths of light are reflected equally.

External and internal reflection
Figure 20.3 illustrates an example of **external reflection**, where the reflection occurs in the *less* dense medium. Reflection may also be demonstrated in the denser medium (Fig. 20.4), when **internal reflection** is said to occur.

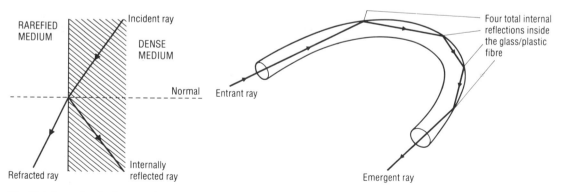

Fig. 20.4 Internal reflection at an interface. If the angle of incidence is greater than the critical angle, total internal reflection occurs and no light is refracted.

Fig. 20.5 The principle of the light pipe. A ray of light entering one end of the transparent fibre suffers successive total internal reflections causing the ray to follow the curved shape of the fibre.

Total internal reflection

If the angle of incidence is greater than a specific value, known as the **critical angle**, no refraction occurs and **total internal reflection** takes place (England *et al.*, 1990). For a glass–air interface, the critical angle is 40°. The phenomenon of total internal reflection is employed in **fibre-optic** technology, where total reflection within a fine transparent flexible glass or plastic fibre causes light to be contained within the fibre. The fibre then acts as a **light pipe** (Fig. 20.5).

20.2 Lenses

Lenses are transparent optical devices designed to refract light rays in a systematic way, bringing them to a common focus. The cheapest lenses are made from plastic. In recent years the quality of the best plastic lenses has improved tremendously, but for optimum results optical glass lenses are still preferred because glass can be worked and polished to finer tolerances than plastic and is more resistant to scratching.

Simple lenses consist of a single element made from only one piece of glass. Better results are obtained from compound or complex lens systems which consist of several components, each of which may be formed from a number of individual lenses cemented together. The lens systems used in diagnostic imaging are usually of this type.

The surfaces of a lens are normally spherical but they may have different shapes (e.g. cylindrical) in special cases. A lens surface may be convex, concave or planar; thus, a number of different types of lens are possible, as shown in Figs 20.6 and 20.8.

Lenses are classified as being either **convergent** (positive) or **divergent** (negative), depending on whether the lens causes parallel light rays to converge or diverge.

20.2.1 *Convergent (positive) lenses*

A convergent lens is thicker at its centre than at its periphery. Thus, at least one surface of a convergent lens must be convex. The lens may be biconvex, plano-convex or meniscus (Fig. 20.6).

Parallel light rays striking the face of the lens are refracted towards its principal axis (Fig. 20.7). Peripheral rays suffer the greatest refraction, while central rays are

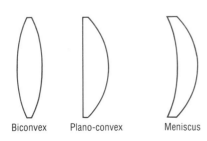

Biconvex   Plano-convex   Meniscus

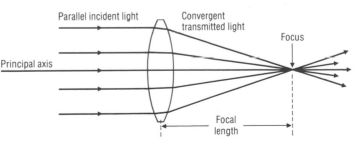

Parallel incident light   Convergent transmitted light   Focus   Principal axis   Focal length

Fig. 20.6 Three types of convergent lens. Each type is thicker at its centre than at its periphery.

Fig. 20.7 The action of a convergent lens in bringing parallel light rays to a common focus.

refracted the least. Those rays which pass through the centre of the lens are not refracted at all. The point of intersection of the convergent rays is known as the focus, and its distance from the lens is known as the **focal length** of the lens.

Convergent lenses can be used to focus an image of an object onto a surface, e.g. a sheet of photographic film, the signal plate of a television camera pick-up tube or the retina of the eye. Images which can be focused onto a surface in this way are known as *real* images. They are positioned on the side of the lens away from the object.

20.2.2   *Divergent (negative) lenses*

A divergent lens is thinner at its centre than at its periphery: at least one surface must be concave. The lens may be described as biconcave, plano-concave or meniscus (Fig. 20.8).

Parallel rays are refracted *away* from the principal axis of the lens (Fig. 20.9). The divergent rays thus created appear to have originated from a focus on the *same* side of the lens as the light source.

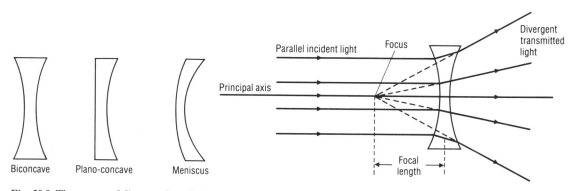

Fig. 20.8 Three types of divergent lens. Each type is thicker at its periphery than at its centre.   Fig. 20.9 The action of a divergent lens. The diverging light rays appear to have originated from a common focus.

Images created by divergent lenses are known as **virtual** images: they cannot be focused onto a surface except by the use of additional convergent lenses, which can transform them into real images.

20.2.3   *Lens equation*

A simple relationship known as the lens equation (or lens formula) exists between the focal length of a lens and the distances of the object and the image from the lens:

$$\frac{1}{u} + \frac{1}{v} = \frac{1}{f}$$

where u = object distance, v = image distance and f = focal length.

This relationship enables the position of an image to be predicted if the focal length and object distance are known. Note that f has a positive value for convergent lenses and a negative value for divergent lenses. A positive value for v indicates that the image is real; a negative value indicates that the image is virtual.

20.2.4 *Magnification*

The ratio of image size to object size determines the magnification factor of a lens or lens system. A system producing an image smaller than the object is known as a **reducing lens system**, while one producing an image larger than the object is termed an **enlarging** or **magnifying lens system**. For a simple lens, the magnification factor depends solely on the relationship between the distances from the lens of the object (u) and its image (v):

$$\text{Magnification factor} = \frac{\text{Image size}}{\text{Object size}} = \frac{\text{Image distance } (v)}{\text{Object distance } (u)}$$

Under different conditions, the same lens or lens system can produce a magnified or reduced image, e.g. a magnifying glass used at close range provides an enlarged image while if held at arms length it gives a reduced (and inverted) image. A **zoom** lens provides a continuously variable magnification factor.

20.2.5 *Lens specifications*

There are a number of descriptive terms which may be applied to a lens to specify its basic characteristics (Jenkins & White, 1957).

Shape: for example, biconvex, plano–concave, etc.

Focal length (f) The focal length of a lens is defined as the distance between the lens and its focus for a light beam travelling parallel to its principal axis. Its value is often quoted in millimetres, e.g. 50 mm, 100 mm, etc.

Power (P) The power of a lens is defined as the reciprocal of its focal length in metres, i.e.:

$$P = \frac{1}{f}$$

where P is quoted in units called **dioptres** ($= \text{m}^{-1}$). Conventionally, P has a positive value for convergent lenses and a negative value for divergent lenses.

Stop or aperture (D) This is a measure of the diameter of the lens. It specifies the size of the opening through which light can pass. It controls light transmission and therefore affects image brightness. In some instances a separate, smaller diaphragm opening is placed in front of or behind the lens, which artificially reduces the value of D. The opening may be fixed or variable in size, as in an **iris** diaphragm which thus controls the amount of light passing through a lens. Aperture size sets a theoretical limit to the resolving power of a lens.

Resolving power The resolving power of a lens is the minimum angular separation of objects that can be detected as separate entities in the image (Fig. 20.10). Resolving power depends on both the lens aperture (D) and on the wavelength (λ) of the light concerned:

$$\text{Resolving power } \alpha \ \frac{\lambda}{D}$$

Notice that resolving power improves as lens aperture increases.

Relative aperture The relative aperture or **speed** of a lens is also an indication of its ability to admit light. It is defined as:

$$\text{Relative aperture} = \frac{\text{Focal length}}{\text{Aperture}} = \frac{f}{D}$$

Its value is quoted as a ratio (1:8, 1:3.5, etc.) or as an '*f*' number (*f*8, *f*3.5, etc.). For example, a lens whose focal length is 50 mm and whose aperture is 25 mm has a relative aperture of 1:2 or *f*2. The smaller the *f* number, the greater the speed and the brighter the image.

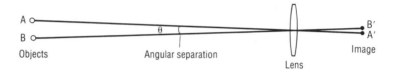

Fig. 20.10 Resolving power of a lens. Two objects, A and B, subtend an angle θ at the lens. If the images A′, B′ of A and B can *just* be distinguished as separate entities, the angle θ is said to be the resolving power of the lens.

Depth of focus When a real image is focused onto the emulsion surface of a film, the positioning of the film is extremely critical. An error in positioning can lead to the image being unsharp or 'out of focus'. However, we know that if unsharpness is kept below a certain level the image will not appear noticeably unsharp. Thus, an acceptably sharp image can be obtained over a small range of positions on each side of the exact focal plane. This latitude of position is known as **depth of focus**. Its magnitude increases as the *f* number of the lens increases (i.e. as the lens aperture gets smaller). Thus, depth of focus can be increased by *stopping down* or reducing the aperture of a lens, e.g. with an iris diaphragm.

Depth of field If a real image of an object is focused onto a film, it is possible to increase or decrease the object distance slightly without the image becoming noticeably unsharp. The maximum variation in object distance while still maintaining an acceptably sharp image is known as the **depth of field**. Its magnitude increases as the lens *f* number increases.

Transmittance The fraction of incident light transmitted through a lens is known as its **transmittance**. Its value is never 100% because:

(1) Some light is absorbed in the lens since it is not perfectly transparent;
(2) Some light is reflected at the lens surfaces.

Reflection can be reduced markedly by the process of **blooming**. This is the application to the lens surface of a transparent film whose thickness is only one-quarter of the wavelength of light. Light rays reflected from the surface of the coating interfere destructively with light rays reflected from the surface of the lens because the wave crests of one set of reflected rays coincide with the wave troughs of the other (Fig. 20.11). Depending on its thickness, the coating produces optimum effect for only one colour (wavelength) of light. Green, being in the middle of the white light spectrum, is generally chosen, thus no green light is reflected and the lenses display a purplish hue by reflected light. The coated surfaces are very delicate and should not be touched.

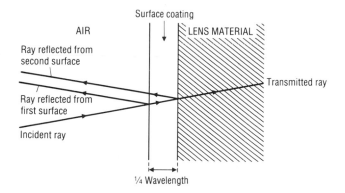

Fig. 20.11 Bloomed lenses. The ray reflected from the second surface has travelled about $\frac{1}{2}$ a wavelength of light further than the ray reflected from the first surface. Because they are out of phase their wave troughs and crests coincide, cancelling each other out. Thus no light energy is reflected from the lens surface.

Blooming is particularly important with multi-element, compound lens systems, where the number of surfaces involved increases the potential losses due to reflection.

20.2.6   *Lens aberrations*

Lenses are not perfect instruments. They suffer from failings known as **lens aberrations**, which lead to unsharpness and distortion of the image (Jenkins & White, 1957). A simple lens exhibits a number of aberrations, which become more intrusive as its relative aperture is increased. To permit the use of the wide apertures needed to reduce patient dose in fluorographic applications, complex lens systems must be employed. Different kinds of glass are combined and radii of curvature accurately computed in order to correct the aberrations inherent in a simple lens. The major lens aberrations are described below:

20.2.6.1   **Monochromatic aberrations**
Those lens defects which are apparent even with light of a single wavelength are known as **monochromatic** aberrations. Four such defects may be noted.

(1) Spherical aberrations The grinding and polishing methods used during lens manufacture produce lens surfaces which are spherical in shape. As a result of this spherical shape, a light beam travelling parallel to the principal axis of the lens has its peripheral rays brought to a slightly different focus from its central rays (Fig. 20.12). This produces a degree of unsharpness over the entire image field.

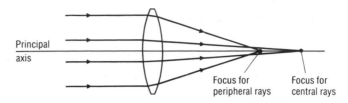

Principal
axis

Focus for
peripheral rays

Focus for
central rays

Fig. 20.12 Spherical aberration. Light rays passing through the periphery of the lens are brought to a different focus from rays passing near its principal axis. This causes image unsharpness which can be reduced by 'stopping down' the aperture of the lens.

(2) Coma Light rays arising from off-axis object points strike the lens obliquely, resulting in a form of unsharpness known as **coma** which gets progressively worse towards the edges of the image field. It derives its name from the comet-like appearance of the image of a point object located just off the principal axis of the lens.

(3) Astigmatism Off-axis rays also produce an aberration known as **astigmatism** in which a point object results in two separate line images, one vertical and one horizontal, at slightly different distances from the lens. Optimum image quality is found between these two distances, where the point object is reproduced as a disc. The visual effect of astigmatism is shown in Fig. 20.13.

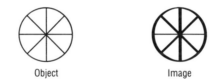

Object

Image

Fig. 20.13 Astigmatism. A wheel having eight spokes of equal thickness is imaged in such a way that only the spokes in one particular direction appear sharp (horizontal spokes in the diagram). Those spokes at right angles to this (i.e. vertical in the diagram) appear blurred and therefore thicker.

(4) Curvature of field A simple lens, free from the above defects, may suffer from an aberration known as **curvature of field**, which means that the plane of sharpest focus is curved rather than flat. In the case of a convergent lens, the image plane is concave (see Fig. 20.14).

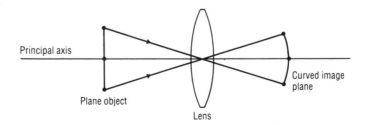

Principal axis

Curved image
plane

Plane object

Lens

Fig. 20.14 Curvature of field. The image of a plane (flat) object is reproduced in focus on a curved surface.

There are two basic approaches to overcoming these monochromatic aberrations:

(1) Stopping down or reducing the aperture with an iris diaphragm positioned just in front of or behind the lens. This restricts the field of view of the lens to a narrower angle, cutting out the off-axis and peripheral rays, thus improving image sharpness. Unfortunately, stopping down limits the amount of light transmitted through the lens, resulting in an image which is less bright.

(2) Modified lens design. Spherical aberrations may be reduced by careful choice of lens shape (e.g. a biconvex lens with its two surfaces of different convexities) or by the use of combinations of lenses.

20.2.6.2   Distortions

Distortion occurs when the magnification of central parts of an image differs from that of peripheral parts. If magnification increases towards the periphery, **pin-cushion** distortion occurs. If magnification reduces towards the periphery, **barrel** distortion is produced (Fig. 20.15).

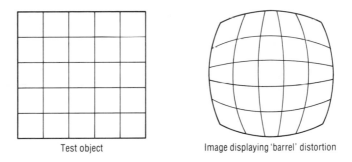

Test object   Image displaying 'barrel' distortion

Fig. 20.15 Barrel distortion in lens systems. Image magnification reduces towards the edges of the image field. The effect is exaggerated in the illustration.

These image distortions tend to occur in the complex multi-element lens systems which are designed to eliminate spherical aberrations. They can be reduced by careful placement of a stop between the separate elements of the lens system or by making use of only the central parts of the image field.

20.2.6.3   Chromatic aberration

We noted earlier (section 20.1.1.1) that different wavelengths of light are refracted by different amounts: e.g. short-wavelength (blue) light is refracted more than long-wavelength (red) light. Thus, when white light is passed through a simple lens, the different colours of the spectrum are focused at different points (Fig. 20.16). The image appears unsharp due to colour fringing effects. There are two solutions:

(1) Use two lenses cemented together, one convergent and one divergent, each one being made of a material with a different refractive index, e.g. crown glass and flint glass. A combination such as this is known as an **achromatic doublet**.

(2) Use two lenses of the same material, but separated from each other. Note that monochromatic images do not suffer from chromatic aberration.

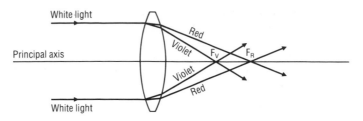

Fig. 20.16 Chromatic aberration. Different wavelengths (colours) of light come to a focus at different points, e.g. violet light focus is at F_V, while red light focus is F_R.

20.2.6.4 Vignetting

The term vignetting is used to describe the reduction in image brightness which is sometimes experienced away from the central axis of the image. It is most likely to occur in a lens system containing aperture stops when a wide field of view is employed or when the object distance is small.

20.3 Mirrors

Mirrors are optical devices designed to reflect light in a systematic way, in some cases bringing the light rays to a common focus. Mirrors consist of an optically smooth, plastic, metal or glass base onto which is applied a highly reflective metallic coating. The base is said to have been 'silvered', although the reflective coat is aluminium rather than silver.

Direct reflection occurs even from transparent surfaces, and in special circumstances highly efficient reflection takes place, e.g. as in the **total internal reflection** described in section 20.1.1.2.

20.3.1 *Front- or back-coated mirrors*

For domestic applications adequate results are obtained by using back-coated mirrors, but examination of Fig. 20.17 shows that with this arrangement light rays must pass through the transparent base before being reflected. Thus, light suffers

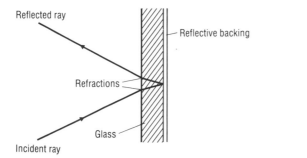

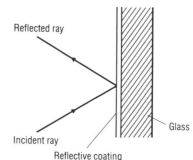

Fig. 20.17 Back-coated mirror. Light is refracted as it enters and exits from the transparent glass base. Unless the light is *mono*chromatic, chromatic aberration occurs and image quality is affected.

Fig. 20.18 Front-coated mirror. Such mirrors do not suffer chromatic aberration because no refraction is involved.

two refractions as it enters and leaves the mirror. As we have seen with lenses, chromatic aberrations are caused by refraction, and back-coated mirrors also suffer from this defect.

For high-quality work it is better to use front-coated mirrors, which avoid refraction and therefore do not suffer chromatic aberrations (Fig. 20.18).

20.3.2 Partially-coated mirrors

For some purposes a mirror may be designed to reflect a specified fraction of the light incident upon it, and to transmit the remainder. In such cases, the base must be transparent and the 'half-silvered' metallic reflecting layer must be so thin as to be semi-transparent. A better alternative is to dispense with the metallic reflector and to apply a very thin transparent coating to the base in order to control direct reflection from its surface in a way similar to that described in section 20.2.5 in relation to bloomed lenses. Such devices are known as **beam-splitting** mirrors and provide a method for distributing the light output from an image intensifier to different image receptors (see section 20.4.2.2).

20.3.3 Mirror shapes and types

Reflecting surfaces may be classified as plane (flat), concave or convex, but plane mirrors are most commonly used in radiography.

20.3.3.1 Plane surface reflection

Plane reflecting surfaces are used to change the direction of a light beam (Fig. 20.19) e.g. the light emerging from the output phosphor of an image intensifier is reflected by a mirror through 90° into a fluorographic camera.

It is also possible to use total internal reflection in a **right-angle prism** to produce the same effect (Fig. 20.20); the luminance of the output phosphor image is monitored by directing a sample of its light via such a prism to a photomultiplier tube (see section 20.4.2.3).

Reflection at a plane surface causes a lateral (left-to-right) or vertical (top-to-bottom) inversion of the image, depending on whether the light beam is travelling in a horizontal or a vertical plane. This may be corrected optically (e.g. by a second reflection) or electronically (e.g. by a television system).

The beam-splitters described in section 20.4.2.2 have plane reflecting surfaces.

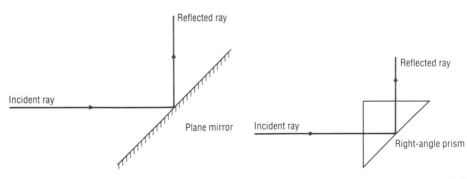

Fig. 20.19 Light beam altered in direction by 90° by reflection at a plane mirror.

Fig. 20.20 Light beam altered in direction by 90° due to total internal reflection in a right-angle prism.

20.3.3.2   Concave mirrors

A concave mirror causes parallel light rays to converge to a focus (Fig. 20.21). It thus behaves in a similar fashion to a convex lens and may be used to produce a real image. Its shape may be spherical, in which case it exhibits spherical aberrations corresponding to those described for lenses, or more complex, e.g. parabolic. An advantage of the convergent mirror over the convergent lens is that it is cheaper to manufacture a large aperture mirror than a lens of equivalent size and it does not suffer chromatic aberration. The **Odelca** fluorographic camera once used for mass chest radiography employed a large concave mirror as a vital part of its image focusing system.

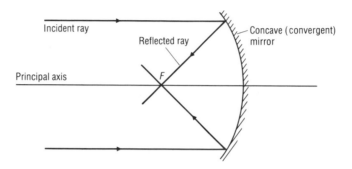

Fig. 20.21 Parallel light rays being brought to a focus (*F*) by reflection from a concave mirror.

20.3.3.3   Convex mirrors

A convex mirror causes parallel light rays to diverge as if from a focus positioned behind the mirror. Its behaviour thus corresponds closely to that of a concave lens. It produces a virtual image. An example of an application of a convex mirror is to provide the X-ray receptionist with a **wide-angle** view of a patient waiting area when direct vision is partly obstructed.

20.4   Fluorographic image focusing

Before it can be displayed on television or recorded on film, the output phosphor image on an image intensifier must be focused onto the TV camera signal plate or onto the emulsion of the fluorographic film (Jenkins, 1980). There are two fundamental requirements:

(1) A focusing system, e.g. using lenses in tandem;
(2) An image distribution system, e.g. using a beam-splitting mirror.

Figure 20.22 illustrates a typical arrangement for satisfying both of these requirements.

20.4.1   Tandem lens system

The tandem arrangement of lenses consists of two separate convergent lens combinations: a collimator lens and a camera or television lens.

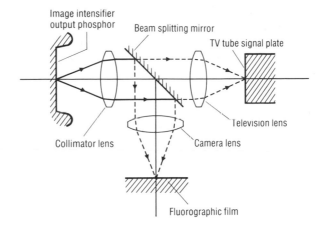

Fig. 20.22 The image focusing and distribution system of a fluorography/fluoroscopy unit. Note that for the sake of clarity the lenses are shown as simple biconvex type. In practice multi-element combinations are used (see text).

20.4.1.1 Collimator lens

The first lens combination is known as a **collimator**. Its function is to render parallel the divergent light rays arriving from the output phosphor image. This is achieved by placing the collimator lens at a distance from the output phosphor equal to its focal length. Because of its large aperture, the depth of field of the collimator is very small and its positioning is extremely critical. An error of a fraction of a millimetre can result in the final image being unsharp. During installation, the lens combination is coupled firmly to the image intensifier and fine adjustments are made before locking it permanently in position. The collimator is a high-quality complex multi-element lens combination, having its entry lens matched in diameter to that of the output phosphor, e.g. 25 mm. Its exit lens is of much larger diameter, e.g. 100 mm. It has a relative aperture of around f 0.75 and a short focal length e.g. 65 mm.

As Figure 20.22 shows, the parallel light rays emerging from the collimator lens may pass directly to the television lens, or be deflected through 90° by a mirror or beam-splitter before reaching the camera lens.

20.4.1.2 Camera or television lens

The function of the second lens combination is to focus the parallel light beam from the collimator lens onto the film in the fluorographic camera or onto the signal plate of the television pick-up tube. The film or signal plate must be placed exactly at the focus of the lens, i.e. at a distance from it equal to its focal length. The depth of focus of the lens is extremely small and it must be positioned with great accuracy in relation to the image receptor if optimum image quality is to be maintained. The coupling of the lens onto the film or television camera is therefore permanent and should only be adjusted by a properly trained engineer. A different lens combination is required for film and television cameras because the dimensions of the signal plate image on the TV pick-up tube (e.g. 25 mm diameter) are much smaller than those of the fluorographic film image (e.g. 65 or 100 mm diameter). For each size of fluorographic film a lens of different focal length is needed, since it is this which determines the size of the image (Jenkins, 1980), e.g. a 70 mm film may require a lens of 200 mm focal length while 105 mm film may need a 300 mm lens. Incorrect choice of lens could result in the image size not matching the film size, causing over- or underframing to occur (Fig. 20.23).

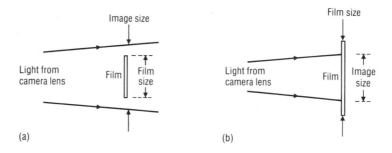

Fig. 20.23 (a) Overframing. The image size is greater than the film size because the focal length of the camera lens is too long. The image is apparently magnified (see text). (b) Underframing. The image size is smaller than the film size because the focal length of the camera lens is too short. The image suffers from vignetting.

Deliberate overframing provides the basis for a method of obtaining a magnified image. However, as the focal length (and image size) is increased, the brightness of the image is reduced. Image magnification by this means therefore requires increased X-ray exposure.

To ensure maximum image brightness and minimum X-ray exposure, television and fluorographic camera lenses always have wide apertures, e.g. *f*1.25 or even faster.

20.4.1.3 Advantages of the tandem lens system

The tandem system permits a mirror or beam-splitter to be interposed between the collimator lens and the camera or television lens.

The mirror can be used to reduce the space needed to accommodate the image intensifier and its attachments, and thus allow the intensifier to be placed beneath the X-ray table top. The beam-splitter enables fluorographic filming and television fluoroscopy to be undertaken simultaneously.

As we have seen, the positioning of the collimator lens in relation to the output phosphor, and the camera lens in relation to the image receptor, are critical. However, the distance separating the collimator lens from the camera lens is not critical. Thus, the attachment of alternative image receptors, with their own lenses, is possible without the need for time-consuming refocusing.

20.4.2 Optical image distributor

Basic fluoroscopic units have an in-line television camera tube directly coupled to the image intensifier via a tandem lens system or a fibre-optic disc. With these methods, the intensified image can only be accessed through the television system, which therefore limits image quality.

A more versatile arrangement is to employ an optical image distributor housed in a **distribution box** between the intensifier and the television camera. This allows the intensified image to be projected onto one or more fluorographic recording cameras, as well as onto the television system (Fig. 20.24).

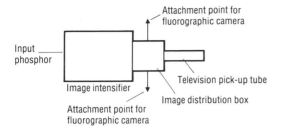
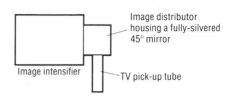

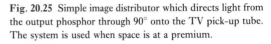

Fig. 20.24 Distribution box showing its relationship to the image intensifier and television camera tube. The diagram illustrates two additional attachment points for fluorographic film cameras.

Fig. 20.25 Simple image distributor which directs light from the output phosphor through 90° onto the TV pick-up tube. The system is used when space is at a premium.

Manufacturers offer a number of different designs of image distributor but all designs include a plane mirror set at 45° to the long axis of the image intensifier. The mirror reflects parallel light from the collimator lens through 90° into the lens of the film camera or television pick-up tube. The designs are of two basic types, depending on whether the 45° mirror is fully- or half-silvered.

20.4.2.1 Fully-silvered mirror

One design incorporating a fully-silvered mirror has a television image as its only output. The mirror enables the television camera tube to be set at right angles to the axis of the image intensifier, thus reducing the overall length of the imaging device (Fig. 20.25).

A more common arrangement is to use an electrically driven mechanism, which enables the mirror to be rotated 90° in either direction from its central position. This directs the light from the collimator lens onto any one of three devices, e.g. a 105 mm cut film fluorographic camera, a 35 mm or 16 mm cine camera, or a television camera (Fig. 20.26). For fluoroscopy, the television system is selected with the mirror in its central position. When a fluorographic record is required, the

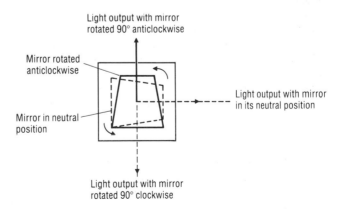

Fig. 20.26 Image distributor with rotating mirror. The diagram shows the appearance viewed along the central axis of light emitted from the output phosphor. The mirror, set at 45° to this axis, can be rotated about the axis to direct light upwards (anticlockwise rotation) or downwards (clockwise rotation) from its neutral position.

mirror is rotated to reflect the light into the appropriate camera. Simultaneous fluoroscopy and fluorography is not available with this arrangement.

20.4.2.2   Half-silvered (beam-splitting) mirror

The beam-splitting mirror does not reflect all of the light that falls upon it; typically only 90% of the light from the collimator lens is reflected, the remaining 10% being transmitted through the mirror into the lens of an in-line television pick-up tube. The reflected light is directed into the camera lens of a fluorographic or cine camera (Fig. 20.27). Less light is distributed to the television system because it is more sensitive than the fluorographic or cine film. The advantage of the beam-splitting image distributor is that film recording can be undertaken simultaneously with television fluoroscopy, which therefore provides continuous real-time monitoring of the intensified image.

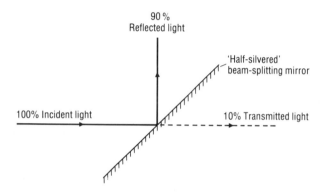

Fig. 20.27 The beam-splitting mirror which both reflects and transmits light. Roughly 90% of the light from the output phosphor is reflected into the fluorographic camera. The remaining 10% is passed to the television system.

20.4.2.3   Automatic brightness control

The distribution box also houses a small right-angle prism which forms part of the **automatic brightness control** (ABC) system. By total internal reflection, the prism diverts a sample of the light from the collimator lens into a photomultiplier tube for the purpose of monitoring the brightness of the output phosphor image. The signal from the photomultiplier tube is fed back to the X-ray generator control system, which modifies the X-ray tube current or kilovoltage to maintain an image of constant brightness.

In the chapter that follows, we describe some of the fluorographic systems and materials currently in use, the image quality which they offer and the ways in which fluorographic images may be presented.

Chapter 21
Photofluorography of the Intensified Image

In previous chapters we saw the way in which images are produced by an image intensifier and learned of the principles involved in its use. In this chapter we will examine the ways in which the images so produced may be recorded and subsequently viewed.

Taking a photograph (whether it be a dynamic cine run or a series of static pictures) of those images produced at the output phosphor of an image intensifier is known as **photofluorography**.

If you refer to Fig. 21.1, you will see the way in which the various camera options listed in Table 21.1 fit into the fluorographic scheme. The image on the output phosphor is focused onto the films by the optical distribution system as well as by any lenses incorporated inside the cameras.

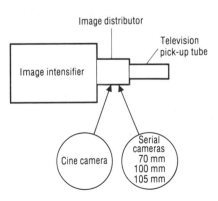

Fig. 21.1 Photofluorography of the intensified image. The various camera options can be connected to the image distribution box. The image on the output phosphor of the image intensifier is focused on to the films by the image distributor optical system as well as any lenses incorporated inside the cameras.

Table 21.1 Camera options.

Camera	Film size
Cine	16 mm or 35 mm
Serial type	70 mm or 105 mm roll film
	100 mm sheet film

21.1   The cine camera

When a cine camera (Fig. 21.2) is used to record images from the image intensifier, the process is commonly known as **cinefluorography**.

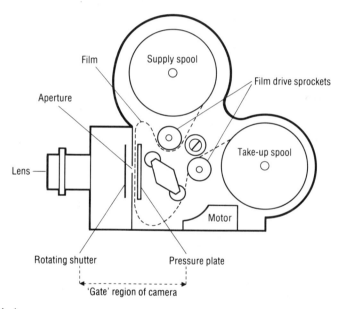

Fig. 21.2 A cine camera.

These cameras take a rapid series of pictures or 'frames' on 16 mm or 35 mm roll film. When the film is processed and played back through a projector at a similar rate, the eye perceives the series of images as *one* moving image.

Applications
These cameras are used in the medical imaging department in conjunction with an image intensifier to record rapidly moving physiological events, e.g. the act of swallowing in a barium contrast examination. However, their principal application nowadays is in the field of cardioangiography, where rapidly-moving blood flow through the heart chambers can be examined in the search for shunts or other abnormalities.

Significance of frame rate on visual perception
The film is exposed at rates usually in excess of 16 frames per second (fps). The

eye's persistency of vision is such that it will accept as continuous, a succession of images which replace each other at a rate of 16 or more per second. Below this figure, the lag is too great for the eye successfully to merge each image into the next, and the images are seen as separate entities rather than as one moving image.

21.1.1 The camera in action

Film travel
The route taken by the film inside the camera – supply spool to exposure area or **gate**, to take-up spool – may be seen in Fig. 21.2. Notice also the slack loop of film above and below the gate. This is necessary because the take-up spool and film-drive sockets run continuously when filming, whilst the film in the 'gate' region has a stop–start motion. The film has to stop, albeit for a fraction of a second, in order to be exposed. The pressure plate holds the film firmly whilst an exposure is made, then a 'pull-down' mechanism inside the gate moves the film fractionally forward so that the next frame can be exposed. The loop of film allows for this differential rate of film movement to take place.

Variable-speed motor
A variable-speed motor drives both the film sprockets and take-up spool and thus governs the number of frames exposed per second (the framing rate).

Different framing rates can therefore be selected. In practice, speeds in excess of 60 fps are seldom used, although the 16 mm camera does permit framing speeds as high as 200 fps; 35 mm cine cameras are capable of 150 fps.

The shutter
This is the mechanism in a camera which controls the duration of an exposure. In the cine camera it takes the form of a shaped disc of metal which continuously rotates between the lens and the aperture when the camera is filming.

The shape can vary but one type is illustrated in Fig. 21.3 and is called a 180°, shutter. The rotation of the shutter is synchronized with the film movement so that when the solid part of the shutter lies over the aperture, the film is advanced. When the aperture is unobstructed during the next 180°, the film is held stationary and exposed.

Thus if the camera is driven at 25 fps, the film is exposed for half of 1/25th (i.e. 1/50th) of a second.

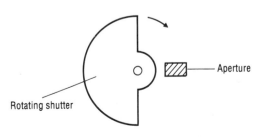

Fig. 21.3 A 180° cine camera shutter. When the solid part of the shutter lies over the aperture the film is advanced. During the next 180° of rotation the film is held stationary and exposed.

The aperture

The size of aperture governs the amount of light allowed through to the film (section 20.2.5).

In cinefluorography, a large aperture is used (e.g. *f*2) in order to admit as much light as possible from the image intensifier output phosphor and thus to minimize the exposure times that will be required. A small aperture would mean that either a correspondingly longer exposure time would have to be allowed (thus limiting the frame rate one could select) or that the brightness of the output phosphor would have to be increased (thus increasing dose to the patient).

Film exposure and X-ray generators

Rapid cinefluorography is demanding on both X-ray generator and tube because the greater the camera's framing speed, the shorter must become the X-ray exposure interval.

Typically, an exposure time of 5–6 ms (0.005–0.006 s) is required for an exposure rate of 48 fps. Consequently, X-ray generators suitable for cinefluorography must offer high output (130–200 kW), short minimum exposure times and high exposure repetition rates.

Cinefluorographic equipment is often pulsed in operation. This means that the X-ray tube is not continuously energized during filming but passes current only during those intervals when the camera shutter is open. To do otherwise would result in unnecessary irradiation of the patient.

21.1.2   Cine film

The 16 mm and 35 mm cine film is usually sold in lengths of 85 or 150 m.

Along one or both edges of the film are rows of regularly spaced 'sprocket' holes (Fig. 5.8, section 5.2.2.2) which assist in the movement of the film through the camera mechanism.

The 35 mm film appears to be the most popular choice because of its superior resolution (offering four times the recording area of 16 mm film).

The spectral sensitivity of cine film needs to be either orthochromatic or panchromatic, so as to match the predominantly green emission of image intensifier output phosphors.

Cine film has a relatively high-speed emulsion in comparison with conventional 35 mm camera film. A fast emulsion thus affords an opportunity to obtain adequate film blackening even when in the presence of low light intensities and brief exposure times, as experienced in cinefluorography.

This combination of fast emulsion and small exposure may produce quantum mottle (section 2.1.1.1). Such a phenomenon would be highly unsatisfactory were it necessary to view each frame individually. However, cine film is played back through a projector, with each image or frame rapidly merging into the next and adding to the overall quality of the image (a case of two or more frames being better than one!). The presence of mottle on each frame is not compounded by merging one frame into another, as might at first be expected. The very random nature of the mottle ensures that its presence will not be detected when the moving film is viewed.

Processing cine film

See section 10.13.1.

21.2   Serial cameras

Such cameras are sometimes referred to as '**spot-film**' or '**rapid-sequence**' cameras. The following types are available:

- 105 mm camera using roll film;
- 100 mm camera using sheet film;
- 70 mm camera using roll film.

All of them record the image intensifier output phosphor picture via the image distribution box in the same way as the cine camera.

Whilst we refer to them as cameras, they are in fact very different from the type of camera that you might use at home! They do not have need of a shutter, for example, since exposure can be controlled simply by the rapid switching of the X-ray generator. No X-rays, no image!

Serial cameras are capable of recording images at the rate of one per second ('single-shot') or a rapid sequence of up to 12 images per second.

Camera features

- Separate supply and take-up magazines.
- Automatic exposure of patient data onto film.
- Automatic recording of serial number of each shot in a sequence.
- A safety mechanism to prevent use if camera runs empty or patient's identity card is not inserted.

21.2.1   *105 mm camera*

The 105 mm camera (Fig. 21.4) uses an orthochromatic, perforated roll film, 105 mm wide and 45 m long, which is loaded into the camera's supply magazine.

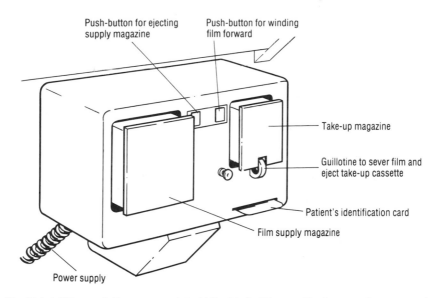

Fig. 21.4 A 105 mm roll film camera made by Philips Medical Systems. For demonstration purposes the camera is shown with both magazines slightly withdrawn.

Some 430 exposures are possible on each roll, although the take-up magazine has only a limited storage capacity (e.g. 130 frames).

Located near the entrance to the take-up cassette is a guillotine, which is used to divide the film and thus allow the cassette to be withdrawn. Variable lengths of film can therefore be processed and examined at any time.

The slot for taking the patient's identification card can be seen in Fig. 21.4. Other features include:

- Orange warning light in operator's console when take-up cassette is nearing maximum capacity;
- No filming possible if patient's identification card is not inserted;
- Up to 12 fps are possible, as well as single-shot;
- Indication on operator's console of amount of unused film remaining.

21.2.2 *100 mm camera*

The 100 mm camera exposes separate sheets of orthochromatic film, each 100 × 100 mm.

Single-shot and rapid-sequence filming is possible, the more expensive cameras being capable of exposing 12 sheets of film per second. The most popular choice of model seems to be one capable of two or three films per second. This is perfectly adequate for most fluoroscopic applications.

Typical capacity of two particular 100 mm cameras
Table 21.2 shows the typical capacity of two 100 mm cameras. Other useful features associated with these cameras include:

- Indication on operator's console of the number of films remaining in the supply magazine;
- Warning neon light on the camera when film supply is down to 20 films;
- The patient's identification, the exposure number and date are automatically exposed onto each film.

Table 21.2 Capacity of two types of 100 mm cameras.

Supply magazine	Take-up magazine
1st type 120 films	100 films
2nd type 70 films	20 films

21.2.3 *70 mm camera*

This camera uses orthochromatic roll film, 70 mm wide and 45 m long.

Some 600 exposures are possible on this length of film and, just as with the 105 mm and 100 mm cameras, the 70 mm camera has a detachable supply and take-up cassette. The capacity of the latter is 5 m of film (60 exposures).

Single-shot or rapid-sequence filming is possible up to a maximum of 6 fps. There is a slot on the camera for insertion of a card with the patient's identification details.

21.3 Processing fluorographic film

An automatic processor for processing all types of roll film, from 35 mm to 105 mm, was described in section 10.13. Such a processor will also take 100 mm sheet film if a special adaptor is first attached.

In a department where these films are used extensively, such a processor is a very necessary requirement. For the less-frequent user or where such a processor breaks down, the roll film can be processed satisfactorily in a standard automatic processor providing that a 'leader' is attached, as in Fig. 21.5. This ensures that the film, which has a natural tendency to curl, remains on track when passing through the processor, instead of winding itself around the rollers.

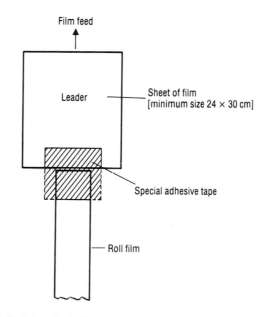

Fig. 21.5 Method of splicing a leader before processing roll film. The two films are placed edge to edge and the chrome splicing tape applied on both sides. The dotted areas should be trimmed before processing.

A suitable tape for attaching the roll film to the 'leader' is Scotchbrand 850 Silver Tape or Scotchbrand Plastic Tape 471.

21.4 Presentation of fluorographic images

Because of their size, fluorographic films are more difficult to handle during the viewing and reporting stage. For this reason, a variety of methods exist to make handling easier and we shall consider just two of them:

- Film-viewing mounts.
- Lamination.

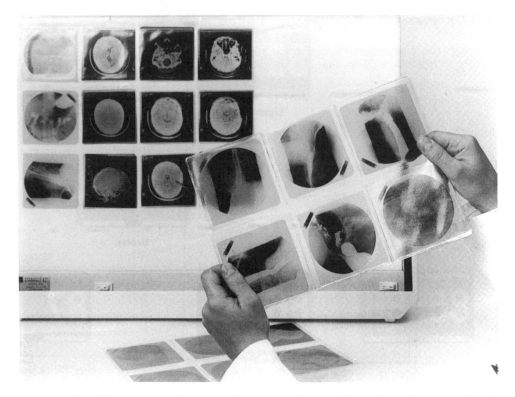

Fig. 21.6 Transparent film packets for mounting 100 mm × 100 mm films. (Courtesy of Wardray Products Ltd.)

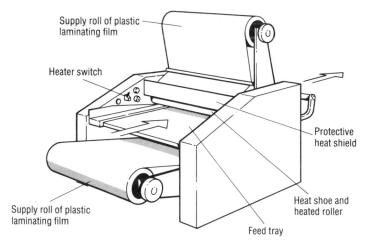

Supply roll of plastic laminating film

Heater switch

Protective heat shield

Heat shoe and heated roller

Feed tray

Supply roll of plastic laminating film

Fig. 21.7 A laminating unit. The film(s) to be laminated are placed on the feed tray and advanced until taken up by a pair of heated rollers. Simultaneously the film is sandwiched between two sheets of plastic supplied by the upper and lower supply rolls and heat sealed. (Courtesy of Laminex International, Mold, Clwyd, UK.)

Film viewing mounts

These are transparent film packets designed to hold four to six 100 mm × 100 mm films (Fig. 21.6) and are made from semi-rigid, clear PVC.

Lamination

This is a procedure whereby the films are mounted between two clear sheets of plastic film, which are then bonded together using a high temperature and pressure provided by specially heated rollers (Fig. 21.7).

In this chapter we have examined those methods by which an image on the image intensifier output phosphor is photographed, the film materials used and their presentation. In the next chapter we shall begin our study of the television image.

Chapter 22
Television and Digital Images

We explained in Chapter 19 that the images produced during image intensifier fluoroscopy are invariably displayed via a closed circuit television (CCTV) system. In this chapter we outline the principles of television, explain how CCTV may be attached to an image intensifier, and describe the characteristics of a television image. Towards the end of the chapter we examine the properties of images generated from digital information.

22.1 Principles of television

Television is a means of transmitting visual images from one place to another through the medium of electrical signals. A television camera containing a **pick-up tube** converts the visual image into an electrical (**video**) signal, while a television monitor containing a **cathode ray tube** is used to convert the video signal back into a visual image (Fig. 22.1).

Domestic television signals are normally transmitted across hundreds of kilometres using an ultra-high-frequency (UHF) electromagnetic radio-wave link. The radio link requires no physical connection between the transmitter and receiver. In radiography, where the distance between the TV camera and monitor is only a few metres, it is more convenient (and cheaper) to provide a cable (closed-circuit) link. In both cases the video signal is communicated at such a high speed that there is no noticeable time delay between its transmission and receipt.

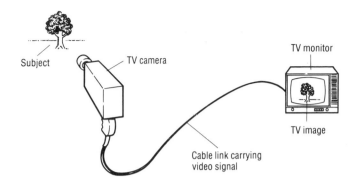

Fig. 22.1 Principles of television. The camera converts a visual image into an electrical 'video' signal. The signal is conveyed via a radio or cable link to a television monitor. The monitor converts the video signal back into a visual image.

22.1.1   Closed-circuit television

We shall describe the principles of closed-circuit television in three parts:

(1) TV pick-up tube;
(2) Video link;
(3) TV monitor.

22.1.1.1   TV pick-up tube

The function of the television pick-up system is to transform a light image into an electrical signal. There are various designs in use, including solid-state **charge-coupled devices** (CCDs), but the **Vidicon** and **Plumbicon** tubes (and their derivatives such as the Chalnicon and Hivicon) are the most common in radiography. Both latter types operate on broadly the same principles (Fig. 22.2). At one end of the evacuated pick-up tube is a 2.5 cm diameter **signal plate** onto which the light image is focused. The signal plate has a photoconductive coating applied whose electrical conductivity varies according to the intensity of the light incident upon it. From an electron gun at the other end of the tube, a fine stream of electrons scans systematically over the photoconductive layer or **target**. This produces an electrical signal whose magnitude varies as the electron beam passes over different parts of the target, e.g. illuminated parts produce a higher current than dark parts. The pattern of light intensities is thus converted into an electrical video signal (Carter, 1994).

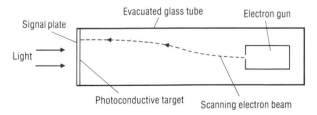

Fig. 22.2 The television pick-up tube. The electric current drawn from the signal plate is higher when the electron beam hits an area which is brightly illuminated, and a video signal is produced. Note that the focusing and scanning coils are omitted from this diagram.

The scanning pattern or **raster** consists of a series of parallel sweeps across the target (Fig. 22.3), sampling the entire image twenty-five times every second. The same raster is used in the television monitor (Forster, 1985).

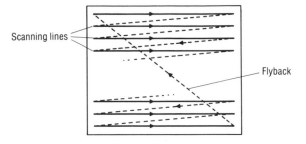

Fig. 22.3 Television scanning raster. The same pattern of horizontal sweeps of the target is reproduced on the screen of the television monitor. The central section of the raster has been omitted to allow the 'flyback' of the electron beam from bottom right to top left of the screen to be more clearly seen.

22.1.1.2   Video link

The video signal from the pick-up tube is very weak and must be amplified before it can be used. Once amplified the video signal is fed through a screened cable to the television monitor and also, perhaps, to a videotape recorder (Fig. 22.4).

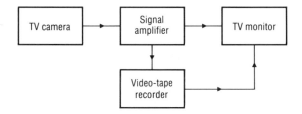

Fig. 22.4 Block diagram showing the relationship between major components of a television system.

22.1.1.3   TV monitor

The function of the television monitor is to transform the video signal back into a visual image. The TV monitors found in radiography departments are based on the vacuum **cathode ray tube** (CRT) (Fig. 22.5). An electron gun at the narrow end

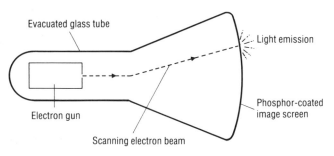

Fig. 22.5 The television cathode ray tube. The brightness of the screen is determined by the electron beam current which, in turn, depends on the strength of the video signal. Note that the grid, focusing and scanning coils are omitted from this diagram.

of the CRT produces a fine stream of electrons which scans systematically over the phosphor-coated image screen at the other end. The scanning raster is identical to and synchronized with that used in the pick-up tube. The intensity of the electron beam is modulated by the video signal and the image screen fluoresces with a brightness proportional to the intensity of electron bombardment. Thus a visual image is created on the screen which matches closely the image which appeared on the signal plate of the pick-up tube.

22.2 Television fluoroscopy

The image produced by the output phosphor of an image intensifier is viewed through the medium of a high-resolution, closed-circuit television chain. The TV pick-up tube is coupled onto the image intensifier tube, while the TV monitor(s) may be ceiling-suspended, wall-mounted or placed on a free-standing trolley. The output phosphor image may be transferred to the signal plate of the pick-up tube in one of two ways.

(1) Fibre-optic coupling
A fibre-optic disc, which contains a bundle or matrix of transparent optical fibres, is fitted with one face immediately over the output phosphor. The TV pick-up tube is attached with its signal plate in contact with the opposite face of the fibre-optic disc (Fig. 22.6). Thus, light is transmitted directly from the output phosphor to the pick-up tube (Stockley, 1986). This is a compact and relatively cheap method of linking the TV system to the image intensifier, making it ideal for the mobile systems often used in the operating theatre. However fibre-optic coupling does not permit direct photographic recording of the intensified image (fluorography).

(2) Optical lens coupling
A tandem system of lenses is used to focus the output phosphor image onto the pick-up tube signal plate (Fig. 22.7). This is often used in conjunction with an image distribution system, which allows simultaneous fluoroscopy and fluoro-

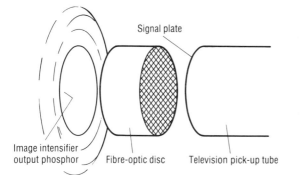

Fig. 22.6 Fibre-optic coupling. The components have been separated to show their relationship more clearly. The fibre-optic disc is normally in close contact with both the output phosphor and the signal plate.

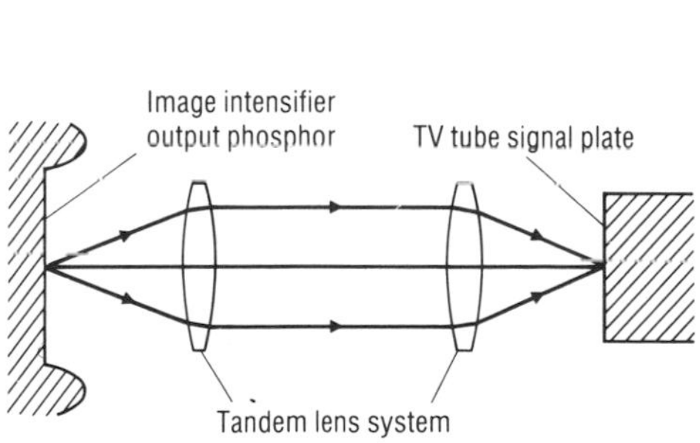

Fig. 22.7 Optical lens coupling. An image distributor is often interposed between the collimator lens and television lens. Note that although simple, single element convergent lenses are shown, in practice multi-element compound lenses are employed.

graphy of the intensified image (see section 20.4.2). Sophisticated lens systems are expensive components and add to the overall size of the image intensifier assembly, but they are capable of producing images of higher quality than can currently be achieved with fibre-optic coupling.

22.3   Television image quality

The convenience of viewing the intensified image via a television chain is achieved at the expense of a potential loss of image quality. The assessment of the quality of television images is a complex subject but there are a number of image characteristics relating specifically to television systems which it is appropriate to describe:

22.3.1   *Resolution*

The unsharpness of the television system has a limiting effect on the spatial resolution of the fluoroscopic image.

22.3.1.1   Vertical resolution
Television image resolution is affected by the scanning pattern or raster employed. Domestic TV screens in the United Kingdom, and many television fluoroscopy systems, display an image consisting of 625 lines. In recent years the manufacturers of radiodiagnostic imaging equipment have developed **high-definition** television systems which employ 1249 or even more lines. The number of lines used sets a theoretical limit to the vertical resolution of the television image. There are a number of techniques for reducing the intrusiveness of the raster pattern, e.g. by deliberately defocusing the image, but there is no consequential increase in image resolution. Indeed, the resolution may be reduced as a result of such raster suppression (Cowen & Coleman, 1986).

22.3.1.2   Horizontal resolution
The horizontal resolution of the television image is limited by factors such as the frequency bandwidth of the video signal, but discussion of such technicalities is beyond the scope of this book (Gunn, 1994).

22.3.1.3   Electron beam focusing
TV image unsharpness, and therefore resolution, is also dependent on the focusing of the electron beam onto the image screen phosphor of the TV monitor. Focusing is often less effective towards the edges of the screen. Additionally, the electron beam tends to become progressively defocused as image brightness is increased because it is difficult to overcome the greater mutual repulsion between the more densely packed electrons in the beam. The image sharpness can thus be improved by reducing screen brightness on the television monitor.

22.3.2   *Noise*

As we saw in section 19.2.2.2, the output phosphor image of an image intensifier may exhibit quantum noise and structure mottle. The inherent unsharpness of the television system masks structure mottle, but quantum noise may be transmitted through to the final TV image.

22.3.2.1 Electronic noise

The television system itself may introduce an additional form of noise created during the process of electronic amplification of the weak video signal from the pick-up tube. This produces on the TV monitor screen a 'snowstorm' effect similar to quantum noise, which is more noticeable when the amplification factor (**gain**) is at its highest. Electronic noise is minimized by the use of high-quality, **low-noise** components in the television system.

22.3.3 Brightness

The terms luminance and brightness are often used when discussing this aspect of the television image. The terms are not synonymous.

Luminance is a physical measure of the light emitted per unit area from a surface. Its value is quoted in candela per square metre ($cd\,m^{-2}$) in SI units, or foot-lambert (ft L) in imperial units (Workman & Cowen, 1994).

Brightness describes the subjective effect of luminance.

Brightness control Television monitors have a brightness control with which the image screen luminance can be varied. When viewing a television image under different ambient lighting conditions, we adjust the screen luminance (with the brightness control) so that the image brightness appears the same, e.g.:

(1) When viewing in a darkened room the luminance can be reduced, yet the image appears acceptably bright;
(2) In strong daylight, when the background lighting is high, it is necessary to increase the luminance to provide adequate screen image brightness.

From our earlier discussion of the effect of luminance on electron beam focusing, we must conclude that optimum television image quality is obtained when the screen is viewed under conditions of reduced background illumination with the brightness control turned down. Note, however, that if the TV screen image is to be recorded photographically (**videofluorography**), there are other factors which may influence the brightness control setting (section 23.4.3).

22.3.4 Contrast

The contrast of the image on a television screen clearly depends on the contrast of the original image focused onto the signal plate of the pick-up tube. But contrast may also become altered within the television system itself. e.g.:

(1) Deliberately, by electronic manipulation of contrast;
(2) Incidentally, due to the inherent characteristics of the television system.

(1) Electronic control of contrast
Television monitors have a contrast control which permits adjustment of the screen image contrast. Altering the contrast control setting results in a corresponding change in the *spread* of luminance values between the brightest and the darkest parts of the screen image. Unfortunately, contrast adjustments cause a change in the *average* screen luminances as well as in the range of luminances, e.g. reducing

the contrast setting also causes a reduction in image brightness and a compensatory adjustment to the brightness control is required to maintain a satisfactory image.

(2) Inherent contrast characteristics

Little, if any, distortion of contrast occurs in television pick-up tubes unless they generate a **dark current**, which represents the production of a video signal from an unilluminated part of the target. Modern television systems have overcome the problem of dark current. Television monitors tend to exaggerate contrast due to the characteristics of the electron gun, but this increase in contrast tends to compensate for the deterioration in contrast that occurs when viewing conditions are poor (Hay, 1982).

Viewing conditions Television image contrast is greatly affected by the ambient lighting conditions. If some of the background illumination falls on the TV monitor screen it is reflected from its surface. Thus, when we view the screen we see not only light emitted by fluorescence from the screen phosphor but also ambient light reflected from the screen. This is particularly noticeable in the darkest parts of the image, where its effect is to increase luminance and therefore reduce overall contrast. This effect on contrast is similar in some respects to that of image fog on a radiograph (section 16.3).

It is difficult to believe, but nevertheless true, that those parts of a television image which appear black are in fact grey: exactly the same grey that the screen appears when the monitor is switched off.

During videofluorography the electronic contrast control provides a useful way of ensuring that the range of screen luminance values lies within the latitude of the film.

22.3.5   Image lag

Lag is the term used to describe the inability of an imaging system to follow rapid changes in its input image.

When a patient is being examined by fluoroscopy, the image produced is rarely static. Even if the patient is able to cooperate fully, there are respiratory movements and involuntary movements of organs such as the heart and gut to contend with. Thus, the imaging system is presented with a *moving* subject. Ideally, the television system should be capable of presenting the observer with a series of images in which rapid movements of the subject are reproduced equally rapidly in the image. In practice, lag is most likely to occur in the Vidicon type of pick-up tube. It results in unsharpness of rapidly moving parts of the image and can therefore lead to a reduction in image quality.

An incidental and beneficial consequence of lag is to reduce the effect on the screen image of the snowstorm appearance of X-ray quantum noise. The graininess of quantum noise is highly dynamic and the unsharpness induced by lag blurs out the effect of noise, at the same time increasing the signal-to-noise ratio.

22.3.6   Bloom, after-image and persistence

It is not uncommon while adjusting beam centring or collimation during fluoroscopy for the image field to extend beyond the edge of the patient, e.g. the lateral abdominal wall, such that the input phosphor of the image intensifier is subjected to the *unattenuated* X-ray beam. Momentarily, this creates an extremely bright image on the output phosphor until the automatic brightness control system compensates by reducing the X-ray exposure factors. The excessive image brightness may overload the television pick-up tube, causing an effect on the image known as **flare** or **bloom**. The pick-up tube may take a second or two to recover. In bad cases, a residual **after-image** may be 'burnt' into its target and remain on screen for several minutes. The retention of such an image on the target of the camera tube is known as **persistence**.

22.3.7 *Distortion*

As we explained in section 19.2.2.4, some distortion of the image may occur in the image intensifier or in the optical coupling system which links its output phosphor to the signal plate of the television pick-up tube. Additionally, the television system itself may introduce further distortion.

The convex shape of the television monitor image screen (Fig. 22.5) contributes to **barrel** distortion, which becomes more noticeable towards the edges of the screen (Fig. 20.15). Recent developments in television technology have allowed manufacturers to produce **flat-screen** cathode ray tubes, in which the convexity of the image screen is much less pronounced.

Distortion also occurs if the screen is viewed obliquely, but this is true of all two-dimensional images and is not a fault peculiar to television systems.

22.3.8 *Positive/negative image modes*

The image focused onto the signal plate of the pick-up tube from the image intensifier is a **positive** image, i.e. radiolucent structures appear bright while radiopaque structures are dark. This is the reverse of the appearance of the image on a radiograph. The television system can reproduce the image on its monitor screen in either the positive or negative mode merely by the pressing of a button or flicking of a switch. The fact that radiologists generally prefer the positive mode during fluoroscopy probably originates at least in part from pre-television days, when no negative fluoroscopic image was available.

22.3.9 *Image inversion and transposition*

Electronic manipulation of the image is not restricted to the positive/negative tone reversal described above. It is a simple matter also to **invert** the image (turn it upside down) or to **transpose** the image (produce a left-to-right reversal or mirror image). These facilities enable true anatomical viewing of the image to be achieved, no matter what the actual orientation of the patient. However, transposition of the image can sometimes lead to confusion in the mind of the observer and an anatomical marker may be required to eliminate doubt.

22.3.10 *Spectral emission*

The spectrum of light emitted from a television screen is determined by the nature of the phosphors employed. If the image is to be viewed by the human observer, phosphors emitting white light are chosen, e.g. P4 or P45 type. If the image is on a display monitor for videofluorographic recording purposes, a blue- (P11) or green- (P24 or P31) emitting phosphor is selected, to which the fluorographic film emulsion is spectrally matched (see also section 23.4.1.1). The spectral emission curves for these phosphors are illustrated in Fig. 22.8.

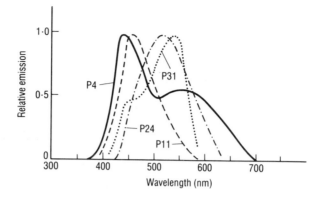

Fig. 22.8 Spectral emission curves for four screen phosphors: P4, P11, P24 and P31.

22.4   Digital television imaging

22.4.1   *Analogue signals*

The video signal generated by a television pick-up tube and fed to the TV monitor may be described as an **analogue signal**. The term is chosen because the variations in amplitude of the electrical video signal follow closely (i.e. are analogous to) the changes in luminance of the image on the pick-up tube signal plate. As the electron beam in the pick-up scans across each line of its raster, the video signal that it produces varies continuously in a way which mimics the changing luminance of corresponding parts of the image (see Fig. 22.9).

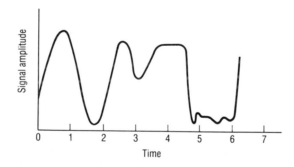

Fig. 22.9 The continuously varying amplitude of a video signal. This type of variation is characteristic of an *analogue* signal.

22.4.2   *Digital signals*

It is possible to convert the analogue video signal into **digital** form by analyzing the signal into a series of numerical values, each one representing the amplitude of the video signal at a particular instant (see Fig. 22.10). A scan line can then be visualized as a finite number of individual, discrete picture elements or **pixels** (see Fig. 22.11). The luminance of each pixel is represented by a **binary code** consisting of a short sequence of zeroes and ones, which can be translated into OFF or ON voltage pulses capable of being passed along a conducting wire (Pizzutiello &

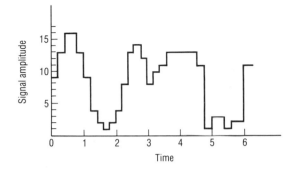

Fig. 22.10 The 'stepped' variations of a digital signal derived from the analogue signal of Fig. 22.9. Five samples of signal amplitude have been taken for each unit of time on the horizontal scale. The vertical scale has been analysed into sixteen discrete values. The analogue to digital conversion has resulted in loss of the finer details of the original signal because of the coarseness of the conversion.

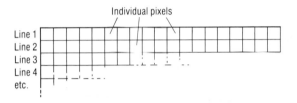

Fig. 22.11 Digitized picture information showing each scan line formed from a number of discrete picture elements (pixels). In the diagram there are 19 pixels per line. In reality there may be 512 or more pixels per line.

Cullinan, 1993). For example, an **eight-bit code** consisting of sequences (**bytes**) of eight binary digits (**bits**) provides $2^8 (= 256)$ different numerical values. This offers the possibility of producing an image containing up to 256 luminances or grey tones, including black and white, i.e. a **grey scale** of 256. Binary codes based on more than eight bit sequences permit an even wider range of values to be represented, e.g. a 12-bit code can represent 4096 (2^{12}) different numbers.

The process of digitization could lead to reduced horizontal resolution of the image compared with the original analogue signal, but the loss is minimized by increasing the frequency of sampling, thus maximizing the number of pixels per line. A typical arrangement is to have 256 (or 512) pixels per line, combined with 256 (or 512) lines, giving a matrix of 256 × 256 (or 512 × 512) pixels. Even the 512 × 512 matrix gives an image which is of lower spatial resolution than that of a traditional analogue system, but the advantages offered by computer image processing may outweigh such a drawback.

The conversation of an original analogue video signal into its digital counterpart is undertaken by an **analogue-to-digital converter** (ADC). The digital signals produced are accepted readily by digital computers, enabling image data to be computer processed. The cathode ray tube of a television monitor cannot accept digital information directly. It is therefore necessary to transform the digital signal back into an analogue form before feeding it into the monitor. A **digital-to-analogue converter** carries out this task, but on the monitor screen each line of the image is formed from individual pixels rather than being a continuous line.

Close examination of the television screen may enable an analogue image to be differentiated from a digital image by the presence of discrete pixels in the latter.

22.4.3   *Image processing*

Computerized image processing is a method by which the detectability of features of interest in an image can be improved. The digital computer carries out two main forms of image processing (Chesters, 1982).

(1) Image enhancement
There are many ways in which digital image processing can be used to enhance an image, but we shall describe here just one aspect: the manipulation of image contrast by control of window width and window level.

Window width (WW) control selects the *width* of the band of luminance values in the digital signal which are to be represented as a full range of perhaps 256 grey tones in the final image, e.g. the operator could choose the complete range of (say) 512 values to be represented (WW = 512) or restrict the range to (say) 128 values (WW = 128) (see Fig. 22.12). Window width control provides a means of compressing or expanding image contrast.

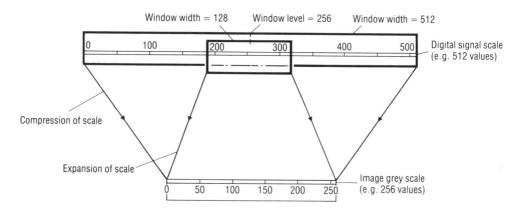

Fig. 22.12 Window width. A window-width of 512 enables a range of 512 digital values to be compressed into an image grey scale of 256 values. The compression involves some loss of information. A window width of 128 allows the 128 digital values inside the window to be expanded onto the 256 grey scale. Digital values outside the window are imaged as black or white.

Window level (WL) control selects the *level* of the displayed band of values within the complete range, e.g. having selected a window-width of 128 the operator could position it to run from 0 to 128 (WL = 64), 192 to 320 (WL = 256) or 351 to 479 (WL = 415) (see Fig. 22.13). Window level control enables the observer to investigate the effects of contrast manipulation on different parts of the image in order to optimize the recovery of diagnostic information.

(2) Image restoration
This is a method of reconstructing an image to correct the degradation (e.g. vignetting) that may have occurred as part of the image-forming process.

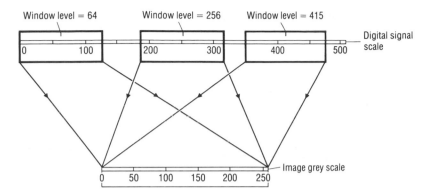

Fig. 22.13 Window-level. Adjustment of window-level allows different sections of the digital signal scale to be displayed, in turn on the 256 grey scale. In the case shown, the same window width (128) has been used, but window levels of 64, 256 and 415 have been selected.

22.4.4 Display of digital images

22.4.4.1 Grey-scale images

Digitally generated images are usually displayed on the cathode ray tube of a television monitor or visual display unit (VDU) as monochrome grey-scale images, in which each pixel is capable of reproducing a range of luminances. The images associated with diagnostic techniques such as ultrasonography, computerized tomography (CT), magnetic resonance imaging (MRI) and digital subtraction imaging (DSI) are all of this type.

22.4.4.2 Bistable images

The images produced during radionuclide imaging (RNI) are rather different. Pixels in the image demonstrate whether or not a γ-ray photon has been detected: each pixel therefore has only two states represented by two luminances: it is either ON (white) or OFF (black). The image thus formed is said to be **bistable**, consisting of black and white with no intermediate grey tones. If the image is to be photographically recorded, its high contrast may demand film emulsion characteristics which are different from those required for recording a grey-scale image (see section 28.8.2.1).

22.4.4.3 Spectral emission characteristics

The cathode ray tube images that we have described can either be observed directly or they may be photographically recorded. Screen phosphors with appropriate spectral emission characteristics must be selected. As we described in section 22.3.10, for direct observation a white-emitting phosphor might be chosen, e.g. a P4 phosphor. For photographic purposes, a blue- (P11) or green- (P24 or P31) emitter is more suitable (see Fig. 22.8).

22.4.4.4 Colour images

The human eye can distinguish only about 100 different tones of grey. However, a diagnostic image such as a CT scan may carry up to 2000 tonal values, most of which would be lost to the observer if presented as a single monochrome image (Chesters, 1982). A possible solution is to use the window width and window level controls to produce a number of images, each one displaying only a part of the full range of grey tones, but which together enable the whole tonal range to be appreciated. A second solution is to use a full colour display. MacAdam (1942) showed that the eye is able to distinguish about 20 000 different shades of colour, thus if tonal values are represented as a range of colours rather than as a grey scale it is possible to present all of the information in a single image. Such colour images are spectacular but it is a matter for debate as to whether the observer is capable of absorbing such a vast quantity of data.

The use of television in conjunction with electronic image intensification revolutionized fluoroscopic procedures from the 1960s onwards. But only since the advent in the 1980s of high-resolution television imaging has the **recording** of television images played a major role. Digital images presented on the screen of a cathode ray tube have rapidly gained in importance since the early 1970s, with the development of computerized tomography and other digital techniques. In the next chapter, we examine the various methods available for making a permanent record of the television or cathode ray tube image.

Chapter 23
Recording the Television Image

In Chapter 21 we examined those methods by which the image appearing on the output phosphor of an image intensifier tube may be recorded. In this chapter we will look at methods of image recording which take place at a point after a TV pick-up tube has been involved in the imaging process.

The imaging methods available are:

(1) Video tape recorder (VTR);
(2) Laser imager.
(3) CRT camera (polaroid or multi-imager);
(4) Video imager or multiformatter;
(5) Dry silver imager.

23.1 The videotape recorder

In the same way as an audiotape recorder is able to record sounds on tape, so a videotape recorder (VTR) is able to record images – in the form of magnetic impulses on magnetic tape. A typical VTR for use in a medical imaging department is illustrated in Fig. 23.1.

In order to explain how these images are recorded we shall look at just three of the principal components of a VTR.

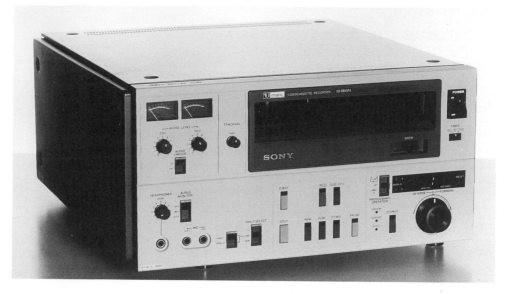

Fig. 23.1 A Sony U-matic videotape recorder. Tape width is 20 mm in contradistinction to domestic VHS format which employs 13 mm tape.

Magnetic tape

Video recording tape is made of plastic and coated with chrome or ferric oxide. It is available in a range of widths, depending on the type of VTR in use. The ordinary domestic VTR uses a 13 mm ($\frac{1}{2}''$) tape, whilst the type of professional model used in medical imaging and illustrated in Fig. 23.2 employs 20 mm ($\frac{3}{4}''$) tape.

The tape is normally held within a protective case or cassette, which contains a supply spool and a take-up spool (Fig. 23.2). When the cassette is inserted into the VTR, a loop of tape is automatically extracted, 'laced' through a system of tensioning rollers and around the recording head–drum assembly ready for use.

Just as with audiotape, videotape may be used for re-recording over and over again.

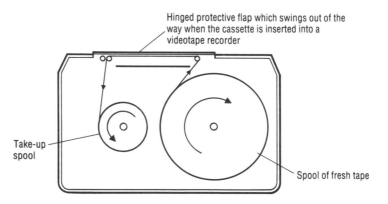

Fig. 23.2 A Sony U-matic videotape cassette. The tape runs from right to left unlike the domestic VHS format where the tape runs from left to right.

The video recording head(s)
A video recording head (Fig. 23.3) has two functions:

- To transfer the incoming video signal onto tape;
- To 'read' the tape on playback and reproduce the same signal.

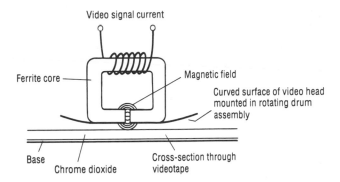

Fig. 23.3 A video recording head. A varying magnetic field is produced across the gap in the head in response to the varying video signal current.

To understand how the head is able to accomplish these tasks we need first to examine its construction. The head comprises a ferrous core around which is wound a coil of wire. A varying video signal is fed from the TV pick-up tube to the coil, producing a varying magnetic field which is concentrated across the gap in the core. The plastic recording tape which passes beneath this gap has a coating comprising millions of particles which can be thought of as potential bar magnets. In their 'normal', unmagnetized state they lie in a random fashion with their axes in all directions (Fig. 23.4(a)). As the tape passes over the recording head during a recording, they become magnetized, aligning themselves in the same direction as the fluctuating magnetic field, the degree of alignment being dependent upon the strength of the field (Fig. 23.4(b)).

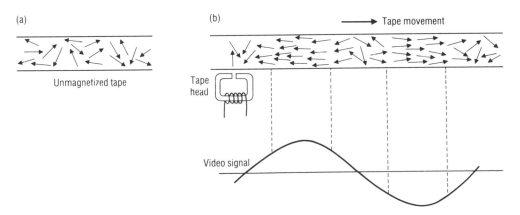

Fig. 23.4 (a) The tape is unmagnetized and the particles of the tape coating lie in a random fashion. (b) The tape head is receiving a varying video signal and this is personified in the way in which the now magnetized particles adopt a position first in one direction, then in the opposite direction. In addition, the degree of alignment achieved by the particles is indicative of the strength of the original field.

During playback, the movement of the magnetized tape across the same recording head is sufficient to produce a varying magnetic field within the core. The lines of force 'cut' the coil, so inducing a varying voltage across the coil. These electrical signals are fed to the grid of a cathode ray tube (section 22.1.1.3).

The recording heads, usually two, are mounted at about 180° to each other within a rotating drum assembly. The recording tape passes around the drum, which is tilted in relation to the tape (Fig. 23.5).

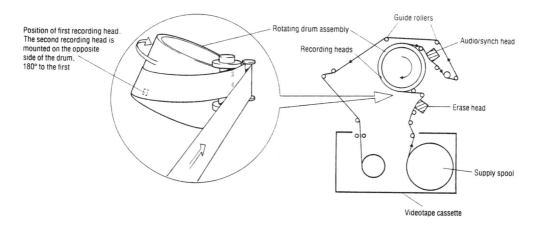

Fig. 23.5 The configuration of tape to head accounts for the slanting video tracks, seen in Fig. 23.6.

Combined audio/sync head

This module consists of two sections, an upper control or sync track section, and below, twin audio heads mounted one above the other. They produce the track recording patterns seen in Fig. 23.6.

The function of the control/sync track is to synchronize the recording head with the recorded track during playback. We shall refer to this again later when examining the way in which a video recording is made.

The paired audio heads provide two audio tracks, thus permitting, if required, a simultaneous recording of the radiologist's commentary as well as the patient's heart sounds for example.

23.1.1 *Video recording*

Those of you who listen to Hi–Fi audio recording will appreciate that the faster the tape speed, the better the recording of high frequencies. The greater the amount of information that one wishes to put on tape (i.e. the greater the frequency), the faster the tape must pass over the head. An analogy is that of a typewriter, where in order for the letters to remain separate on the page the carriage must move in relation to the typist's speed. The faster the input of characters, the faster the carriage has to move.

In our video recorder this problem becomes apparent when you consider how fast the tape would need to pass over the tape head in order to record a video signal

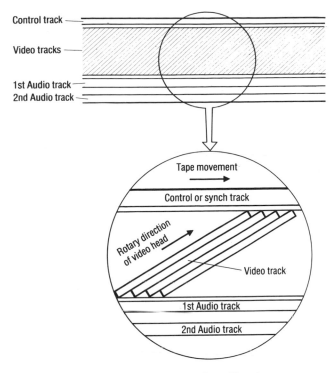

Fig. 23.6 The pattern of the various track recordings made on U-matic tape.

(5 000 000 Hz), as opposed, say, to an audio recording of middle C on the piano (256 Hz).

There are two solutions, either moving the tape faster or moving the tape heads. The former is not practical since only 5 min of recording would require nearly a mile of tape! The latter is the method adopted. The drum assembly containing the two video heads is made to rotate at 1500 rpm whilst the tape moves in the same direction at a more modest 9.53 cm/s. This provides an effective tape-to-head speed of > 8 m/s!

This is not the whole story, since the method just described would still be wasteful in terms of the length of tape required. The answer is to have the tape travel diagonally around the drum. The result is that the recorded tracks are at an angle to the long axis of the tape (Figs 23.5 and 23.6). Such a configuration ensures that more information is recorded per length of tape than would be the case if the recorded track ran parallel with the tape edge. This type of recording is known as **helical scanning**, since the tape follows a helical or spiral course around the drum.

Each pair of recorded tracks represent one frame or 625 lines of TV image. One of the video heads 'writes' one field ($312\frac{1}{2}$ lines), whilst the second head following behind compiles a 'frame' by 'writing' the other $312\frac{1}{2}$ lines.

Besides the video and audio tracks, there is a 'control' or 'sync pulse' track which is recorded at the same time as the others and which we mentioned previously. The function of this control track is to provide a reference for the recording head–drum assembly during playback and so enable each of the video recording heads to line up precisely with the individual video tracks for which they had originally been responsible for 'writing'.

23.1.1.1   Advantages of VTR over cineradiography

(1) Immediate playback.

(2) No processing required.

(3) No special projection equipment needed.

(4) The tape is reusable.

(5) Contrast and brightness are adjustable on the TV monitor during playback.

(6) Sophisticated 'search' and replay facilities exist on the higher priced 'professional' VTRs, which enable the operator to find any part of the recording quickly and easily. In addition, the VTR can be programmed to replay continuously a particular recorded sequence, a facility very useful for teaching purposes.

(7) The radiation dose involved in producing a videotape recording is less than that required in cinefluorography. This is because the same radiation exposure required to produce a picture for viewing on the monitor simultaneously produces a video recording. Cine recording requires a quite separate exposure to that being used to produce a monitor image.

The dose rate with cine recording is approximately 0.1–0.4 mGy per frame, whereas with video recording it is only 0.25–1.0 mGy/s. So if we compare a 10 s cine run (on a pulsed cine unit) at a framing rate of 25 fps (and dose rate of 0.4 mGy per frame) with a 10 s video sequence (and dose rate 1.0 mGy/s) we find the following:

$$\text{Cine for } 10 \text{ s} = 100 \text{ mGy}$$
$$\text{Video for } 10 \text{ s} = 10 \text{ mGy}$$

The cine dose rate is ten times higher!

23.1.1.2   Disadvantages

Even with the best VTRs, some disadvantages still remain.

(1) Image resolution is inferior to that recorded on film. With cine recording the image is taken directly from the output phosphor of the image intensifier. The VTR image, however, is made up of many scanning lines due to the involvement of the TV pick-up tube. The vertical resolution, as it is called (section 22.3.1.1), is therefore dependent upon the number of scanning lines of which the image is composed. The greater the number of lines, the better the resolution. However, with 1249 line TV systems (instead of 625 lines), this disparity between video and cine is negligible.

(2) The quality of 'still' frame viewing, particularly on the cheaper domestic type VTRs, can be very poor due to the inability of the video head to retrace precisely the original track when the tape is stationary. Instead, the head may cross over to 'read' part of an adjacent recorded track (Fig. 23.7). Secondly, because the tape is stationary and the video heads are rotating, both video heads are reading the same track. So, whilst the one head originally responsible for that track is making a real contribution, i.e. reading one half-frame ($312\frac{1}{2}$ lines), the other is merely replaying noise.

(3) If a great deal of 'still' frame playback is used, then tape/head wear may become a problem.

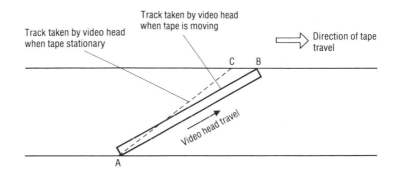

Track taken by video head when tape is moving

Track taken by video head when tape stationary

Direction of tape travel

C   B

Video head travel

A

Fig. 23.7 One reason for poor quality still frame images. A–B is the video track created during a video recording. However, when still-frame playback is selected, the tape will be stationary and the video head will travel along line A–C instead of A–B. This discrepancy occurs because during recording the tape will have moved a distance of C–B during the time it takes the head to travel from A–B. So the path followed by the head during recording is longer than it will be when the tape is stationary. This inability of the tape head to follow exactly the original track and its encroachment on an adjacent track results in a band of noise across the image.

23.2 The laser imager

The laser imager (Fig. 23.8) provides a hard-copy image by using the infrared beam from a laser to expose the film.

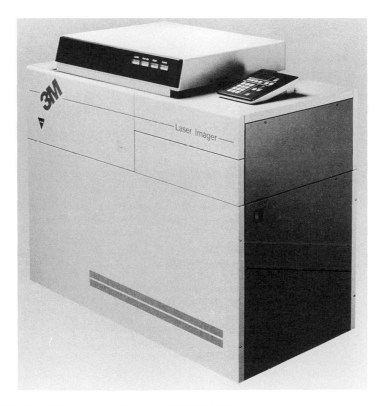

Fig. 23.8 The 3M laser imager. (Courtesy of 3M UK Ltd.)

The unit may be connected to several imaging modalities simultaneously, such as computerized tomography, magnetic resonance imaging, digital fluoroscopy and computed radiography to provide one common source of hard-copy images (Fig. 23.9). This avoids the expense of providing various imagers for each modality.

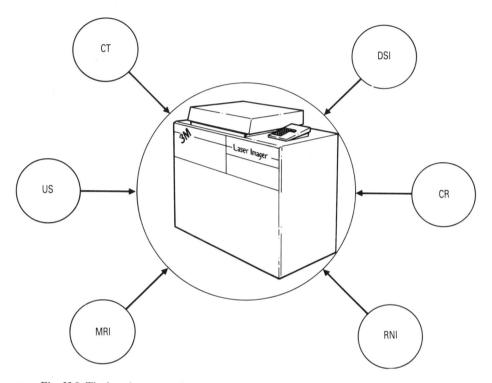

Fig. 23.9 The laser imager may be connected to several imaging modalities.

23.2.1 Imager construction

The imager in Fig. 23.8 comprises a film-supply magazine capable of holding 125 35 × 43 cm films at one end, a middle 'staging' and exposure section, and a film take-up magazine at the opposite end (Fig. 23.10).

Instead of using the take-up magazine, the imager may be connected via a 'docking' unit to an automatic processor, thus providing a full daylight processing facility.

The laser used in the 3M imager is a solid–state diode emitting an infrared beam with a wavelength of 850 nm. A sophisticated optical system, comprising lenses and polygonal mirror, focuses and moves the laser beam across the film during the scanning sequence.

A control panel on the front of the imager and an operator's key pad enable a range of operating functions to be selected, as we shall see later. The key pad may be used remotely.

23.2.2 The laser imager in use

The radiographer working at a computerized tomography console, for example,

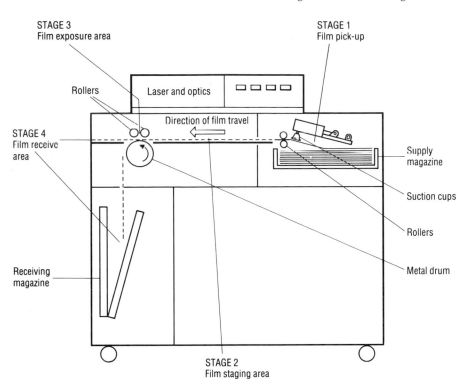

STAGE 3
Film exposure area

STAGE 1
Film pick-up

Rollers

Laser and optics

Direction of film travel

STAGE 4
Film receive
area

Supply
magazine

Suction cups

Rollers

Receiving
magazine

Metal drum

STAGE 2
Film staging area

Fig. 23.10 The 3M laser imager. (Courtesy 3M UK Ltd.)

selects those images required for recording on film. Using the special key pad provided, the chosen images are relayed in the form of a video signal to an analogue-to-digital converter within the imager. Up to 12 digitized images (512×512 matrix) may be stored in the imager's internal memory. (This memory capacity may be expanded if required.)

The images selected can be arranged in any position on the film at the discretion of the radiographer. Once this formatting has been chosen, a print can be obtained simply by pressing the 'print' button on the key pad. This initiates the following sequence of events.

A film is conveyed to the middle 'staging' area, automatically checked for correct alignment and then advanced into the exposure area. In this position, it is scanned by the laser in a direction at right angles to the line of film travel (Fig. 23.11).

In just the same way as an electron beam inside a cathode ray tube (CRT) produces an image on its screen phosphor, so the laser beam produces a latent image on the film in response to a similar input signal. In other words, the intensity of the laser beam varies (modulates) in proportion to the intensity of signal being received by the memory store. In this way, the various densities which go to make up the eventual image are determined.

The laser beam scans the film at a rapid 600 lines/s. The scanning motion is achieved by focusing the laser beam onto a rotating polygonal mirror, which thus provides a continuously changing angle of reflection (Fig. 23.11), whilst at the same time moving the film perpendicular to the direction of scanning.

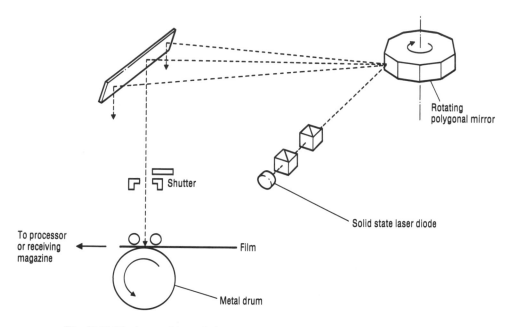

Fig. 23.11 The laser and its optical system.

The whole sequence – from supply to take-up magazine – takes only 23 s (the printing cycle takes only 8.5 s).

23.2.3   *Why a laser?*

There are three principal advantages of using a laser beam rather than a conventional light spot to put the image on to the film:

● The light is of one wavelength;
● The light beam is parallel and not divergent;
● The light is of high intensity.

These features mean that a very sharp, intense point of light no greater than 85 μm can be used to scan the film (equivalent to 11.8 spots of light/mm!). On a 35 × 43 cm film, this means that the image comprises 4000 × 5000 light spots or pixels, which results in an image of very high resolution.

In addition, because laser light is naturally parallel, a less complex optical system is required to focus the beam onto the film than would be the case with ordinary light, with its divergent characteristic.

The laser imager illustrated in Fig. 23.8 uses a solid-state laser with a pure infrared emission of 850 nm. (The laser has an expected life span of 770 years!)

23.2.4   *The film*

The film used is 35 × 43 cm, single-sided, with an infrared sensitive emulsion to match the 850 nm laser emission. A graph of the film's spectral sensitivity may be seen in Fig. 23.12.

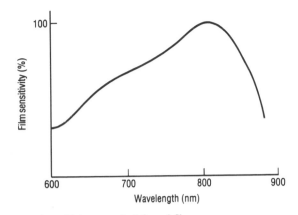

Fig. 23.12 The spectral sensitivity curve for infra-red film.

The notch in the film is used by the imager to check mechanically the film for perfect alignment as it passes through the 'staging' area.

The film can be processed using the same chemistry as for conventional radiographic films and with a standard 90 s processing cycle. However, because of its extended spectral sensitivity, infrared film should be handled either in complete darkness or with a green filter over the safelight, e.g. the Kodak No. 7 filter.

23.2.5 *Advantages of using a laser imager*

There are many advantages associated with the use of a laser imager:

(1) Very-high-resolution images: the images produced have 20 times the resolution of a 1000 line cathode ray tube (CRT). In addition, there is no phosphor noise or lens distortion to mar image quality, so the images are much sharper than those obtained from photography of a cathode ray tube.

(2) Improved grey scale: each 35×43 cm image produced by the 3M laser imager contains 4000×5000 pixels, with each capable of recording any one of 256 shades of grey. But note the reservation in section 23.4.5.

(3) Less image distortion: image magnification is done electronically, so avoiding the distortion that can occur with optical systems.

(4) Choice of format: 1, 2, 4, 6, 9, 12, 15 or 20 images on one film.

(5) Images may be placed in any preferred position on the film.

(6) Choice of positive or negative image.

(7) Choice of clear or black borders to the film. A black border can help to minimize glare from the illuminator when the film is being viewed.

(8) The imager can be interfaced with several imaging modalities (e.g. ultrasound, computerized tomography, magnetic resonance, radionuclide imaging, etc.) at any one time, so obviating the need for separate imagers for each modality.

(9) The unit can be controlled remotely: the selection of images to be stored in the equipment's memory and the initiation of a hard-copy print are all controlled from a key pad in the imaging room.

(10) Any number of identical copies may be made rapidly and without any variation in image quality.

(11) The imager is self-monitoring, so that any equipment fault may be identified and corrected quickly.

(12) No cassettes to insert every time a film is required.

(13) The imager may be linked directly to an automatic processor.

23.3   CRT cameras

CRT cameras basically consist of a single lens connected via a custom-designed mount to the CRT screen, and a rear component known as a multi-imaging back designed to take a specific size and type of film (Fig. 23.13).

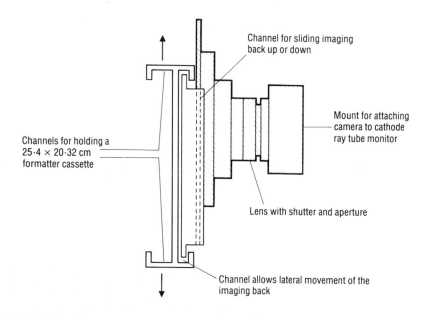

Channel for sliding imaging back up or down

Mount for attaching camera to cathode ray tube monitor

Channels for holding a 25·4 × 20·32 cm formatter cassette

Lens with shutter and aperture

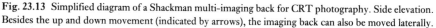

Channel allows lateral movement of the imaging back

Fig. 23.13 Simplified diagram of a Shackman multi-imaging back for CRT photography. Side elevation. Besides the up and down movement (indicated by arrows), the imaging back can also be moved laterally.

Just as with any camera, there is an aperture and shutter control facility present, although in some of them there may be a fairly limited range of apertures ('*f* stops') and speeds available.

They are commonly identified by the type of 'back' or film-holder employed at the rear of the camera, i.e. Polaroid, Shackman, etc. In the case of the 'Shackman' back, a 25.4 × 20.32 cm (10 × 8″) cassette (Fig. 23.13) is mounted inside a framework which can be moved up or down and side to side by the operator to obtain up to six images on the one film.

The camera lens

This is usually of fixed focal length. When the camera is initially set up, the lens is focused on a ground-glass screen positioned in place of the CRT. Once this has been done, the glass screen is removed and the camera is ready for use.

Aperture

Typical aperture sizes vary from $f1.9$ to $f11$. Remember that the smaller the 'f' number, the larger the aperture (section 20.2.5). However, the larger the aperture, the more critical the focusing needs to be, and vice versa. An aperture of $f8$ or $f11$ is ideal.

Exposure time

The aperture size (or f number) that we select will have a bearing on the exposure time needed, since total film exposure depends on aperture *and* exposure time.

In the UK there is one TV frame (625 lines) displayed every 1/25th of a second, therefore photography of a TV image will necessitate an exposure time longer than 1/25th of a second or otherwise only part of the TV picture will be captured! Suitable speed settings are 1/8th or 1/15th of a second.

A shutter-release cable is usually provided to help make the exposure, since finger pressure on an exposure button may cause movement between the camera body and the CRT, with consequent image unsharpness.

23.4 Video imagers or multiformatters

Video imaging cameras are variously described as **video imagers, hard-copy units** or in some cases **multiformatters** which enable several images to be recorded on a single sheet of film (Fig. 23.14). They are available from a number of manufacturers and in a wide range of designs and models. The more expensive models offer high-quality images, accept a variety of film sizes and offer many image formats. The cheaper models may still provide high-quality results but with less flexibility of film size and image format.

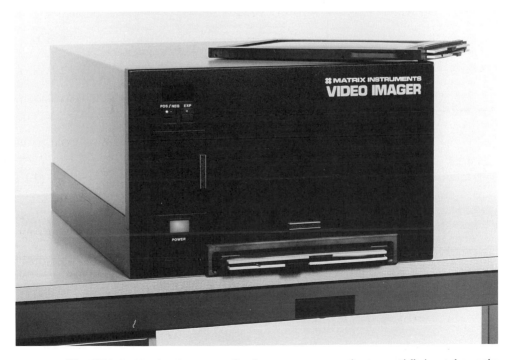

Fig. 23.14 A video imaging camera. One formatter cassette can be seen partially inserted near the bottom of the imager, while a second rests on the top.

23.4.1   *Design features*

Automated self-contained video imagers consist of a number of essential features:

(1) Cathode ray tube;
(2) Optical system;
(3) Film platform;
(4) Control system and electronics; and in many cases an additional feature;
(5) Multiformat option.

There are many designs of video imager but a typical arrangement is illustrated in Fig. 23.15.

We shall examine each of the design features in more detail (Cowen & Coleman, 1986).

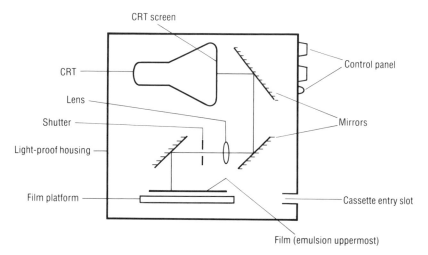

Fig. 23.15 Video imaging camera. In this example the film platform is in the base of the unit and the optical system consists of one lens and three mirrors.

23.4.1.1   Cathode ray tube

We discussed the principles of operation of cathode ray tubes in section 22.1.1.3 but there are a few points which are particularly relevant here.

Raster pattern

With any CRT imaging camera system, the CRT screen display must be of very high quality and high resolution. Typically, a basic raster pattern of 625 (or 1249) lines is employed, but in the high-technology video imagers currently under discussion a system of **multiple interlacing** may be offered to suppress the intrusive appearance of the raster scan-lines. With this facility the position on screen of the raster scan-lines is displaced slightly in successive image fields. The cumulative effect after a number of fields have been displayed is to reduce the spaces between lines to a point where they are no longer perceptible. After two, or sometimes four successive fields the scan lines return to their original positions and the cycle is repeated.

Screen size

The CRT screen is of the **flat-face** design to avoid the problems of **barrel distortion** associated with a curved screen. It has a diameter of 15–17 cm, although typically only a 12 cm diameter central region of the image, where electron beam focusing is at its optimum, is actually recorded on film. This ensures that image distortion and unsharpness are minimal.

Brightness and contrast

The **brightness** and **contrast** of the CRT image may be controlled to obtain optimum image quality. Conventional television monitors and domestic TV receivers have brightness and contrast controls that are interactive e.g. adjustment of the contrast control affects image brightness as well as contrast. Some video imagers offer truly independent control, where adjustment of one parameter has no effect on the other. In general, sharper images are obtained if brightness and contrast are not excessive (see section 22.3.1.3).

Spectral emission

Screen phosphors are commonly of the P11 (blue) or P45 (blue-green, often known as 'white') types, intended for use with monochromatic or orthochromatic films.

Accessibility

The image screen of the CRT carries an electrostatic charge which causes it to attract dust particles. The screen should therefore be accessible for cleaning purposes, to prevent the dust from producing artefacts on the recorded image.

23.4.1.2 Optical system

The CRT image is focused onto the photosensitive film by means of a high-quality optical system using lenses and mirrors (Fig. 23.15). The design of the optics varies between different models, e.g. one manufacturer offers a system with a single lens and three mirrors, another design has no mirrors, while yet others employ a multiple lens array with four, six or even nine lenses to allow multiformatting. One or more mechanical exposure shutters are incorporated into some optical systems, while others use an electronic shutter.

Whichever system is employed it should preferably be free from aberrations, vignetting and distortion (see Chapter 20), although sophisticated units provide a degree of automatic electronic compensation in the CRT for some of these optical defects.

Over a period of time the surfaces of optical components collect dust, which may degrade image quality. The lenses and mirrors (if present) should be accessible for cleaning when required.

23.4.1.3 Film platform

Sheet film is the most popular type of photographic material used, but at least one manufacturer offers a camera which accepts roll film. Sheet film is inserted into the imaging camera via a specially designed cassette. Once the cassette slide is removed, the film is held ready for exposure using the cassette as a supporting platform. The cassette may be movable, allowing different sections of the film to be exposed sequentially in a multiformat mode. Roll film is fed from a supply spool through an exposure area or **gate** onto a take-up spool. A guillotine enables the exposed film in its take-up spool to be cut and removed from the imager, ready for processing. The use of roll film avoids the need for frequent loading of film cassettes into the imager.

Dust is often inadvertently carried into the camera on the film or cassette. It is therefore desirable that the film platform be situated *below* the optical system and the CRT screen so that dust cannot fall onto any of these components.

Both sheet and roll films are available in a wide range of different sizes, using both metric and imperial measurements: e.g. 8 × 10″, 18 × 24 cm and 11 × 14″ sheet films, and 70 mm, 105 mm and 8″ roll films. Some imagers are available in versions which can accept more than one film size.

23.4.1.4 Control system and electronics

Apart from the electronic system which generates and monitors the CRT raster, modern video imagers employ microprocessor control of various functions, such as:

(1) Automatic exposure control;
(2) Contrast and brightness adjustment (see below);
(3) Selection of white-on-black or black-on-white CRT images;
(4) Self monitoring; any faults are immediately identified by an LED displayed code;
  and with multiformatters:
(5) Automatic image advance and thus prevention of double exposure on the same part of the film;
(6) LED displays such as those showing the number of exposures made.

Brightness and contrast controls

Brightness and contrast settings are controlled through the microprocessor. The settings for an ultrasound image are likely to be quite different from those required for a gamma camera image because the basic characteristics of the two images are so different (see section 28.8.2.1). Film characteristics also vary and may require different settings to be selected, e.g. a high-contrast film is likely to require a lower contrast setting on the CRT than would a low-contrast film. On some imaging cameras, the settings appropriate to a particular type of image or film may be stored in memory and recalled at will. This avoids the need to set up the CRT controls from scratch each time the imager is switched from (say) computed tomography to radionuclide imaging.

Exposure timing

A third control that is necessary is exposure time: the length of time for which the film is exposed to the light from the CRT screen. In general, longer exposure times are used than are found in conventional radiography. It is usually preferable to select a long exposure time and a reduced brightness setting rather than a short time and increased brightness, since excessive brightness leads to a loss of sharpness in the CRT image. Exposure timing may be achieved either by the opening of a mechanical shutter for a predetermined time or by displaying a specific number of complete television image frames on the CRT screen (e.g. 50 frames).

23.4.1.5 Multiformatting facility

The multiformatting option is a feature of most modern video imagers. It enables the user to record a sequence of images, juxtaposed on a single sheet of film, e.g. a sheet of 8 × 10″ film may be used to record either a single image occupying its entire area or 2, 4, 6, 9, 12, 16 or even 25 separate miniature images (Fig. 23.16). The optical system must be able to adjust the image size to match the film area available.

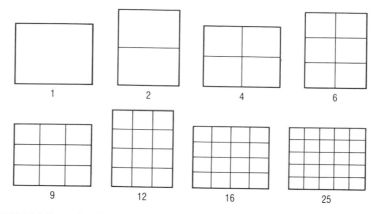

Fig. 23.16 Multiformatting. The diagram shows how an 8 × 10″ film can be formatted to record 1, 2, 4, 6, 9, 12, 16 or 25 images.

Several different methods are used by the manufacturers to achieve multi-formatting, e.g.:

(1) The CRT and optical system may be fixed while the film platform is moved to bring the appropriate section of film into the exposure frame. An advantage of this method is that the axis of the optical system can be maintained in line with the centre of the CRT screen.
(2) The CRT may be fixed but two or more off-axis optical systems are provided, each able to project an image onto a different part of the film. The film platform may also be moveable, thus increasing the variety of formats available. A possible drawback of this multiple lens array is that the off-axis optical arrangement makes image distortion more likely.
(3) The CRT and optical system may be moveable, possibly in conjunction with a movable film platform. If the CRT and optical system move as a single unit, the advantage of in-line optics is retained.
(4) The image may be displayed in different positions and in different sizes on the CRT screen. This eliminates the need for complex mechanical transport systems and adjustable optical components and may perhaps offer greater reliability, but image resolution may be reduced.

23.4.2 *Benefits of using a multiformat video imager*

Compared with the CRT camera discussed in section 23.3, a video imager offers the advantages of:

(1) Greater choice of image format;
(2) Automatic exposure control;
(3) CRT-settings memory;
(4) Automatic image advance;
(5) Double exposure prevention;
(6) Ease of use.

23.4.3 *Setting up the CRT display*

Whenever a new multi-imager is installed in a medical imaging department or a change is made in the type of CRT film or imaging modality being used with it, a check should be made to ensure that satisfactory film images are being obtained.

This is not an easy matter since judgement is to some extent dependent upon the personal preference of the radiographer or radiologist who regularly views those films, and this can vary from one individual to the next.

The objective in any adjustment exercise is to set the monitor's contrast, brightness and exposure time controls so that all of the important clinical information seen on the monitor screen is recorded within the straight-line portion of the film's characteristic curve.

On installation an engineer will first use an electronically generated grey-scale image to help adjust the monitor, and later take some more familiar clinical images for the user to look at. Some fine adjustments can then be made, if required, to suit the personal preferences of the radiographer or radiologist.

Effect of brightness adjustment Increasing the monitor's brightness has the effect of increasing all film densities, but particularly those at the lower end of the characteristic curve. Reducing monitor brightness lowers the overall density of the film image.

Effect of contrast adjustment Increasing the monitor's contrast primarily affects the maximum density of the film image. Such control has proportionately less effect on the minimum density. Reducing monitor contrast reduces the film density in the darker regions of the image.

Effect of exposure time adjustment Increasing the duration of the film's exposure to the monitor image produces an overall increase in all densities, and vice versa.

On some video imagers, brightness and contrast controls are *not* independent of each other. Altering one has an effect on the other and this makes monitor adjustment that much more difficult. Add to that the fact that different imagers vary in the degree to which one control affects another, and you can appreciate that it is impossible to lay down strict guidelines that are applicable to all types of video imager.

The description that follows, while based on the setting-up procedure for one particular imager, demonstrates principles which are widely applicable.

23.4.4 *Procedure for monitor adjustment*

Remember! There are three parameters:

- Contrast;
- Brightness;
- Exposure time.

Change only *one* parameter at a time!

(1) Make a note of the present parameter settings and expose a film (e.g. $8 \times 10''$) with these factors. This will be known as the **control** film.
(2) Set contrast on a low setting and make a series of exposures with different brightness factors. Ensure that each image can be identified, along with its respective factors.

(3) Examine the images and select one where minimum density is approximately gross fog + 0.10. Note the brightness setting responsible for this image.
(4) Keeping the above brightness setting, make a series of exposures with a variety of contrast settings. Ensure once again that each image or frame can be identified with its respective factors.
(5) Examine the images produced and select the frame that produced a maximum density of around 1.6.
(6) Using these new settings, produce one 8 × 10″ film and compare it with the control image.
(7) If satisfactory, write on the film the parameter settings used and retain for future reference.

23.4.5 *Laser imager or video imager?*

The decision whether to purchase a laser imager or a video imager is not an easy one to make. Image resolution is one important consideration.

As we have seen, the **laser imager** (section 23.2) is also capable of producing multiformat images from a video signal. The laser imager employs a fixed number of scan lines to cover the complete film area. If a single full-sized image is recorded, the resulting resolution is very high. However, if a multiformat mode of (say) 20 images is used, each individual image is produced from less than one-quarter of the total number of scan lines and resolution is reduced.

In the case of most video imagers, each image is formed from the same number of scan lines, whatever the type of formatting used. For example, in the 25 image, multiformat mode, each individual small image is recorded using the same number of scan lines as is used for a single, full-sized image. In video imagers it is the optical system rather than the television raster that produces variations in resolution between different image sizes.

At present, therefore, the advantage in image resolution of laser imagers over video imagers is most pronounced when a single image or a small number of images are recorded on one film. Moreover the time taken to expose the film in a laser imager is much longer than in a video imager, e.g. 20–30 s compared with 1–5 s. Nevertheless, laser imagers appear to be increasing in popularity in the 1990s, whereas the popularity of video imagers is declining.

23.4.6 *Video signal interfacing*

Both laser imagers and video imagers operate from a video signal input but unfortunately there is no universally accepted standard specification for video signals. It is vital, therefore, that the signal output from (say) an ultrasound unit is fully compatible with that required at the input of the video or laser imager. Some imagers offer more flexibility than others in this respect, i.e. they may provide a facility to interface with different video signal standards, though not necessarily at the same time. They may also offer a number of input channels, enabling the imager to be linked permanently to more than one imaging system.

It is essential before purchasing an imager to confirm with the supplier that its video input specification is compatible with the output standard of the medical equipment to which it is to be attached, both now and in the future.

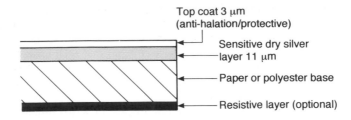

Fig. 23.17 A cross-section through a sheet of dry silver film.

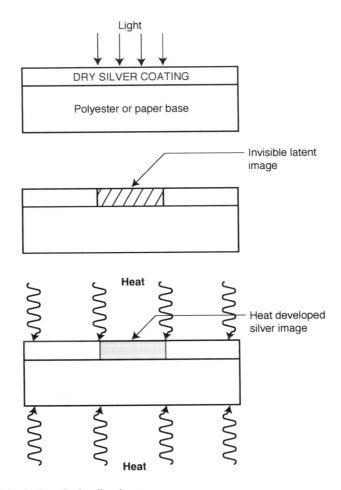

Fig. 23.18 Production of a dry silver image.

23.5 Dry silver imager

Dry silver imaging was pioneered by the 3M Company in the late 1960s as a method of photographing television monitor images, and was used mainly in conjunction with paper-based materials. More recently, the company has developed a dry silver imaging *film* with a transparent polyester base intended for use with laser imagers. The development of the dry silver image on film, like that on paper-based material, is an application of the principle of **photothermography**.

A specialized light-sensitive emulsion containing a silver halide is coated onto a base of either paper or polyester (Fig. 23.17). The top coat fulfils two functions: to prevent halation, and to protect the sensitive emulsion layer. Depending on the type of processing it is to undergo, the paper may also have a carbon deposit backing known as a **resistive layer**.

When light from a CRT image display or laser exposes the emulsion, a latent image is created which is subsequently made visible by using heat as a reducing agent (Fig. 23.18). In the case of film, or where paper with *no* resistive backing is used, heating is by means of an electrically heated plate (Fig. 23.19). Where paper *with* a resistive backing is used, the material is heated by passing an electric current through the backing layer via carbon brushes in contact with its surface (Fig. 23.20). The latest emulsions have a spectral response ranging from ultraviolet to near infra-red, and a resolution exceeding 400 lp/mm. Until recently, archival permanence has been a problem with some of the paper-based material, but this problem has now been resolved and both paper and polyester film materials are as reliable as conventional photographic materials, providing they are stored at temperatures not exceeding 35°C.

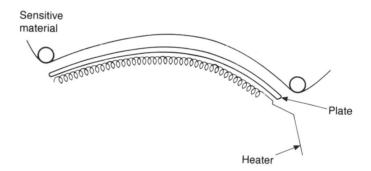

Fig. 23.19 The dry silver development process using heated plate method. (Courtesy of 3M (UK) Ltd.)

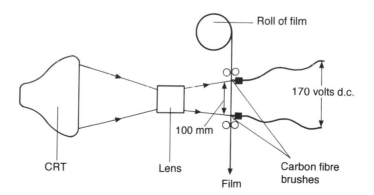

Fig. 23.20 The dry silver development process using resistive backing layer. Heat is generated within the resistive backing of the film by passage of electric current between the carbon brushes in contact with the film.

Advantages

The principal advantage of this latest technology lies in the fact that no wet chemical processing is required. Laser imagers are therefore able to produce high quality film images without the need for an associated automatic processor.

Our study of the television image and its recording is now complete. In the next series of chapters we shall examine some of the more specialised imaging techniques undertaken in a modern department of diagnostic imaging.

Part 5
Special Imaging Techniques

Chapter 24
Duplication of Radiographs

There are several ways in which a radiograph may be copied, e.g.:

(1) In miniature form, on 100 mm film;
(2) In digital form;
(3) As a facsimile (same size) replica or duplicate;
(4) As an enlargement copy.

Miniaturization and digitization were discussed in Chapter 15 in relation to the storage of radiographs. We shall not consider the production of enlargement copies because it is a procedure rarely undertaken in imaging departments. However, the creation of facsimile radiographs (duplication) should be within the capabilities of most departments and it is on this procedure that we shall concentrate in this chapter.

24.1 Reasons for duplication

Duplicate copies of radiographs may be required for a number of reasons:

(1) For transfer with the patient to another hospital. This allows the original radiograph to be retained in safety at the parent hospital.
(2) For display in exhibitions, or as part of a film archive or X-ray museum, perhaps as an example of a rare pathology.
(3) For publication in a book or learned journal.
(4) For teaching purposes in a radiography or medical school.

The production of a facsimile avoids the patient having to undergo a repeat examination in order to get a second radiograph. It therefore helps to minimize the radiation dose to the patient.

24.2 Principles of duplication

The method used in X-ray departments to make a facsimile radiograph is called

contact copying. The radiograph to be copied is placed in intimate contact with a special film material known as duplicating film. The duplicating film is exposed to light through the original radiograph (Fig. 24.1) and the result after processing is a facsimile radiograph identical to the original.

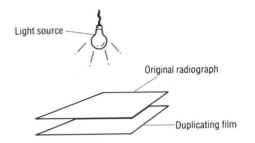

Fig. 24.1 Contact copying of radiographs. Light passes through the original radiograph onto the duplicating film beneath. In practice the radiograph and duplicating film are placed in intimate contact with each other.

24.2.1 *Duplicating film*

Radiograph duplicating film is single-coated film using an emulsion exhibiting reversal characteristics (see Chapter 4, section 4.5.5.3). Like most single-coated film materials, it incorporates an anti-halation backing which dissolves away during processing. One edge of the base is notched to facilitate identification of the emulsion side of the film. It is available in a range of sizes similar to standard X-ray film, e.g. 24 × 30 cm, 30 × 40 cm, 35 × 43 cm, and it is suitable for rapid automatic processing. It can be handled in the same darkroom safelight conditions as monochromatic and orthochromatic X-ray film.

Reversal The response to exposure of duplicating film is the opposite of normal X-ray film since its density *reduces* with increasing exposure. The mechanism by which this occurs is still not fully understood. It is believed that the exceptionally high exposure required to trigger reversal may result in the release of excess bromine into the emulsion. At the end of the exposure the bromine recombines with the free silver formed at the sensitivity specks, reconstituting silver bromide and thus inhibiting development of the latent image. The greater the exposure, the more bromide is released and the greater is the number of exposed halide grains protected from development (Jenkins, 1980).

Duplicating film is treated during manufacture to bring it to the point where any further exposure will result in a density reduction. Thus, during the copying process light rays passing through translucent parts of the original radiograph expose the duplicating film, causing it to become translucent after processing. Light cannot penetrate the blackened parts of the original, so the duplicating film beneath is unexposed and remains black. The densities of the original image are therefore reproduced in the facsimile.

Figure 24.2 shows the characteristic curve of a typical duplicating film.

24.2.2 *Reproduction of contrast*

Ideally, the contrast of the original radiograph should be reproduced exactly in the

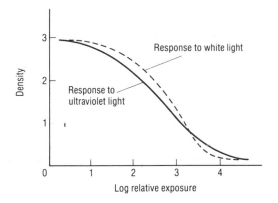

Fig. 24.2 Characteristic curve of duplicating film. The film operates in reversal mode in which increased exposure leads to reduced density. Exposure to ultraviolet light gives an image contrast which is similar to the original. Exposure to white light produces an image with increased contrast.

copy. This requires that duplicating film has an average gradient of −1, representing a characteristic curve with a slope angle of 45° to the left. In practice, this condition may not be achieved exactly, but is approached most closely when the exposure is made with ultraviolet light rather than visible light. Exposure to white light from an incandescent tungsten lamp modifies the characteristic curve (Fig. 24.2) and causes an increase in contrast of up to 30% compared with the original image. Kodak recommend an 8 W BLB (Black Light Blue) fluorescent lamp as an ultraviolet source (Pizzutiello & Cullinan, 1993), and a 275 W Photoflood bulb for white light when using their X-OMAT duplicating film, though a domestic 100 W pearl lamp can be used as an alternative to the Photoflood if necessary. Note that if a radiograph is lacking in contrast, a copy produced using a white light source can provide a welcome improvement in contrast.

24.2.3　Reproduction of density

The density of the copy is controlled to match that of the original by varying the exposure time. In considering exposure time it must be stressed that excessive density in a copy is the result of *underexposure* while insufficient density is due to *overexposure*. It is all too easy to forget that reversal films contravene the rules that we apply when judging radiographic exposures.

The duration of ultraviolet or white light exposure required to make a successful copy depends on:

(1) The mean density of the original radiograph: e.g. an over-penetrated radiograph requires a longer exposure during copying to produce a duplicate of correct density. By adjusting the exposure time carefully, an experienced operator can produce a good-quality duplicate even if the original radiograph is slightly over- or under-penetrated.
(2) The brightness and nature of the light source used: e.g. the exposure times used with an ultraviolet source are appreciably longer than with a white light source.
(3) The distance between the light source and the duplicating film being exposed: for this reason it is recommended that a constant source–film distance is used.
(4) The sensitometric characteristics of the duplicating film.

The exposure time required to make a good copy of a radiograph can be determined by trial and error, but this may be wasteful of time and materials. In such cases, a sheet of duplicating film should firstly be cut into small strips under safelight conditions. A series of test exposures can then be made, one on each film strip, each using a different exposure time. For each exposure, the film strip should be positioned across the main area of diagnostic interest in the original radiograph.

The manufacturers of duplicating film usually provide suggested exposure times, which can be used as long as the exposure conditions match those indicated by the manufacturer.

The best results are probably achieved by an experienced radiographer or processing technician who undertakes the task frequently and therefore becomes skilled at judging the exposure time required.

24.3 Duplicating equipment

The duplicating film and the original radiograph must be held in close and uniform contact while the exposure is made. The contact needs to be maintained by firm pressure evenly applied over the surfaces of the films. The consequence of poor contact is a noticeably unsharp image, similar to that which results when a radiograph is exposed under the conditions of bad film–screen contact (see section 7.2). It is also essential for light from the ultraviolet or white light source to reach the duplicating film while it is held in contact with the original radiograph. Some equipment is therefore required to ensure that these conditions are satisfied. The choice lies between a simple, home-made contact printing assembly and a purpose-built or commercially manufactured desk-top or floor-mounted duplicating unit.

24.3.1 Simple contact printer

A typical version consists of a 35 × 43 cm baseboard (e.g. 10 mm chipboard), the upper surface of which is covered with a thin (~ 6 mm) layer of polyfoam sheet. The baseboard rests on the darkroom benchtop. A piece of optically clear 6 mm plate glass slightly larger than the baseboard is used to maintain good contact between the radiograph and duplicating film.

24.3.1.1 Procedure

(1) Under safelight conditions, a sheet of duplicating film is placed, *emulsion side upwards*, on the polyfoam-covered baseboard.
(2) The original radiograph is laid with its normal viewing aspect uppermost on top of the duplicating film so that the edges of the two films coincide.
(3) The glass sheet is carefully rested on both (see Fig. 24.3).
(4) A suitable light source, suspended about 1.2 m above the assembly, is used to make the exposure. **NB** Care must be taken that no photosensitive material is inadvertently fogged when the exposure is made.

24.3.2 Purpose-built duplicating unit

Such units can be desk-top type or floor-mounted, free-standing or built into the darkroom bench. However, all versions consist essentially of a light-proof, box-like

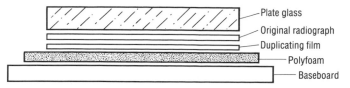

Fig. 24.3 Simple contact printer. The weight of the plate glass maintains good contact between the duplicating film and original radiograph. The polyfoam ensures contact is maintained evenly over the entire area of the film.

structure with internal light sources. The hinged 'lid' of the box is used to apply firm pressure to the duplicating film and radiograph, which are supported on a glass sheet at the top of the box (Fig. 24.4). There may be up to three internal light sources:

(1) A **safelight** to enable the original radiograph and duplicating film to be positioned accurately. The safelight is extinguished automatically when either of the other light sources are switched on.
(2) A **white light source** (e.g. 40 W tungsten lamp) to enable contrast-amplified copies to be produced. The white light may be dimmer-controlled to provide additional flexibility.
(3) An **ultraviolet source** (e.g. 8 W BLB) to produce identical contrast copies.

Switches enable the appropriate light source to be selected, while exposure is controlled by a digital timer adjustable typically between 0.2 and 90 s.

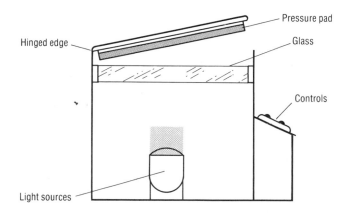

Fig. 24.4 A purpose-built duplicating unit. The duplicating film is placed on top of the original radiograph and located on the glass sheet.

24.3.2.1   Procedure

(1) The radiograph to be copied is placed on the glass sheet with its normal viewing aspect downwards so that the copy, when viewed, will be seen from its non-glossy, emulsion side.
(2) Under darkroom safelight conditions, a sheet of duplicating film of the same size as the radiograph is placed, *emulsion side downwards*, in contact with the radiograph and in registration with it.

(3) The lid of the unit is closed and the catches (if any) are fastened.
(4) The required light source and exposure time are selected and the exposure initiated (a typical ultraviolet light exposure is around 12 s). A warning light indicates that the exposure is in progress.
(5) When the exposure is ended, the duplicating film is removed and processed. The result is a facsimile radiograph from the original.

The reader should note that most commercially available duplicating units are light-tight, thus other work in the darkroom does not have to cease when copying is in progress. Duplicating units can also be used for photographic subtraction purposes (section 25.1). In this case, a white light rather than ultraviolet exposure would be required.

24.4   Image quality of facsimile copies

We have mentioned that by careful choice of exposure factors during the copying process, minor improvements may be made to the image such that the contrast and density of the copy may be more acceptable than those of the original radiograph. We must stress, however, that major errors in the contrast or density of the original cannot be corrected. The photographic duplication technique that we have described is very limited in its ability to modify the characteristics of a radiographic image. Much greater scope is provided by the electronic and digital archiving systems that we considered in Chapter 15.

The process of producing facsimile radiographs always results in some loss of image sharpness because although the adjacent surfaces of the original radiograph and the duplicating film may be in perfect contact, their emulsion layers are not.

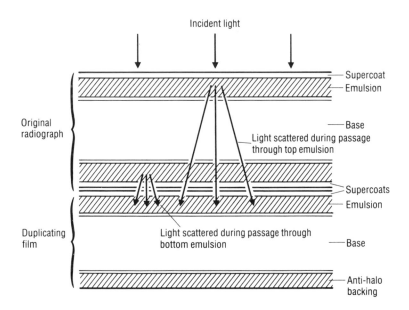

Fig. 24.5 Scattering of light during the process of copying. The gaps between the image-carrying emulsion layers of the original radiograph and the emulsion of the duplicating film allow the spread of light and therefore loss of sharpness.

The finite thickness of the emulsion layers, the supercoat of each film, and the base of the radiograph introduce gaps (see Fig. 24.5) in which scattered light can result in a loss of resolution. In practice, the increased unsharpness is not apparent at normal viewing distances and therefore is not a source of real concern. More serious degradation can arise, however, if a copy is made from a radiograph which is itself a copy, or even a copy of a copy. Thus, whenever possible it is preferable to make a copy from the original radiograph.

In the next chapter we shall investigate the process of image subtraction and describe the various subtraction techniques available in a modern imaging department.

Chapter 25
Image Subtraction Techniques

Subtraction is a technique employed to remove unwanted images from a radiograph and thereby leave important diagnostic information more readily visible.

Its primary application is in angiographic procedures, where bony and soft tissue detail may be subtracted from a radiographic image leaving the contrast-filled blood vessels clearly outlined.

We shall examine two types of subtraction:

(1) Photographic subtraction;
(2) Digital subtraction.

25.1 Photographic subtraction

Figures 25.1 and 25.2 represent two radiographic images, the first with six metal numerals, the other with seven. By applying photographic subtraction it is possible to remove the original six numerals, leaving the seventh (the figure 7).

Let us examine the principal steps in this process.

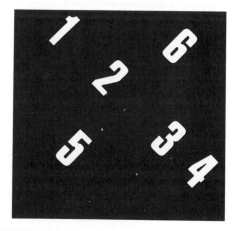

Fig. 25.1 The first 'radiographic' image.

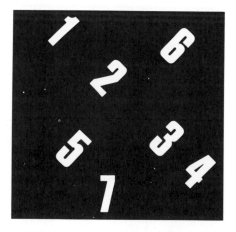

Fig. 25.2 The second 'radiographc' image containing an extra numeral.

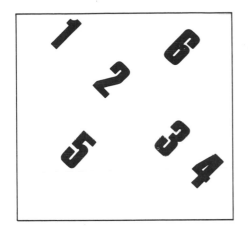

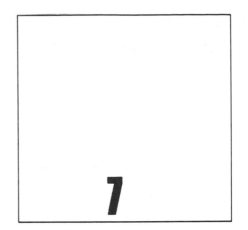

Fig. 25.3 The 'mask' which has been made by contact printing the first image. The 'mask' is the reverse or positive image of the first film.

Fig. 25.4 The subtracted image. The result of superimposing Fig. 25.3 on Fig. 25.2 and making a contact print.

Step 1

Produce a film known as a **mask**. This is done by placing the image in Fig. 25.1 in contact with a fresh unexposed film and giving the two films a brief exposure to light (known as **contact** printing). In this way, a reverse or positive image will be obtained. This is called the mask (Fig. 25.3).

Step 2

Place the mask image on top of the film with the added numeral (Fig. 25.2), carefully superimposing the two films until all the numerals on one film correspond

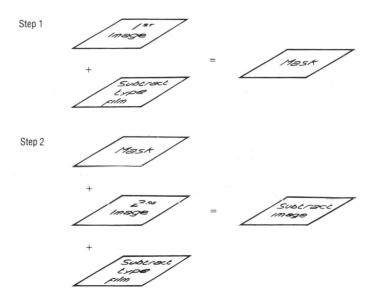

Fig. 25.5 Photographic subtraction. Step 1 – production of the mask. Step 2 – using the mask to produce a subtracted image.

with all the numerals of the other. It will be seen that whilst all the lead numbers that were common to both images will no longer be visible, the added one will be shown clearly. A final contact print can be made of this by placing the two superimposed films on top of a third unexposed film, so producing the image in Fig. 25.4.

These steps can be illustrated by the use of a simplified diagram, such as that seen in Fig. 25.5.

This subtraction process can also be followed in the case of a cerebral angiogram (Figs 25.6–25.9).

25.1.1   Equipment for photographic subtraction

The equipment is the same as that used for the duplication of radiographs and which was described in Chapter 24. Whilst the duplication process uses an ultra-violet light source, photographic subtraction requires a white light in order for sufficient image contrast to be maintained, particularly when making the final print, a point we shall return to later when discussing film materials.

25.1.2   Film materials for photographic subtraction

Any type of duplitized X-ray film may be used for producing both the control and angiographic images. However, two specialized films are available for producing the mask and final print:

(1) Subtraction mask film;
(2) Subtraction print film.

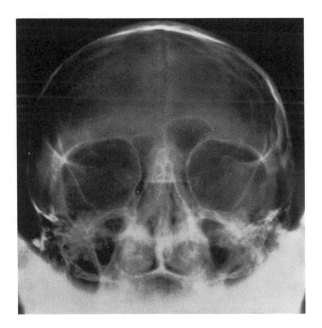

Fig. 25.6 Radiograph prior to the injection of contrast agent. This is the basic radiograph in the subtraction procedure.

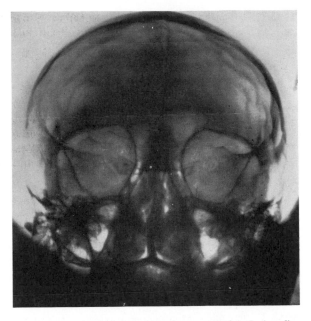

Fig. 25.7 The radiographic mask, which is a positive image copy of the basic radiograph.

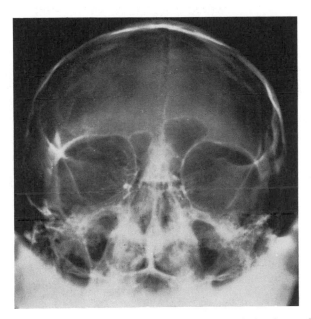

Fig. 25.8 Radiograph made after the injection of contrast agent in a cerebral angiogram. The radiograph is identical with that in Fig. 25.6 except for the presence of contrast agent.

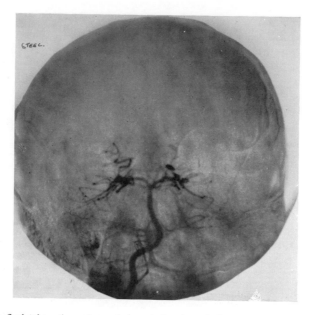

Fig. 25.9 The final subtraction print made by printing through the superimposed radiographic mask and the image with contrast agent.

25.1.2.1 Physical characteristics of subtraction films

- Single-sided emulsion to minimize photographic unsharpness.
- Anti-halation backing for the same reason as above.
- Polyester film base.
- Suitable for automatic processing.
- Available in 24×30 cm and 35×43 cm formats.
- Single notch in mask film and double notch in print film, to facilitate film and emulsion surface identification.

25.1.2.2 Sensitometric characteristics of subtraction films

- Both types of film have a monochromatic emulsion.
- Average gradient $(\overline{G})$ of subtraction mask film is 1.
- $\overline{G}$ of subtraction print film ~ 1.75.

In other words, subtraction print film has slightly more contrast than the mask film.

The reason for this is that each of the two stages in the subtraction process – production of mask and production of final print – results in a gradual loss of image contrast. Because images with higher contrast always appear more sharp (section 2.1.1.3), the use of a higher-contrast film for the final print is sometimes regarded as advantageous in that it can help restore some of this lost contrast.

Unfortunately, using a relatively high-contrast film at the end of the process also enhances the noise that each production stage inevitably introduces into the image. As a consequence, perceptibility of very small contrast-filled vessels within the image may become difficult. This is why many radiographers prefer to use the lower-contrast mask-type film for both mask and final print.

25.1.2.3   Average gradient of subtraction mask film
The significance of having a film with a $\overline{G}$ of 1 can be explained as follows.

Imagine that you have a control film with three different density values, e.g. 0.7, 1.2 and 1.7 (Fig. 25.10(a)). In order for the difference between these densities to be eliminated in any subtraction process, it will be necessary for the subtraction mask film to be able to reproduce those density differences exactly. Let us assume that the subtraction film does just that (Fig. 25.10(b)). The corresponding densities on the mask are 1.5, 1.0 and 0.5.

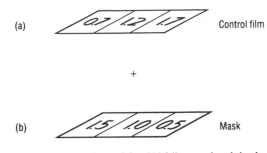

(a)   Control film

+

(b)   Mask

Fig. 25.10 The film used to produce the mask has faithfully reproduced the density differences of the control film. Therefore superimposing mask and control film results in one uniform density – in our example $D = 2.2$. In other words the three original densities of the control film have been subtracted because there is zero contrast.

You can see that by superimposing mask on control film and adding together the densities, one uniform density results. In other words, there is no contrast in the image and the three original densities on the control film have been effectively subtracted.

This feature of subtraction mask film to reproduce similar density differences arises because it has a $\overline{G}$ of 1. Look at the characteristic curve for subtraction mask film in Fig. 25.11(a) and you will see that each density difference in the original image corresponds to similar density differences in the subtraction mask image. If a film with a $\overline{G}$ greater or less than 1 was used (Fig. 25.11(b)), then the same density changes in the original image would not be reproduced faithfully in the mask. In such a case, superimposing mask on control film would result in an image still being present because subtraction was incomplete.

25.1.3   The subtraction procedure in practice

(1) Take the 'control' film (a radiograph taken before the injection of a contrast agent) and an identical film following injection.
(2) Place the control film in contact with the emulsion surface of a sheet of subtraction masking film.
(3) The two films are placed on the glass surface of the copier (section 24.3.2), with the subtraction film uppermost.
(4) Expose the film to a tungsten light source, (e.g. 40 W bulb at 1 m for 3–5 s). A series of masks may have to be made using different exposure times before the correct exposure is found. Process the film.
(5) Take the selected mask and carefully superimpose it on the radiograph that has contrast agent present, taking great care to ensure that all identical bony

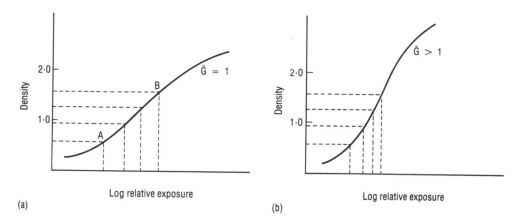

Fig. 25.11 (a) Subtraction mask film characteristic curve. Note the limited density range A–B over which the average gradient equals 1. This is why the density range of the control film should be restricted to ensure that it can be accommodated by the mask film. The $\bar{G}$ of 1 means that comparable density differences in the original correspond to similar density differences in the mask. (b) An imaginary subtraction mask film. The average gradient is greater than 1 and consequently density differences in the original are not faithfully reproduced but instead amplified.

landmarks in each image precisely coincide. Use a few small pieces of sellotape to keep the film edges in position.

(6) Place the two films on the glass of the printer so that the conventional viewing aspect of the film with contrast agent is in contact with the glass.

(7) Place a sheet of subtraction print film on top of the two films, with its emulsion surface in contact with them. Make an exposure as before. (This final print may be made using subtraction mask film instead of subtraction print film.) Process the film.

'Black' or 'white' blood vessels

By following the above method, you will find that the blood vessels will be shown in 'black'. If preferred, instead of making the mask from the 'control' film, it may be made from the film containing contrast material. This mask (showing the blood vessels as black) is then superimposed on the 'control' film and a final print made, as before. This will show the vessels as white on a dark background.

25.1.3.1   Second order subtraction

The method of photographic subtraction that we have just described is sometimes referred to as 'single order subtraction'. In most situations this method is perfectly adequate. It is a fact, however, that the higher the contrast of the film from which the mask is to be made, the more difficult it is to produce a mask in which density differences will be comparable with that of the control. The result is that when superimposition of mask and contrast image is done, subtraction will be incomplete.

The problem can be overcome by 'second order subtraction' in which a second mask is made from the superimposition of the first mask and the control film (Fig. 25.12).

When the subtraction film is being made, *both* masks are used together (Fig. 25.13). Those densities that cannot be subtracted by the first mask will now be subtracted by the combined effect of the two mask images.

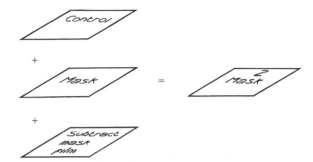

Fig. 25.12 Second order photographic subtraction. Producing the second mask.

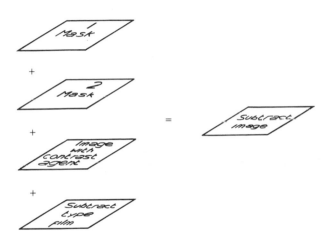

Fig. 25.13 Second order subtraction. Using the two masks to produce a subtracted image.

Whilst second order subtraction is a useful 'tool' to have in one's armoury, it does have certain disadvantages.

Disadvantages

(1) The extra film involved in the subtraction process makes the process of accurately superimposing all the images that much more difficult.
(2) The added densities provided by the second mask will mean that a strong light is required in order to view the films whilst they are being superimposed.
(3) The extra step in the process means additional noise introduced into the image.

It should be remembered that when carrying out photographic subtraction the best results are obtained using single order subtraction and a control film that is sharp and not too high in contrast.

25.2 Digital subtraction

This is an electronic method of subtraction known by several different names, the most common being:

- Digital subtraction angiography (DSA);
- Digital subtraction imaging (DSI).

As we saw in Chapter 22, the conversion of analogue video signals to digital ones enables us to manipulate images, e.g. as with 'window width' and 'window level' controls (section 22.4.3). Subtraction is another manipulative process made possible by having the image available in digital form.

During an angiographic investigation, the analogue video signal from the television pick-up tube (Plumbicon) is first amplified before being fed through an **analogue-to-digital converter** (ADC) (section 22.4.2). The digitized images are then stored in one of two data storage devices known as 'frame stores' (Fig. 25.14).

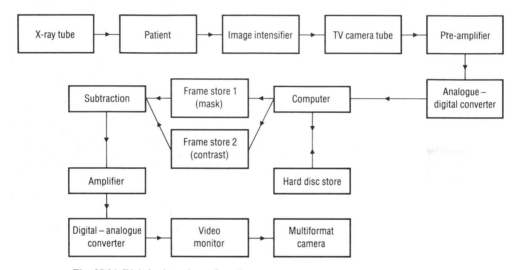

Fig. 25.14 Digital subtraction – flow diagram.

The radiographer carefully times the imaging sequence so that the first image will be taken *before* the arrival of contrast agent at the site of interest. This will be the 'mask' and, once digitized, it will be fed to the first frame store. Subsequent images from the angiographic 'run' are digitized and stored in the second frame store. These latter images will be the ones containing the contrast medium. It thus becomes possible to subtract arithmetically the mask from each of the contrast images, with the resulting 'difference' signals converted back into analogue form by means of a **digital-to-analogue converter** (DAC).

The subtraction is immediate, with the subtracted images appearing one by one on a high-resolution TV monitor as the angiographic sequence progresses.

Later, when the investigation is complete, the radiographer carries out computer 'processing' of the stored images, selecting and where necessary enhancing the subtracted images electronically on a CRT monitor prior to making hard-copy images of them (Fig. 25.15).

In this chapter we have looked in detail at image subtraction techniques, both photographic and digital. In Chapter 26 we shall examine the method of producing magnified images by the technique of macroradiography.

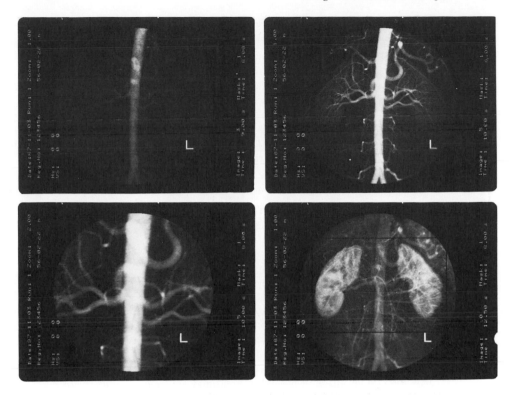

Fig. 25.15 Digital subtraction. The final formatted images from an angiographic examination.

Chapter 26
Macroradiography

In section 3.1.2.1 we noted that X-ray beam divergence causes the image of an object to be larger than the object itself. Macroradiography is a radiographic technique for producing magnified images by taking advantage of this natural consequence of the divergence of the X-ray beam. Produced under optimum conditions, the magnified image enables fine anatomical details to be seen more easily than on an image of normal size and may thus aid accurate diagnosis.

In this chapter we shall outline the fundamental principles on which macro-radiography is based, examine the important criteria which limit the quality of the magnified image, and indicate some of the applications of the technique.

26.1 Principles of macroradiography

Figure 26.1 illustrates the principal dimensions relating to the production of a radiographic image. Knowledge of the geometry of similar triangles allows us to determine, quantitatively, the relationship between the sizes of an object and its image:

$$\frac{\text{Image size}}{\text{Object size}} = \frac{\text{Focus} - \text{film distance}}{\text{Focus} - \text{object distance}} = \frac{\text{FFD}}{\text{FOD}}$$

26.1.1 Magnification factor

The ratio of image size to object size is known as the **magnification factor**. Its value is normally assessed by measuring the focus–film distance (FFD) and the object–film distance (OFD). The focus–object distance (FOD) is then obtained by subtraction:

$$\text{FOD} = \text{FFD} - \text{OFD}$$

Thus:

$$\text{Magnification factor} = \frac{\text{FFD}}{\text{FFD} - \text{OFD}} = \frac{\text{FFD}}{\text{FOD}} \quad \text{(Kreel, 1981)}$$

For a routine examination of the hand (dorsipalmar projection), the relevant dimensions are typically: FFD = 100 cm, OFD = 1 cm. This gives a magnification factor of 100/99 = 1.01. Thus, a 10 cm long finger gives an image which is 10.1 cm in length. In practice, such a small degree of magnification can be ignored.

For a lateral projection of the lumbar spine, the relevant dimensions are typically: FFD = 100 cm, OFD = 25 cm (spine–table-top distance + table-top–film distance). This gives a magnification factor of 100/75 = 1.3. A true measurement of 10 cm in the spine is reproduced as 13 cm in the image. This magnification *is* significant if measurements are to be taken from the radiograph, and it may have implications in terms of geometric unsharpness (see section 3.1.2.3).

In both examples quoted above, magnification is an *incidental* consequence of the radiographic techniques undertaken. Macroradiography is the *deliberate* introduction of magnification in the radiographic image.

For macroradiography, it is usual to arrange the FFD and OFD to give a magnification factor of at least 1.5. Typically, a magnification factor of 2.0 is achieved by positioning the structure under examination half-way between the X-ray tube focus and the film, i.e. FFD = FOD × 2 (see Fig. 26.2). In practice, the FOD is often maintained at its normal value but the FFD is increased, i.e. the X-ray tube and patient are positioned normally but the film is moved further from the patient.

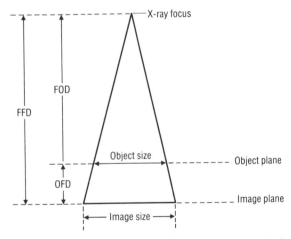

Fig. 26.1 Principal dimensions in radiographic image production. FOD = focus–object distance; FFD = focus–film distance (or focus–image distance); OFD = object–film distance (or object–image distance).

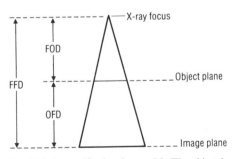

Fig. 26.2 A magnification factor of 2. The object is halfway between X-ray tube focus and image plane (film). Thus FOD = OFD = $\frac{1}{2}$ FFD.

26.2 Factors limiting image quality

As we have seen, the criteria that determine the magnification factor are the focus–film distance and the focus–object or object–film distance. However, the quality of the magnified image is also an important consideration, which may be affected by modifications to the FFD, FOD and OFD.

26.2.1   Geometric unsharpness

In section 3.1.2.2 we saw how the finite size of the X-ray source (focal spot size) creates geometric blurring of the image:

$$\text{Geometric unsharpness} = \frac{\text{Focal spot size} \times \text{Object–film distance}}{\text{Focus–object distance}}$$

We stated that increasing the object–film distance (and thus reducing the focus–object distance) causes a loss of sharpness and that the patient should therefore be placed as close as possible to the film. In undertaking macroradiography, we are deliberately defying this principle. It is thus essential that the focal spot size is as small as possible in order to avoid noticeable geometric image unsharpness. In practice, a 0.6 mm focus permits a magnification of 1.5 times, while a 0.3 mm ('ultrafine') focus is needed to allow a magnification factor of 2. Higher magnifications can be produced with a 0.1 mm 'microfocus', but X-ray tube rating may then take precedence over geometric unsharpness as the limiting factor.

It is interesting to note that it is not the object–film distance *per se* but its relationship to focus–film distance which determines geometric unsharpness. Thus, for a given magnification factor (M), geometric unsharpness (U_G) depends only on focal spot size (f). It can be shown that:

$$U_G = f(M - 1)$$

from which we can see that geometric unsharpness increases with magnification. In effect, the penumbra is magnified with the image.

26.2.2   X-ray tube rating

To limit geometric unsharpness and still achieve substantial magnification requires the use of an ultrafine focus. Such a small focus sets serious constraints on the output of the X-ray tube. For example, even a high-speed tube offering an output of 80 kW on its broad (0.8 mm) focus, may barely achieve a 30 kW output on its fine (0.4 mm) focal spot (Siemens, 1986). This may well be manifested as a reduction in maximum tube current e.g. from over 1000 mA on broad focus to less than 400 mA when fine focus is selected, and consequently, exposure times become longer than desirable. Unless great care is taken, motional unsharpness is the result.

Motional unsharpness problems can be alleviated by:

(1) Taking positive measures to immobilize the patient;
(2) Using fast film–screen systems, if necessary (see section 7.6.3).

The radiographer must judge whether the reduced movement unsharpness which results from the shorter exposures possible with high-speed screens outweighs the increased photographic unsharpness associated with such screens (see below).

Macroradiography of the extremities is often highly successful because the required X-ray exposure is small and effective immobilization is possible: thus, high-resolution screens can be used. Under adverse conditions, macroradiography may prove impossible, e.g. for many abdominal structures the large exposures necessary and the problems of involuntary movement may exclude macro-radiography as a viable technique.

Problems due to limited tube rating are exacerbated by the use of excessive focus–film distances. Conversely, minimizing the FFD may ease rating problems but the radiographer must be alert to the increased radiation dose to the patient associated with a short focus–skin distance.

26.2.3   *Photographic unsharpness*

Although included here for the sake of completeness, the resolution of the film or film–screen system is not normally a critical limiting factor in carrying out macroradiography. Whatever degree of magnification is used, photographic unsharpness (U_P) remains constant because it is not the *recorded* image that is magnified. Thus, as magnification is increased and as geometric unsharpness (U_G) rises, a critical point is reached where U_G becomes approximately equal to U_P. Under these conditions, minimum total unsharpness is achieved. If magnification is increased further, geometric factors prevail. Even with low-resolution, high-speed film–screen systems, this critical point occurs at a relatively low level of magnification.

At magnifications of ×3 and above, the positive benefits arising from the reduced exposure required by high-speed film–screen systems probably outweigh any disadvantages. Only under the most favourable conditions is the use of slower, high-definition systems justified, e.g. a single-screen, single-emulsion film vacuum pack has been used in conjunction with a 0.1 mm focus for ×3 macroradiography of the extremities.

26.2.4   *Scattered radiation*

The large object–film distance used in macroradiography creates a welcome reduction in the amount of forward-scattered radiation reaching the film from the patient (see 'air-gap', section 3.1.1.3). Consequently, it is not necessary to employ a secondary-radiation grid, even for regions such as the skull or spine where, with orthodox techniques, a grid would be essential. The absence of a grid makes it unnecessary to increase exposure to overcome attenuation in the grid.

Collimation of the X-ray beam and provision of back-scatter protection for the film help to maintain optimum contrast on the macroradiograph.

26.3   Applications of macroradiography

Macroradiography is a specialized technique. Its use is limited to a few specific regions of the body, where the problems we have described can be overcome successfully. The list below is by no means exhaustive but it includes the more common applications of macroradiography:

(1) Carpal bones of the wrist (especially the scaphoid bone);
(2) Bones of the hand, e.g. for early detection of metabolic bone disease;
(3) Temporal bone;
(4) Lacrimal drainage ducts during dacrocystography;
(5) Chest for lung pathology;
(6) Cerebral angiography.

For a detailed description of macroradiography, the reader is referred to the standard texts on radiographic technique (e.g. Kreel, 1981) and to articles in the relevant journals (e.g. Bramble & Templeton, 1987).

Macroradiographic principles are not restricted to conventional radiographic procedures, e.g. they can be applied to fluoroscopic procedures using an image intensifier. In such cases, a gap is maintained between the patient and the input phosphor of the intensifier. An advantage of this technique is that the constraints on X-ray tube rating are partially relieved by the electronic amplification of image brightness, as described in Chapter 19.

The reader should note that there are other methods available for producing magnified images (e.g. the use of a **dual-field** image intensifier (section 19.2.3) or **photographic** enlargement of the radiograph). However, these are not examples of macroradiography since they do not use the divergence of the X-ray beam to create magnification.

In the next chapter we shall examine how stereoscopic, 'three-dimensional' radiographic images can be produced, which demonstrate an illusion of depth.

Chapter 27
Visualization of Depth

Radiographic images are essentially two-dimensional in character because they are formed on the flat surface of a film, screen or other image receptor. The anatomical features which they depict are three-dimensional structures. We are therefore unable to represent the third dimension (depth) directly in a single radiographic image. In this chapter, we shall outline methods by which radiographic images can be produced which convey depth information and describe how such images can be observed to best effect.

The most common method of recording depth information is the routine radiographic practice of taking two radiographic projections at right angles to each other. For example, when an antero-posterior (A-P) and lateral projection are taken, depth information absent from the A-P radiograph is depicted on the lateral and the position of structures can be localized in three dimensions (Fig. 27.1). However, specialized techniques have also been developed by which depth information is portrayed in a single radiographic image or projection.

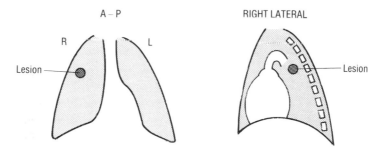

Fig. 27.1 Localization of depth. The position in three dimensions of the chest lesion can be determined by reference to two projections (A–P and lateral) taken at right angles to each other.

There are many ways in which we obtain a sensation of depth from non-radiographic visual images, e.g. the effect of perspective, and the effect of distance on colour. But our perception of the solidity and depth of a structure is influenced most strongly by the effects of parallax and by binocular vision. Let us examine how these effects can be applied to radiographic images.

27.1   Parallax

When we view a scene containing objects at differing distances from us, the relationship between the positions of the objects appears to alter if we change our viewpoint. In Fig. 27.2, when viewed from A the lamp post L appears immediately in front of the telegraph pole T. If we change our viewpoint to B by moving left, L now appears to be on the right of T. The extent of the apparent shift in the positions of L and T provide us with information about their relative distances from us. Near objects are shifted more than distant objects. This **parallax** effect is vividly demonstrated when we observe the scene from the window of a moving railway carriage. Features nearby, such as the fencing or trees by the lineside, appear to race across our field of view, while more distant objects move past at a slower pace. By comparison, features far away, such as the hills on the horizon, appear almost stationary.

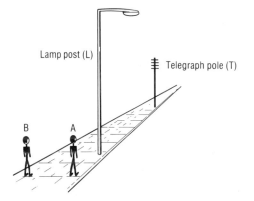

Fig. 27.2 Parallax effect. Viewed from position A, the lamp post appears directly in front of the telegraph pole. Viewed from position B, the lamp post appears to be on the right of the telegraph pole.

But how is it possible to make use of the parallax effect to localize the depth of a structure inside a patient? Two radiographic exposures are made without disturbing the patient or film. For the first exposure, the X-ray tube is displaced laterally to the left, for the second exposure it is displaced to the right, (see Fig. 27.3). The result is that each structure in the patient is projected onto the film in two slightly different positions. The distance between these positions is dependent partly on the depth of the structure in the patient. Knowledge of the focus–film distance and the total tube shift employed, together with the change in image position measured on the radiograph, enables the distance of the structure above the film (and therefore its depth in the patient) to be calculated (Clark, 1956). The parallax or **tube shift** technique was developed early in the history of diagnostic

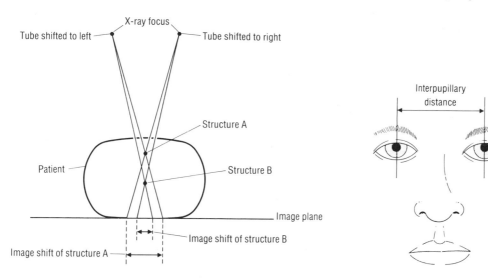

Fig. 27.3 Parallax technique in radiography. The shift in image position of structure A is greater than that for structure B. A is therefore further from the film than B.

Fig. 27.4 Interpupillary distance in man is typically around 6 cm. Each eye sees the world from a slightly different viewpoint creating the three-dimensional effect of binocular vision.

radiography and was used extensively in the Great War of 1914–1918 as a means of localizing the position of bullets and shell fragments. A modification of the parallax technique, for localization of intra-ocular foreign bodies using the Sweet localizer (Todd, 1951; Clark, 1956), was still in use in the 1970s.

27.2 Binocular vision

When we look at a scene an image is focused onto the retina of each of our two eyes. Study of the parallax effect described above shows that the image formed in the right eye is not the same as that formed in the left eye because each eye views the scene from a slightly different position, separated by a distance of about 6 cm, the mean **interpupillary** distance (Fig. 27.4). The human brain compares the two images and extracts from them information about the third dimension. Other depth information is obtained from the effects of perspective and colour. The images from the left and right eye are combined by the brain into what we perceive as a single image conveying a strong impression of depth (Gregory, 1980). The process of viewing a scene with both eyes and mentally fusing the two images into one is described as **binocular vision**. The impression of depth which results is known as the **stereoscopic effect**. The radiographic application of this effect can be achieved by the technique of stereoradiography.

27.2.1 *Principle of stereoradiography*

The radiographic procedure adopted is similar in many respects to that for the parallax technique described earlier. The X-ray tube is centred over the part to be radiographed and two exposures are made; one with the X-ray tube shifted to the left, and one with a right shift but a different cassette is used to record the second image. It is essential that no movement of the patient occurs between the two exposures. The result is a pair of radiographs whose images appear almost identical. The one obtained with the X-ray tube displaced to the left is known as the **left-shift** radiograph and the other is the **right-shift** radiograph. Note that this nomenclature is based on the direction of tube shift *as seen from behind the X-ray tube* (Fig. 27.5). It is *not* determined by the anatomical orientation of the patient.

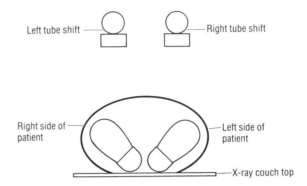

Fig. 27.5 Tube shift terminology. The direction of tube shift is defined as seen from the bottom (foot end) of the X-ray couch. It is *not* related to the patient's right and left side, e.g. if the patient were turned into the prone position the tube shift would remain as shown.

The radiographs are viewed such that the left-shift image is presented only to the left eye of the observer, while the right-shift film is seen only by the right eye. The two images become fused in a single impression which appears, to the observer, to be three-dimensional. A sense of depth and 'reality' is perceived which enables the levels of structure, otherwise superimposed on a plain radiograph, to be differentiated. For an antero-posterior projection, anterior structures (e.g. the facial bones of the skull) appear nearer to the observer than posterior structures (e.g. the occipital bone). The anatomical features seem to have depth.

A total X-ray tube shift of ∼ 6 cm is usually recommended (i.e. a 3 cm right shift and a 3 cm left shift). Reducing the tube shift markedly leads to loss of the stereoscopic effect, while a significant increase in tube shift exaggerates the effect (Harris, 1969).

27.2.2 *Viewing stereoradiographs*

There are two ways in which a pair of stereoradiographs can be presented for viewing by an observer: direct vision and binocular stereoscope.

27.2.2.1 **Direct vision**
With perseverance and practice, many people can develop the ability to 'see' stereoradiographs in three dimensions without the aid of special equipment.

The radiographs are displayed side by side on the X-ray illuminator with their edges touching. The observer faces the radiographs and trains the left eye on the left-shift image and the right eye on the right-shift image. There are two methods of achieving this.

Convergent vision (Fig. 27.6(a)) This method requires the left-shift film to be placed on the right-hand side of the illuminator, and the right-shift film on the left-hand side. Each film is positioned with its tube side **facing** the observer. The observer then induces convergence of his lines of sight so that each eye focuses on the correct radiograph.

Divergent vision (Fig. 27.6(b)) The left-shift film is placed on the left-hand side of the illuminator and the right-shift film on the right hand side. Again, each film is positioned with tube side facing the observer. The observer then induces divergence of his lines of sight, enabling each eye to focus on the correct radiograph.

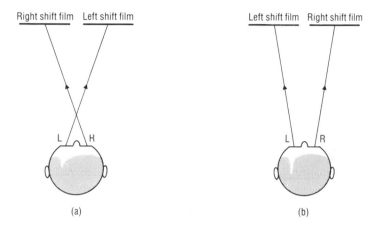

Fig. 27.6 (a) Convergent vision method of viewing stereo radiographs. Arrows indicate lines of sight for right (R) and left (L) eyes. (b) Divergent vision method of viewing stereo radiographs.

Whichever technique is chosen, the observer then attempts to superimpose the two images. With practice, the observer is able to 'lock on' to the superimposed image and obtain the impression of depth. If difficulty is experienced in successfully fusing the two images, the observer should try moving closer to or further from the radiographs. A very similar technique is required to view the computer-generated *Magic Eye* 3-D art which first became popular in 1993 (Liardet, 1994).

27.2.2.2 Binocular stereoscope

Stereobinoculars are similar in appearance to opera glasses. The films to be viewed are placed side by side on the X-ray illuminator, with the right-shift film on the right. The observer faces the radiographs and focuses the binoculars. Prisms in the binoculars both reflect and refract the light, to direct the image from each film into the correct eye. The process of reflection of light in the prisms causes anatomical transposition of the images, which is corrected by placing the radiographs on the illuminator with their tube sides facing *away* from the observer.

It is possible that some radiography departments may still possess apparatus known as a Wheatstone Stereoscope, which was designed for viewing stereoscopic pairs of radiographs by means of two 45° mirrors. Though of historical interest, this equipment was cumbersome and inconvenient and is no longer commercially available.

27.2.3   Marking of stereoradiographs

Appreciation of the three-dimensional effect from stereoradiographs is only achieved if the right- and left-shift films are correctly positioned for viewing. If the right-shift film is viewed by the left eye, a confusing reverse-depth impression is produced in which the most distant structures appear closest. Incorrect positioning of stereoradiographs for viewing is a common reason for failure to gain any impression of depth. To avoid such confusion, it is therefore vital that the right- and left-shift radiographs are unambiguously marked. A radiopaque right (R) or left (L) marker could be used to identify the tube shift, but this may be confused with the R or L anatomical marker unless a standard protocol is adopted, such as always placing the anatomical marker in front of the shift marker (e.g. LR indicates a right-shift radiograph of the left side of the patient). It is better to employ a more complete legend, e.g. 'R shift' or 'R stereo' to provide unequivocal evidence of the tube shift.

27.2.4   The role of stereoradiography

Historically, stereographic methods were used to advantage in imaging the skull, thorax, abdomen and pelvis, but the popularity of such techniques has declined and stereoradiography is now little more than an interesting curiosity. One problem has been that a significant number of radiographers and radiologists either experience extreme difficulty in interpreting three-dimensional radiographic images or even fail completely to gain any impression of depth. However, the technique is simple to carry out and the reader is invited to produce pairs of stereoradiographs of a skull phantom or dry skull and attempt to visualise the third dimension using one of the viewing techniques described.

Two new techniques have been developed which allow the visualisation of depth in diagnostic imaging; three-dimensional reconstruction in computerized tomography (CT) and magnetic resonance imaging (MRI), and holographic image recording. We shall outline briefly the nature of these techniques.

27.3   Three-dimensional CT and MRI images

A comparatively recent development is the ability to construct 3-D images during CT and MRI. The process of 3-D image acquisition is not very different from routine CT or MRI scanning. The patient is scanned and a series of adjacent slices is produced through the relevant anatomy. Using a special software program, a 3-D image is constructed from the scanning data. The data processing may take several minutes. The image appearing on the display monitor employs perspective and shading rather than a stereoscopic effect to create a sense of reality and depth. The technique can be used to generate bone or selected soft-tissue images, which can be rotated or tilted to provide different views of the structure under investigation (Imhof, 1989).

27.4   Holographic images

Of all the techniques available by which three-dimensional images can be created, the one that generates the greatest sense of depth and reality is holography. At present, the application of holographic techniques to radiography is in a very early stage of development, but its potential is enormous (Roberts & Smith, 1988). In contrast to stereographic images, holograms permit a whole range of different aspects or projections of a subject to be recorded simultaneously. Additionally, the recorded holographic image can be viewed and examined from many different angles, each viewing angle revealing a new aspect of the original subject.

But how is a hologram produced? Let us look at the basic principles on which holography is founded.

27.4.1   *Principles of holography*

When a solid object is exposed to light, it reflects and scatters the light in many different directions. When we produce an image of the object by conventional means, e.g. by using a convergent lens, only a minute fraction of this light enters the lens and is used to form the image (Fig. 27.7). Thus, such an image records only a very small sample of the information available about the subject.

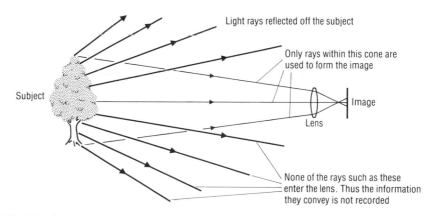

Fig. 27.7 Conventional imaging in two dimensions. The subject is viewed from a single aspect only. Most of the light reflected off the subject fails to enter the imaging system (e.g. lens) and the information it carries is lost.

The hologram works on a different principle. It records a much greater proportion of the network of light rays reflecting off the subject, by 'freezing' the light rays in the photosensitive emulsion layer of a holographic plate. Each part of the plate receives and stores information about every part of the subject in its view. For example, in Fig. 27.8 rays from points A, B and C on the subject all reach points X, Y and Z on the holographic plate, but the information recorded at X relates to a different view of the subject from that recorded at Y or Z. Under the correct lighting conditions, the original patterns of light rays are exactly reconstructed and the subject appears to be in its original position behind the plate, (Fig. 27.9). The first holograms were produced by illuminating the subject with laser light and a similar light source was required in order to view the image. Currently, holograms can be made which do not need lasers for their production or for viewing purposes.

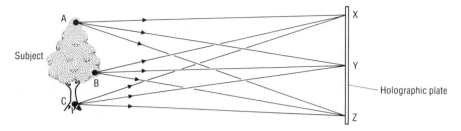

Fig. 27.8 Principle of holography. Light rays recorded at X relate to a different view of the subject from those recorded at Y or Z. Thus an infinite number of viewpoints are present simultaneously on the hologram.

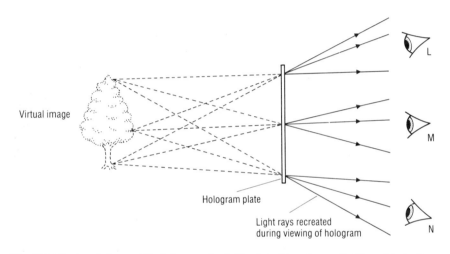

Fig. 27.9 Viewing a hologram. The hologram plate is illuminated in such a way that the original patterns of light are recreated. A virtual image behind the plate is formed. Viewing from different points (L, M, N) presents the observer with different views of the subject. Binocular vision creates a most convincing illusion of depth.

27.4.2   Some properties of holographic images

(1) The image is truly three dimensional: it appears exactly as if the subject were being observed through a window the size of the holographic plate. A change of viewing position gives a different view of the subject. Structures hidden behind an object can be made to come into view by adopting a different viewing position.

(2) Parts of the image which appear more distant are out of focus when the eye is concentrating on apparently near features. Thus, the holographic image demonstrates the same **depth of field** (section 20.2.5) as the original subject.

(3) Every part of a hologram contains some information about the whole subject. If the plate is broken into fragments, each fragment is capable of producing a complete image, although the 3-D effect is reduced.

27.4.3 Limitations of holography

The exposure conditions for producing a hologram are very restricting. In particular, there must be absolute immobilization of the subject, the holographic plate and the light source during the exposure period. Unlike a photograph or radiograph, any relative movement during the exposure of a hologram results not in a blurred image but in the total loss of the image! This effectively rules out, at least for the present, the possibility of undertaking direct holography of a living subject.

The photosensitive holographic emulsions are capable of extraordinarily high resolution, because they must record interference patterns whose details are of the same order of magnitude as the wavelength of light. Resolutions of several thousand line-pairs (lp) per millimetre are necessary (compared with < 10 lp/mm for a typical X-ray film–screen system).

27.4.4 X-ray holograms?

Holography is still in its infancy and direct X-ray holography of patients is not yet feasible. However, techniques have been developed with which the information on a sequence of radiographic images can be condensed into a single hologram. Work has been done on the recording of a series of contiguous slices obtained from a computerized tomography scan. Each slice image is positioned at a different distance from the hologram plate on which it is to be recorded, e.g. if the slices were 5 mm apart in the patient, the images would be recorded 5 mm apart holographically (see Fig. 27.10). Viewing the hologram then gives a pseudo-stereoscopic effect, in which the CT images and the features that they depict are seen in the correct spatial relationship to each other.

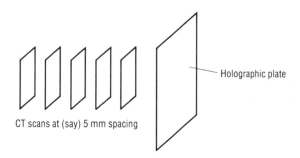

Holographic plate

CT scans at (say) 5 mm spacing

Fig. 27.10 Holographic recording of CT images. The relationship between the scan images for holographic recording is the same as that between the anatomical sections they represent in the patient.

The production of true 3-D X-ray holograms may depend on the development of X-ray lasers. If such holograms become possible, one exposure could provide a radiographic image which the radiologist or clinician could examine from different angles, each viewing angle presenting a different radiographic projection to the observer.

In the next chapter we shall outline the principles of fundamentally different imaging technologies, such as ultrasonography, computerized tomography, computed radiography and radionuclide imaging, and we shall examine how their images are recorded.

Chapter 28
Other Imaging Technologies

Increasingly conventional radiography has been supplemented and in some cases replaced as a diagnostic tool by other imaging technologies such as:

(1) Ultrasound scanning;
(2) Computed tomography;
(3) Radionuclide imaging;
(4) Magnetic resonance imaging;
(5) Digital fluorography and angiography;
(6) Computed radiography;
(7) Xeroradiography.

The reader should refer to specialist texts for detailed descriptions of these diagnostic imaging procedures, but in this chapter we shall confine ourselves to a brief outline of the principles on which each technology is based and a discussion of the different characteristics of the images and their influence on the choice of recording medium.

With the exception of xeroradiography, these imaging techniques are computer-based and generate a digital output which can be stored on magnetic or optical disk (see section 15.2.1.4). The images can be displayed on a TV monitor and recorded as hard copy either with a laser imager or from the cathode ray tube of a video imager.

28.1 Ultrasound scanning

Diagnostic ultrasound is an essential service offered by most imaging departments in the United Kingdom. It provides a means by which images of soft-tissue structures can be produced without the risks associated with the use of contrast agents and ionizing radiation.

28.1.1 *Principles of ultrasound*

Ultrasound imaging is an application of the **pulse-echo** principle (Evans, 1988). Pulses of high-frequency sound waves are transmitted into the patient and the echoes returning from various tissue boundaries (**interfaces**) are detected (Fig. 28.1). The time interval between transmission and detection of each pulse is measured. Since the speed of sound in tissue is known, the depth of each tissue interface can be calculated. The spatial relationships between the various interfaces encountered by the ultrasound beam can thus be determined and are displayed in visual form on the screen of a cathode ray tube.

There are several ways in which the spatial information can be displayed.

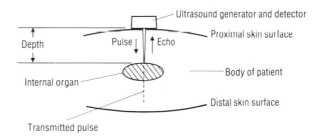

Fig. 28.1 Ultrasound pulse-echo principle. The section through the body shows the ultrasound echo returning from a tissue interface. The time interval between the generation and detection of each pulse is an indication of the depth of the interface.

28.1.1.1 A-scan (amplitude mode)

This is a graphic display showing the distances between the tissue interfaces. It is used for the purposes of measurement, e.g. the biparietal diameter (BPD) of the foetal skull as an assessment of foetal maturity.

28.1.1.2 B-scan (brightness mode)

This display provides a two-dimensional image representing a specific plane of section through the body. Not only are spatial relationships demonstrated, but also different types of tissue are distinguished using a grey-scale representation.

Most modern ultrasound apparatus produces B-scan images in **real time**, i.e. a sequence of grey-scale images is displayed in rapid succession such that a moving 'live' image is perceived. If required, the image may be 'frozen' on screen to facilitate detailed examination. Real-time grey-scale B-scanning is used to image a wide range of structures, particularly in the abdomen, and is used extensively as an obstetric monitoring technique.

28.1.1.3 M-scan (motion mode)

M-scans portray the way in which the positions of tissue interfaces alter with time.

Each interface produces a moving trace on screen; stationary interfaces generate a straight line, whilst moving interfaces produce wavy lines. Applications of M-scans include the display of movements of the flaps of heart valves in the adult and the detection of foetal heart movements in early pregnancy.

28.1.1.4   Doppler ultrasound

Ultrasound waves reflected from a moving interface suffer a **Doppler shift**, a change in frequency compared with the original ultrasound pulse. If the interface is *approaching* the ultrasound probe, frequency is increased; if the interface is *receding*, frequency is reduced. The *magnitude* of the frequency shift is proportional to the speed of approach or recession. Information about Doppler shift is superimposed onto a real time B-scan image and displayed in colour. For example, in **colour flow mapping** of the heart, different shades of red and blue are used to represent different blood flow rates towards and away from the ultrasound probe (Evans, 1988).

28.2   Computed tomography

Computed tomography (CT) provides a means of producing transverse axial tomographic images of a patient.

28.2.1   *Principles of CT*

An X-ray tube rotates on a special gantry around the patient while the transmitted beam is monitored by an array of sensitive detectors (Fig. 28.2). Raw data from the detectors are computer-processed and a grey-scale image is constructed from the digital data and displayed on a CRT monitor. While CT image spatial resolution does not yet rival that possible with conventional radiography, the digital nature of the system permits image enhancement to be carried out, enabling far better dif-

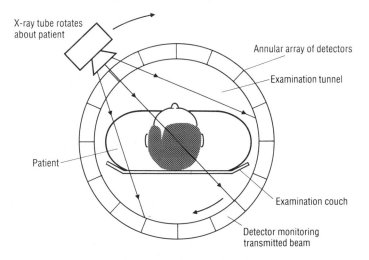

Fig. 28.2 Computerized tomography. As the X-ray tube rotates about the patient an array of detectors measures the transmitted beam. A computer processes the data obtained and constructs a transverse sectional slice image.

ferentiation of soft-tissue structures to be achieved. Measurements of the attenuation coefficients of different tissues are also possible.

Imaging departments with CT facilities have found the technique to be an invaluable weapon in the diagnostic armoury. For example, CT has a vital role to play in the examination of accident and emergency cases, where its ability to produce high-quality images with minimal disturbance to the patient is particularly valuable. However, for some applications, its role has been successfully challenged by MRI.

28.3   Radionuclide imaging

28.3.1   *Principles of radionuclide imaging*

Radionuclide imaging (RNI) is the technique by which diagnostic images are produced following the introduction into the patient of a pharmaceutical preparation 'labelled' with a radioactive isotope. The radiopharmaceutical is often labelled with the nuclide **technetium 99 m**, whose activity decays at a convenient rate (half-life = 6 h) and which emits gamma rays of an energy (140 keV) eminently suitable for imaging purposes. Radionuclide imaging enables images to be produced with little discomfort to the patient and with radiation doses much lower than those associated with conventional radiography. By careful choice of radiopharmaceutical it is sometimes possible to 'target' the agent to a specific organ and to monitor quantitatively the physiology of the organ.

The most popular imaging equipment for RNI is the **gamma camera** (Sharp, 1989), which employs a large scintillation crystal monitored by an array of photomultiplier detectors to measure the gamma ray emissions from the patient (Fig. 28.3). The spatial distribution of gamma ray emissions from the patient is computed and a two-dimensional image reconstructed on a CRT. Each photon detected is reproduced as a bright point of light on the screen. It is possible to produce dynamic as well as static scans, enabling an analysis to be made of the blood flow through an organ such as the heart or brain.

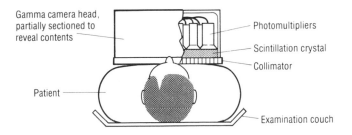

Fig. 28.3 Radionuclide imaging with a gamma camera. Gamma ray photons from the radionuclide in the patient pass through holes in a lead collimator causing scintillation in the crystal. Photomultipliers detect the light flashes and a computer constructs an image of the spatial distribution of the radionuclide.

The resolution of RNI gamma camera images is relatively low and the technique is often used as a preliminary investigation, e.g. prior to CT. In some instances, such as the early detection of bone metastases, RNI provides diagnostic information which cannot be obtained in any other way.

28.4   Magnetic resonance imaging

28.4.1   Principles of MRI

Like ultrasound, MRI is an imaging technique which does not employ ionizing radiation. It is an application of the principle of nuclear magnetic resonance (NMR) in which the distribution of hydrogen atoms in the patient's tissues is examined (Bushong, 1988).

The spinning proton forming the nucleus of each hydrogen atom has magnetic properties which cause it to align with an externally applied magnetic field generated by a powerful cryogenic (very low temperature) electromagnet around the patient. Exposure of the tissues to a short pulse of high-frequency radio waves disturbs the alignment of the hydrogen nuclei. As the protons re-align, they emit weak radio signals which can be detected by suitably placed receiver coils (Fig. 28.4). The signal strength is a measure of proton density, while the time needed for re-alignment gives an indication of the chemical bonding of the hydrogen atoms.

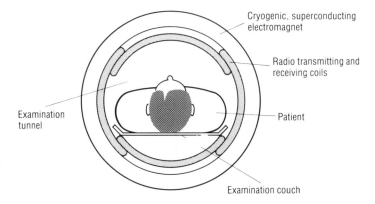

Fig. 28.4 Magnetic resonance imaging. The cryogenic electromagnet is used to align the spin axes of hydrogen nuclei in the patient's tissues. Radio coils transmit and detect radio signals (see text).

Computer analysis of the radio signals detected allows the spatial distribution of hydrogen atoms and their chemical bonds to be determined and the data displayed on a CRT as a two-dimensional grey-scale slice image. While MRI scan times are significantly longer than those for CT, and image resolution is appreciably poorer, soft-tissue differentiation is excellent and it is often possible to distinguish abnormal from normal tissue.

28.5   Digital fluorography

In Chapter 22 we described the production of television images and identified the benefits to be gained by using digital rather than analogue signals from which to derive an image. Digital fluorography is an imaging system which realizes many of these advantages and is now a common sight in modern imaging departments. The principles involved in digital fluorography were described in Chapter 25 under the heading of **digital subtraction**. An advantage claimed for this procedure is that it is possible to carry out DSA arterial studies using intravenous rather than intra-arterial injection of contrast agent. Furthermore, some DSA investigations can be undertaken with smaller quantities of contrast agent than with conventional techniques. Thus, DSA investigations tend to be less invasive and the risk to the patient is reduced.

28.6   Computed radiography

In this recent development, diagnostic X-ray images are acquired in a digital format using phosphors which exhibit **photon stimulated luminescence**. A phosphor-coated **imaging plate** replaces the screen–film system as the image receptor in the cassette. The imaging plate has high sensitivity to X-rays, good resolution, and offers a novel method of image formation with potential for further development (Workman & Cowen, 1992).

28.6.1   *Principles of computed radiography (CR)*

The imaging plate within the cassette looks similar to a conventional intensifying screen but is coated with a phosphor such as a europium activated barium fluorohalide. The radiographer exposes the full sized cassette containing the imaging plate in the normal way. When exposed to X-radiation, the phosphor stores the pattern of energy absorbed from the X-ray beam as a **latent image**. When, later, the phosphor is stimulated, the stored energy is released as visible light rather in the manner of a thermoluminescent phosphor.

After exposure, the imaging plate is unloaded from its cassette into an image reader unit where its phosphor is scanned by a 100 μm diameter light beam from a red emitting (633 nm) helium–neon laser. Exposure to the laser beam stimulates the phosphor to release its stored energy, luminescing in the blue part of the visible spectrum with a brightness proportional to the original X-ray exposure it received. As the latent image on the phosphor is scanned, a photomultiplier system monitors the luminescence and generates an electrical signal which is amplified and then digitized. The digital signal is used to construct a grey-scale image which is computer processed, displayed on a TV monitor, and recorded as hard copy with a laser imager. Image data can be permanently stored on a high capacity optical disk; e.g. a 3.6 Gb (gigabyte) optical disc can hold about 1800 images from a 35 × 35 cm imaging plate.

When the imaging plate has been scanned, any residual latent image is erased by further exposure to red light. The plate is then loaded into its cassette ready for reuse. One manufacturer claims the imaging plates can be used up to 1000 times. Figure 28.5 shows the main components of a CR system.

28.6.2   *Imaging plate construction*

Imaging plates are available in a range of familiar sizes from 18 × 24 cm to 35 × 43 cm (and their imperial size equivalents), and in two grades corresponding to regular and high-definition conventional intensifying screens. The *standard* grade imaging plate has a 210 μm thick phosphor layer with a reflective backing on a polyester base. The surface of the phosphor layer has a protective transparent supercoat applied. The *high-resolution* imaging plate possesses a thinner (140 μm) phosphor layer and smaller phosphor particles which effectively reduce its quantum detection efficiency. It has no reflective layer. The limiting resolution of CR

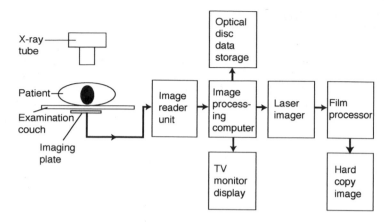

Fig. 28.5 The main components of a computed radiography (CR) system. The image plate in its cassette is positioned and exposed by the radiographer in the same way as a conventional film–screen system. However, the image is retrieved in a fundamentally different way (see text).

images varies with the size of the imaging plate, ranging from about 5 lp/mm for 18 × 24 cm plates, to 2.5 lp/mm for the 35 × 43 cm size.

28.6.3 Advantages of CR

(1) Objective and subjective evaluations have shown that CR is capable of image quality comparable to that produced by conventional rare earth screen–film systems.

(2) CR is far more tolerant of over- or underexposure. The system compensates automatically for exposure variations so that images of optimum density are consistently produced (but see disadvantage (3) below).

(3) Significant reductions in exposure factors without loss of density have been reported with CR, but these may be accompanied by an increase in quantum noise.

(4) Computer processing of raw image data can provide an image of conventional appearance (looking like a 'normal' radiograph), or with contrast or sharpness enhancement.

(5) A CR system is compatible with most conventional X-ray units and can therefore be introduced without the need to replace existing equipment.

28.6.4 Disadvantages of CR

(1) High initial cost.

(2) Slower processing time than conventional screen– film systems. It takes about 4 minutes to produce a CR hard copy image, compared to 90 seconds for screen– film systems.

(3) Radiographers receive no direct feedback on the accuracy of their exposure selection because the resulting CR images are of consistent density regardless of the X-ray exposure used. This may lead to undesirable and undetected over-exposure of the patient.

28.7 Xeroradiography

Xeroradiography is an X-ray image-forming process based on xerography, an electrostatic document-copying system invented in 1937. It is not a process requiring any specialized X-ray equipment but is a method of X-ray image recording which is fundamentally different from the conventional photographic processes associated with the use of X-ray film. Its most common application has been for soft tissue radiography of the female breast (mammography).

28.7.1 Principles of xeroradiography

Xeroradiography is a completely dry, non-chemical process. At its heart is an electrically charged selenium-coated aluminium plate, which reacts to X-ray exposure by leaking the charge from exposed areas, while retaining the charge on unexposed areas. Fine powder, which is blown across the surface of the plate, adheres to the charged areas in amounts proportional to the quantity of charge present. The pattern formed by different concentrations of powder deposited on the plate is transferred and fused onto a plastic-coated paper receptor. The resulting xeroradiographs are quick to produce using automated machinery, and exhibit permanent, high-definition images with exceptional contrast characteristics. The selenium plates are reusable (Xerox, 1974/75).

28.7.2 Xeroradiographic image characteristics

Xeroradiographic images differ from conventional radiographic images in three important respects:

(1) Contrast – xeroradiographs exhibit high edge contrast due to a phenomenon known as **edge enhancement**. However, the overall contrast of xeroradiographs is low.
(2) Print image – xeroradiographic images are prints, whereas conventional radiographs are transparencies; thus, xeroradiographs are viewed by reflected rather than transmitted light. This is generally accepted to be a more convenient way of viewing images, since no special illuminator is required.
(3) Positive image – for mammography, the most common clinical application of xeroradiography, it was usual to produce **positive-mode** images in which the parts of the image receiving the greatest exposure have the lowest density. This is the reverse of the conventional radiograph, which is a negative-mode image.

We shall now consider the special contrast properties of xeroradiographs in more detail.

28.7.2.1 Edge contrast

On a xeroradiograph, the contrast at the boundaries between different structures is exaggerated by edge enhancement. The effect of this high edge contrast is to facilitate the perception of anatomical detail and thus is a valuable aid to radio-diagnosis. In mammography, it accentuates the boundaries of a mass and of microcalcifications. It is an important reason for undertaking xeroradiography.

Edge contrast is a result of the particular way that toner powder is distributed over the charged xeroradiographic plate during development. The abrupt change in electric charge at a boundary on the latent image is shown in Fig. 28.6. The electric field in the region above such a boundary is distorted by the charge

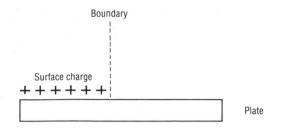

Fig. 28.6 Edge enhancement is caused by the effect on toner distribution of a sudden change in charge at a boundary in the xeroradiographic latent image.

difference, causing an excess of toner powder to accumulate on one side of the boundary during development, while a paucity of toner is created on the other side of the boundary (see Fig. 28.7). This toner pattern on the plate produces the characteristic edge enhancement which enables fine edge detail to be recorded on the xeroradiograph.

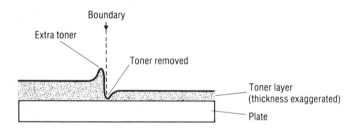

Fig. 28.7 Distribution of toner powder on the xeroradiographic plate at a boundary. Toner is removed from one side of the boundary but creates an excess on the other side thus amplifying the edge contrast in the image.

28.7.2.2   Overall contrast

The overall continuous contrast of the xeroradiographic image is low. This feature enables the nipple, the skin surface of the breast, and the thoracic wall to be visualized with a single mammographic exposure. In the lateral projection of the neck, the soft-tissue structures of the pharynx, larynx and trachea are demonstrated together with the cervical vertebrae (Fig. 28.8). Such great latitude is of benefit when imaging any region possessing an extreme range of tissue thickness or tissue type.

The low overall contrast is created because during development the amount of toner adhering to the plate over large areas is determined more by the density of the powder cloud than by the value of charge on each area. Thus, there is a tendency for the gross distribution of toner on the plate to be uniform. Abrupt charge differences are accentuated (by edge enhancement) but gradual charge differences are suppressed.

28.7.2.3   Xeroradiographic image unsharpness

The unsharpness of a xeroradiograph arises from three major sources:

(1) Geometric factors (see section 3.1.2.2).
(2) Movement factors (see section 16.1.3).

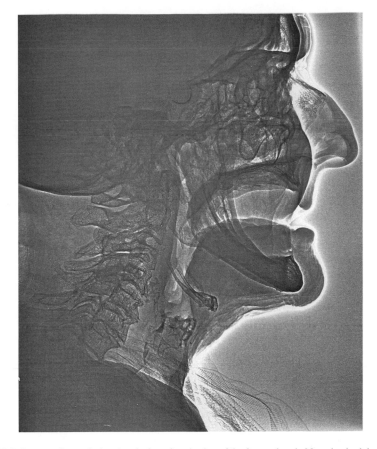

Fig. 28.8 A xeroradiograph showing the lateral projection of the face and neck. Note that both bony and soft tissue details are demonstrated. The image is in positive mood.

(3) Factors related to the inherent characteristics of the image recording process, in this case the xeroradiographic system.

Unsharpness intrinsic to the xeroradiograph occurs at the imaging stage and at the processing stage.

Imaging stage
The resolution of the latent image or charge pattern on the selenium plate is related to the thickness of the selenium layer because the charge patterns at different depths in the selenium are not necessarily identical and may not be exactly in register. The thickness of the selenium layer must therefore be limited to ensure minimum unsharpness. Predictably, however, the radiosensitivity of the plate depends on the thickness of the selenium layer. Thus, the actual coating thickness of 0.12 mm is a compromise between the conflicting demands of resolution and sensitivity.

Processing stage
Powder development may limit resolution due to:

(1) The size of the powder particles: in practice, individual toner particles are small enough not to create significant structure mottle, but clumping of particles could produce a visibly granular image.
(2) The electric charge acquired by the particles as they are aspirated into the developing chamber: good resolution is dependent on each particle carrying a high specific charge, a state which is achieved when a low powder concentration is used.

The intrinsic unsharpness characteristics of the xeroradiographic system are not within the immediate control of the radiographer but, in a well maintained and correctly operated system, intrinsic unsharpness should not be a dominant influence on overall image resolution.

28.7.2.4   Image transposition

Because of the way in which the powder image is transferred onto the final paper hard-copy, the xeroradiographic image is a mirror transposition of the subject. Since the image is a print rather than a transparency, the transposition cannot be corrected by viewing from the reverse side. It is therefore essential that the radiographer employs clearly identifiable anatomical markers.

28.7.2.5   Image artefacts

There are a number of artefacts peculiar to the xeroradiographic system. They include:

(1) Discharge artefacts – caused by abnormal electrical discharge occurring within the cassette.
(2) Image smear – commonly due to premature discharge of the cassette electrode via its charging clips.
(3) Ghosting – the retention on a plate of traces of a previous image, which then interfere with a subsequent image.
(4) Blemishes – isolated spots which may occur on the image due to faults in the selenium coating on the xeroradiographic plate.

28.7.3   *Applications*

Since its introduction as a diagnostic imaging technique, the xeroradiographic process has been used for a very wide range of diagnostic procedures. But it is generally agreed that xeroradiography made its most valuable contribution in the field of soft-tissue imaging, where edge enhancement enables images of superior quality to be produced. In particular, xeroradiography has been recognized as offering a number of advantages over conventional imaging for mammography. It is not necessary to employ very low tube kilovoltages (e.g. 20–30 kVp) for xeromammography because the effects of edge enhancement provide adequate contrast at higher voltages. Xeromammography can therefore be achieved without a specialized mammographic X-ray unit.

However, the development of high-speed, high-resolution, single-coated film–screen systems, together with the availability of dedicated mammography units, has enabled high-quality mammograms to be produced with less radiation dose than is possible with xeromammography. Consequently the provision of mammography as a mass screening service in the United Kingdom, following the recommendations of the Forrest Report, depends on conventional image recording rather than xeroradiographic techniques.

Xeroradiography is a most interesting high-quality imaging system which has played a restricted but, nevertheless, significant role in radiodiagnostic imaging.

In many of the imaging systems we have outlined a video signal is output which may be recorded directly on videotape or on a laser imager (see section 23.2), or the image may be displayed on the screen of a cathode ray tube and may be recorded photographically by a CRT camera, video imager or multiformatter (see section 23.4). We shall next describe the photographic materials which may be used to carry these hard-copy CRT images.

28.8 The photographic material

There is a range of material available on which hard-copy images can be recorded, but the materials fall into one of two broad categories: paper base material and film base material.

28.8.1 *Paper*

The attraction of recording images on paper-based material is that no special facilities are needed to view the image. The images are examined by reflected rather than transmitted light. However, there are problems inherent in the use of paper hard-copy. Reflected light images exhibit a greatly reduced tonal range compared with transparency images: in particular, it is not possible to produce a perfect black because there is always some light reflected or scattered from even the darkest part of the image surface. On the other hand, the dark parts of a transparency image can be totally opaque. The result is that contrast is reduced on a paper copy image and information is lost. This may be considered too heavy a price to pay for the extra convenience of viewing by reflected light. See also polaroid film (section 5.2.2.3) and dry silver images (section 23.5).

28.8.2 *Film*

Video imaging film is available in sheet form or in rolls. In both cases, the basic film construction is the same. The film is similar in many respects to the photo-fluorographic film described previously (section 5.2.2.2). The film has a single emulsion layer coated on a polyester base. An anti-curl layer containing anti-halation pigment is coated onto the reverse. This gives a medium-speed film offering high-resolution capabilities (well over 100 line pairs per millimetre). Sheet film is notched to enable the emulsion side to be identified easily.

The spectral sensitivity of the emulsion is matched to the emission characteristics of the CRT screen phosphors employed and is most commonly orthochromatic in its response.

28.8.2.1 Film contrast

Of the sensitometric properties of imaging film, the emulsion contrast is probably the most important. Imaging film is generally a high-contrast type with maximum gamma between 2.0 and 3.0 (Coleman & Cowen, 1987). It can be argued that the film contrast should be lower for ultrasound imaging than for the other modalities because with ultrasound, the image background on the CRT screen is dark and thus there is less scattering of light within the imaging camera. Scattered light would tend to fog the film and reduce the contrast of the final image. Ultrasound images suffer less reduction in contrast from this cause and therefore do not need as much contrast amplification during the image recording process. Hence, a lower-contrast emulsion is acceptable. It can also be argued that gamma camera images which are bistable (black and white with no grey tones) are best served by a high-contrast emulsion.

Notwithstanding these arguments, in practice it seems that if the controls of an imaging camera are correctly adjusted for each of the different image types that it handles, perfectly acceptable results can be obtained using just one type of film. Indeed, this has been common practice for many departments.

28.8.2.2 Processing

Imaging film is suitable for rapid machine processing and can often be processed successfully in one of the main departmental automatic processors. It is likely, however, that better results would be obtained if a processor dedicated to imaging film were to be used. In practice, such a processor would probably be considered a luxury.

We have now completed our discussion of how diagnostic images are formed and recorded, and the various characteristics they exhibit. In the final chapter we shall investigate how such images are perceived by the observer, and the influences that affect his interpretation of them.

Part 6
Perception and Interpretation of Images

Chapter 29
Visual Perception and Interpretation

Formation of the retinal image
Response of the retina
Interpretation of the perceived image
Receiver operating characteristics

Before studying this chapter the reader may wish to review a description of the eye, such as that provided in a standard textbook of human anatomy and physiology such as Williams *et al.*, 1989.

In previous chapters we have examined the methods available for producing optimum-quality diagnostic images and presenting them to an observer. It is our task in this final chapter to investigate how these images are perceived by the observer, and the influences that affect his interpretation of them. Over the past decade, it has become increasingly common for radiographers to mark radiographs, e.g. with a red dot, if they observe any abnormality (Berman *et al.*, 1985; Bowman, 1990). Such action is particularly helpful in casualty X-ray departments where there is no radiologist present, and where radiographs may be examined by quite junior and therefore inexperienced medical staff. In these cases, the radiographer indicates to the casualty officer the existence of an abnormal appearance without necessarily making a diagnosis. The radiographer may provide more detailed comments during a subsequent discussion with the casualty officer. In other areas, such as ultrasound, nominated radiographers may go further, and provide a written professional opinion on the images they have produced, including a suggested diagnosis. Such developments in the radiographer's role demand that the study of the perception and interpretation of diagnostic images be given a high priority in the education of radiographers.

The human visual system is highly complex and is still not fully understood. It consists of an optical focusing system, a delicately balanced guidance system and an ultrafine matrix of photoreceptors which convert light images into sequences of electrical impulses. These are monitored and interpreted by the brain and presented as visual images in our consciousness. We shall describe the process in three stages:

(1) The formation of an image on the retina of the eye.
(2) The response of the retina to the image and the factors influencing an observer's perception of the retinal image.
(3) The interpretation of the perceived image.

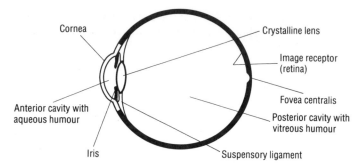

Fig. 29.1 The optical components in the human eye.

29.1   Formation of the retinal image

The eyeball houses a highly developed optical system which gathers light from the subject and focuses it on the photosensitive retina. Figure 29.1 shows the general arrangement of optical components in the human eye. The anterior cavity forms a positive (convergent) compound lens system of variable focal length. It also incorporates a variable-aperture iris diaphragm. Figure 29.2 shows that light passing through the lens system is refracted at four interfaces:

(1) Air to cornea;
(2) Cornea to aqueous humour;
(3) Aqueous humour to crystalline lens;
(4) Crystalline lens to vitreous humour.

The first interface exhibits the highest refractive index because of the great difference in density between air and the corneal tissue.

    We will now examine each feature of the optical system in detail.

29.1.1   *Cornea and aqueous humour*

Light from the subject enters the eye through the transparent convex **cornea** into

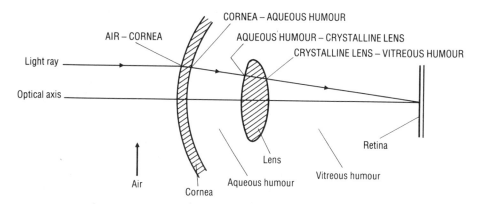

Fig. 29.2 Optical interfaces in the eye. Four interfaces are identified of which the first (air-cornea) produces the greatest refraction.

the aqueous humour. Most of the convergence of light required to focus the image on the retina takes place at this air–liquid interface. It has a fixed focal length of about 23 mm.

29.1.2   *Pupil and iris*

Light then passes through a circular opening (the **pupil**) in the pigmented, variable-aperture **iris**. The iris controls the amount of light entering the eye. At low light levels the pupil dilates, while in bright lighting the pupil constricts. Constriction also occurs when the eye focuses on near objects, thus improving depth of field and image definition (see section 20.2.5). When the pupil is dilated (about 8 mm diameter), 16 times more light is admitted than when it is contracted (about 2 mm diameter). But note that the eye can operate over a much greater brightness range than this, e.g. from starlight to full sunlight (an intensity range of about $100\,000\,000\,000{:}1$). It is therefore unlikely that control of image light intensity is the primary function of the iris (Gregory, 1976).

29.1.3   *Crystalline lens*

On leaving the pupil, light is transmitted through a transparent variable-focus biconvex lens. The function of this lens is to provide the fine adjustment of focus, known as **accommodation**, needed for the observer to focus on objects at different distances. For near vision, the lens becomes more convex, while for distant vision the convexity is reduced. For distant vision its focal length is ~ 60 mm. The focal length of the compound lens formed by the cornea and the crystalline lens is then ~ 17 mm. The radius of curvature of the anterior surface of the crystalline lens can vary between 6 and 12 mm (Lamb *et al.*, 1986), the change of shape being achieved by varying the tension on the suspensory ligament around the lens. With increasing age, the lens begins to lose its elasticity and the eye behaves more like a rigid, fixed-focus lens. Its ability to accommodate to different distances is then reduced and spectacles may become necessary for near vision.

29.1.4   *Vitreous humour*

Convergent light rays from the lens are finally transmitted through the transparent jelly-like vitreous humour before being focused as a miniature, inverted, real image on the retina.

29.1.5   *Quality of the retinal image*

The image formed by the lens system of the eye suffers many of the limitations and aberrations described in Chapter 20. Optimum image definition is achieved on the principal axis but deteriorates rapidly towards the peripheral field. The relative aperture or f number of the eye ranges from about $f0.8$ (pupil constricted) to $f0.2$ (pupil dilated) and, as with other lens systems, stopping down the aperture (constricting the pupil) improves image definition. The image also suffers chromatic aberration, which limits definition even in the central field.

The retinal image is both inverted and reduced in size compared with the subject, e.g. a 43×35 cm radiograph viewed from a distance of 1 m produces an image of only about 7×6 mm in size. It is a sobering thought that our visual appreciation of the external world is gained from so tiny an image.

29.1.6   Eye movements

A finely balanced muscular guidance system maintains the eyes in continuous movement (Gregory, 1976):

(1) When the eyes are searching for and trying to locate an object, they move in a series of small rapid jerks called **saccades**.
(2) When the eyes eventually 'lock on' to their target, they follow its movements with a smooth action.
(3) When concentrating on a fixed object they display a high-frequency low-amplitude tremor (see section 29.2.2.1).

Eye movements are also required to permit binocular vision (section 27.2), in which both eyes must be directed towards an object. With a near object the gaze must be convergent, while for distant objects the eyes are directed parallel to each other. The degree of convergence of the gaze, sensed by proprioceptors in the controlling muscles, conveys depth information to the brain.

We shall now outline the main features of the retina and the manner in which it responds to the patterns of light focused upon it.

29.2   Response of the retina

Figure 29.3 shows the main structures forming the retina, the light-sensitive layer in the posterior cavity of the eyeball. The retina is a specialized extension of the surface of the brain which has become sensitive to light. For reasons related to the evolutionary development of the eye, the retina is 'inside out' in the sense that light must travel through layers of blood vessels, nerve fibres and supporting cells before it reaches the photosensitive receptors (rods and cones) which lie at the *back* of the retina. Exposure to visible light causes the photoreceptors to generate nerve impulses, which travel to the inner surface of the retina and are then conducted away along fibres of the optic nerve. Also, lateral cross-connections are present between adjacent photoreceptors, enabling local processing of visual signals to be carried out.

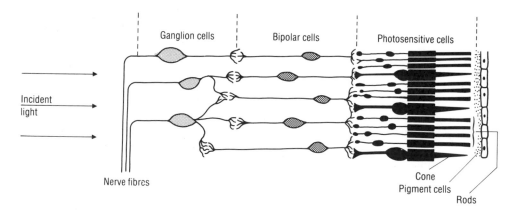

Fig. 29.3 The retina of the eye. This magnified section through the retina shows the relationship between its main structures. The centre of the eyeball is to the left. Incident light approaches from the left (see text).

29.2.1 Rods and cones

The light-sensitive part of the retina is formed from a mosaic of photoreceptors. Under the microscope, two distinct types of receptor are seen, known as rods and cones.

29.2.1.1 Rod vision

The 100 million or so rods are stimulated by low levels of illumination. Rods have a single peak of sensitivity at a light wavelength of about 500 nm (blue–green) (Fig. 29.4). They provide the colourless grey tones of **scotopic** vision, such as is experienced in moonlight. Rods are extremely light-sensitive, responding to as few as half a dozen photons of light (Chesters, 1982). Rods lose their sensitivity and cease to respond in bright light. The screen phosphors once used for direct (naked eye) fluoroscopy were chosen to provide a spectral emission matching the spectral response of rods because the fluoroscopic image brightness was only sufficient to stimulate scotopic vision.

29.2.1.2 Cone vision

The 7 million or so cones are responsible for colour vision and function in bright light or daylight conditions producing **photopic** vision.

Three kinds of cone receptors are normally present, each having a different spectral response. The peaks of the cone responses correspond to wavelengths of 445 nm (blue), 535 nm (green) and 570 nm (yellow), but there is considerable overlap between the responses of the three types of cone (Fig. 29.5) and the eye is sensitive to light over a range of about 400 nm (violet) to 700 nm (red). Full colour vision is achieved by comparing the relative responses of the blue-, green- and yellow-sensitive cones. Colour vision is so sensitive it can discriminate between wavelengths only 3 nm apart (Lamb *et al.*, 1986). Cones do not respond at all in dim light.

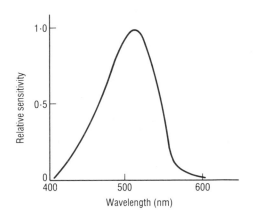

Fig. 29.4 Spectral sensitivity of rod photoreceptors. Maximum sensitivity occurs at just over 500 nm (blue–green).

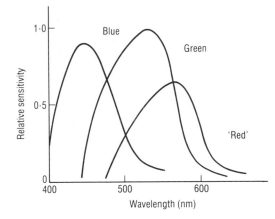

Fig. 29.5 Spectral sensitivity of cone photoreceptors. The three types of cone have peak sensitivities at 445 nm (blue), 535 nm (green) and 570 nm (yellow). The latter cones are commonly known as 'red' sensitive.

29.2.2   Fovea centralis

The fovea is the central area of the retina, $\sim 6\,\text{mm}$ diameter, which provides the best colour vision and the greatest **visual acuity** (visual acuity describes the appreciation of fine detail in a visual image). The fovea is the region most densely packed with cone photoreceptors, some of which are only $\sim 1\,\mu\text{m}$ across (Gregory, 1976). When closely examining an object, the eyes are directed so that the image of the object falls on the fovea of each eye.

29.2.2.1   Adaptation

The sensitivity of cones varies to match the prevailing light conditions, e.g. sensitivity is reduced in bright sunlight compared with indoor artificial lighting. However, the process of adjustment or **adaptation** may take a short time to complete. Additionally, the adjustment is based on the *average* intensity of light over the image field. Thus, a small radiograph displayed on an unmasked X-ray illuminator presents the eye with difficult viewing conditions (section 14.5.2). The glare from unshielded areas of the illuminator upsets the process of adaptation and the sensitivity of the cones is reduced below the level necessary for optimum appreciation of the radiograph. The result is a radiograph which appears to be overexposed and of reduced contrast.

There is a second consequence of adaptation. If an image is held fixed in relation to the retina, vision fades after a few seconds because the receptors adapt to the light incident upon them and cease to signal to the brain the presence of the image. The saccadic movements of the eye (section 29.1.6) prevent such visual 'fatigue' by sweeping the image over the receptors so that their level of adaptation is continually being adjusted.

29.2.3   Extrafoveal retina

Away from the fovea centralis there are fewer cones, but the concentration of rods increases. Relative to the fovea, the extrafoveal region is thus an area of reduced visual acuity but increased sensitivity, particularly at low light levels. In bright light conditions, the light-absorbing pigment ('visual purple') essential to the action of the rod receptors is bleached, rendering the rods inoperative. In darkness, the pigment slowly regenerates and the sensitivity of the rods gradually returns, thus restoring scotopic vision. This process of **dark adaptation** may take up to half an hour to complete. With practice, the process appears to be accelerated; thus, an experienced darkroom technician adapts rapidly on entering the darkroom while an occasional visitor is incapable of seeing anything for several minutes, although this phenomenon may be explained partly by the technician's greater familiarity with the surroundings. Because rod receptors are insensitive to red light, the wearing of red-tinted goggles allows the process of dark adaptation to proceed in normal lighting and was a practice commonly adopted by radiologists prior to the start of a direct fluoroscopy screening session.

A few millimetres medial to and below the fovea is the optic papilla, on which nerve fibres from all parts of the retina converge to form the optic nerve. Retinal blood vessels also enter and leave the eye at this point. The optic papilla is an area devoid of photoreceptors and is thus insensitive to light. It is commonly known as the **blind spot**.

29.2.4 *Edge enhancement*

Edge enhancement is an important characteristic of the response of the eye, which enables the boundaries between adjacent parts of an image to be detected with great sensitivity. The existence of the lateral cross-connections between neighbouring photoreceptors in the retina permits immediate comparisons to be made between the brightness of adjacent parts of the image. It appears that it is primarily information about brightness differences or **edge contrast** which is signalled to the brain. The brain gives priority to such contrast information, often at the expense of perception of constant densities. A commonly experienced consequence of this is the illusion created when viewing a step-wedge image such as that shown in Fig. 29.6. Even though objective measurements show that density is uniform across each individual step, in the region near a boundary between adjacent steps an observer's subjective assessment of the image suggests that density is not uniform. On the lighter side of the boundary, density appears to reduce close to the boundary, while on the darker side density appears to increase (see Fig. 29.7). This phenomenon is known as the **Mach effect** and results in enhancement of edge contrast and the ability of an observer to detect such visual boundaries is increased

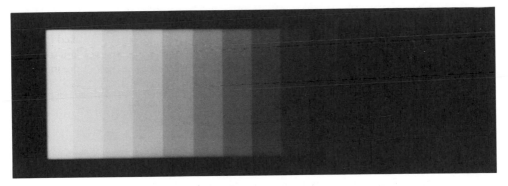

Fig. 29.6 The Mach effect. The density of the steps appears to vary as a step boundary is approached, giving an effect of edge enhancement. Objective measurements show the effect to be illusory.

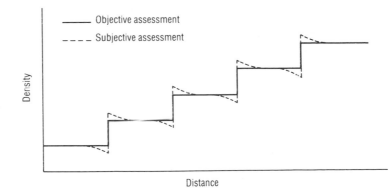

Fig. 29.7 The Mach effect. The continuous line is a trace of density across a step wedge image, as measured with a densitometer. The broken line is a trace of the subjective assessment of density showing exaggerated contrast at each density boundary.

(Chesters, 1982). Note that the edge enhancement exhibited by computer processed and xeroradiographic images is a *real* effect which can be confirmed by objective measurement of the image, while the Mach effect in Fig. 29.6 is a result of the behaviour of the human visual system.

29.2.5   *Visual noise*

Our perception of visual images depends ultimately on the neural signals received by the visual cortex of the brain. In a perfect system, under conditions of total darkness, the retina would be completely inactive and no signals would be transmitted to the brain. In practice, the retina and optic nerve are never entirely free of activity and there is always some residual random electrical activity (known as **dark current**) transmitted to the brain (Chesters, 1982). Additionally, at low light levels, random variations in the number of incident light photons detected by the retina may introduce a random element due to **quantum noise** in the visual signal generated.

The combined effects of spurious neural activity and quantum noise produce **visual noise**. Under good viewing conditions, the amplitude of such noise is negligible compared with the true visual signal: the signal-to-noise ratio (SNR) is high. In poor illumination, the signal and noise may be of similar orders of magnitude and the SNR is low. The brain is able partly to overcome this problem by integrating the visual signals over a longer period of time, thus visual response time is longer when light levels are low.

29.2.6   *Resolution*

The theoretical limit to the resolution of the visual system is determined by a number of factors.

Resolution of the original diagnostic image (e.g. the radiograph or fluoroscopic image)
We have described the factors such as unsharpness, contrast and noise, which contribute to the quality of these images, earlier in the book.

Viewing conditions
We described viewing of radiographs in Chapter 14, fluorographs in Chapter 21 and television images in Chapter 22. Important influencing factors include:

(1) Ambient light level;
(2) Glare;
(3) Viewing distance.

The effects of glare and excessive ambient light levels cause a loss of image contrast as perceived by the observer. The term **subjective contrast** is often used to describe the assessment of perceived image contrast in order to differentiate it from **objective** image contrast as measured directly from the radiograph or television screen. Such loss of contrast, whether objective or subjective, results in reduced image resolution.

For each diagnostic image there is an optimum distance from which it should be viewed. If the image is observed from too short a distance (or with too great a degree of magnification), image noise becomes intrusive, e.g. structure mottle on a radiograph or raster pattern on a television screen. Observation from too great a distance causes the retinal image to be reduced in size to such an extent that resolution is limited by the characteristics of the retina itself (see below). In practice, an experienced radiographer or radiologist adjusts viewing distance according to the type and size of image under investigation in order to provide maximum perception of anatomical detail.

It has been claimed by Jenkins (1980) that at a viewing distance of 40 cm no difference can be detected between the resolution of a radiograph produced using a high-resolution intensifying screen system and one produced using direct-exposure X-ray film, but differences in image quality may well become apparent on closer examination.

It should be noted that when observing images for details near the limits of resolution great care should be taken since the brain may identify recognizable patterns in what are in reality random features of the image (Gregory, 1980). We shall refer to the problem of pseudo-pattern recognition later in this chapter (section 29.3.5).

Resolving power of the optical system of the eye

As we saw in section 29.1.5, the optical focusing system of the eye is not perfect. It suffers many of the defects or aberrations exhibited by the lens systems described in Chapter 20. Optimum resolution is achieved close to the principal optical axis of the eye and under conditions in which the pupil is constricted. Additionally, individuals may suffer from one or more forms of impaired vision e.g. myopia (short-sight), hypermetropia (long-sight) or astigmatism. The use of artificial aids, such as spectacles or contact lenses, can often restore the sight to a satisfactory level of performance. Because of the nature of their work, it is vital that the vision of radiographers and radiologists is as near perfect as possible. Indeed, it has been suggested that tests of visual acuity and resolution should form part of the selection procedure for prospective radiographers (Adrian-Harris, 1979).

Structure of the retina

The rod vision operating under conditions of low light intensity provides very coarse image resolution because rods act in relatively large groups. Thus, high-resolution images were not possible in conditions such as those which prevailed during direct fluoroscopy.

Cone vision offers higher resolution, optimum results being achieved in the fovea centralis where cone photoreceptors are most densely packed. Thus, adequate image brightness is necessary to obtain maximum resolution. Image intensification enables cone vision to be employed during screening and hence produces higher-resolution images than direct fluoroscopy.

The spacing of the cones sets a theoretical limit to image resolution: under optimum conditions, detail forming a retinal image $< 2\,\mu m$ across can be distinguished (Lamb *et al.*, 1986). This represents a structure $\sim 50\,\mu m$ (0.05 mm) across, viewed from a distance of 40 cm. Such a level of resolution falls only slightly below the theoretical maximum and is the origin of the widely quoted statement that an unsharpness of less than about 0.1 mm on a radiograph is not normally visible to the unaided eye (see section 2.1.1.3).

29.2.7 Visual pathways

The neural signals leaving the retina are conveyed along the million or so nerve fibres of the optic nerve to the lateral geniculate nucleus of the thalamus and thence to the higher visual centre or **visual cortex** of the occipital lobe of the brain.

Signals from the left half of each retina (carrying data about the *right* half of the visual field due to the inversion and transposition of the retinal image) pass to the left visual cortex via the left lateral geniculate nucleus. Those from the right half of each retina (carrying data about the *left* half of the visual field) pass to the right visual cortex via the right geniculate nucleus (Fig. 29.8).

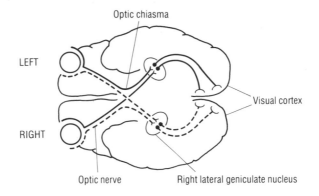

Fig. 29.8 Visual pathways. Neural signals from the right side of each retina (shown as broken line) pass through the right lateral geniculate nucleus to the right visual cortex. (See text.)

29.2.8 *Visual data processing*

Processing or modification of visual information occurs at three locations on the visual pathway described above.

(1) Retina and optic nerve
As we noted in section 29.2.4, local cross-connections between nerve fibres in the retina enable initial modification of the visual signals to be made. Thus, each single optic nerve fibre receives information from a small, circular area of retina rather than from a single photoreceptor. The area may be as small as 0.1 mm in diameter in the fovea but up to 2 mm in diameter at the periphery of the visual field (Lamb *et al.*, 1986). This arrangement produces an effect known as **lateral inhibition**, which suppresses signals due to diffuse, general illumination of the retina while transmitting signals due to contrasts in illumination.

(2) Lateral geniculate nucleus
Further lateral inhibition occurs here, such that the neural signals eventually received by the brain are so modified that the higher visual centres are concerned more with boundaries between different parts of the image than with general levels of illumination.

(3) Visual cortex
Cortical cells are classified according to the type of stimulus to which they respond (Hubel & Wiesel, 1968), e.g.:

(1) **Simple** cells are sensitive to the spatial orientation of the stimuli, e.g. one cell may respond strongly to a vertical stimulus but give no response to a horizontal stimulus. Thus, such cells act as edge detectors.
(2) **Complex** cells are also orientation-sensitive and respond best to moving edges.

(3) **Hypercomplex** cells detect moving stimuli of a particular orientation and also respond to particular shapes, such as strips, corners or angles.

It is the existence of such highly specialized receptors which enables the visual system to detect complex logical patterns in the signals it receives. The analysis of incoming visual signals into combinations of recognizable patterns is fundamental to the process of visual perception and conscious recognition of the significance of what we see.

We shall now examine aspects of how we interpret the meaning of diagnostic images and the factors which influence the accuracy of our interpretation.

29.3 Interpretation of the perceived image

Interpretation of an image is largely a matter of searching the image for familiar identifiable patterns or combinations of patterns (Wackenheim, 1987). The success (or failure) of this process depends on a number of factors which we shall describe below.

29.3.1 *Knowledge*

To extract meaning from a radiographic image requires a knowledge of radiographic anatomy and pathology. We need to be familiar with the normal and abnormal appearances of the structures under investigation. We need to be aware of the spatial relationships between structures and their relative sizes and shapes. We need to know something about their different X-ray attenuating properties. In other words, we need a bank of experience which we can call on to compare with the patterns on the diagnostic image before us.

Such knowledge must be learnt and committed to memory both formally, as part of an organized programme of training, and informally, as a consequence of natural inquisitiveness and observation. Most radiographers will recall times, early in their training, when they completely overlooked much of the subtle (and not so subtle!) appearances on a radiograph because their store of experience was inadequate.

Radiology atlases and radiograph collections act as useful additional 'external' memory banks, particularly for radiographic appearances that are rarely encountered.

Adherence to standardized, widely accepted radiographic projections facilitates diagnostic interpretation by limiting the variety of different appearances that the observer must memorize.

29.3.2 *Understanding*

Acquiring an understanding of normal and pathological processes often enables the significance of an unfamiliar appearance on a diagnostic image to be identified. Thus, interpretation is not *only* a matter of recalling the appropriate information from memory or from a book. A process of extrapolation from the familiar to the unfamiliar is sometimes involved.

29.3.3 *Practice*

Reading diagnostic images is a skill which requires constant practice to maintain proficiency. Radiographers may recall experiencing some difficulty in checking radiographs for a short while after a prolonged absence from work, e.g. due to annual leave or illness.

29.3.4   *Context*

In order to gain maximum information from a diagnostic image it is necessary to have access to the clinical background and context in which the image was produced. On a chest radiograph, an image artefact produced by a barium sulphate stain on a patient's gown is less likely to be misinterpreted as a pathological lung lesion if the observer is aware that the patient had just undergone a barium meal.

It is also true, however, that knowledge of the clinical history of a patient may occasionally hinder the process of diagnosis. The provisional diagnosis indicated on the radiological request form may distract the observer to such an extent that the true diagnosis is overlooked. It is often the case that we see what we *want* to see and are blind to the unexpected. To avoid this danger it may be advisable to make an initial unbiased examination of the image *before* reading the clinical details. Following a systematic and well practised visual search pattern covering the whole of the image also helps to ensure that no aspect of the image is overlooked.

29.3.5   *Optical illusion*

Human visual perception is prone to error and ambiguity. There are many well-known examples of apparently simple images which are open to quite different interpretation: the ellipse shown in Fig. 29.9 could represent a side view of an elliptical object, or it could represent an oblique and therefore foreshortened view of a circular disc. Further information is required before an unequivocal judgement can be made. Equally, many radiographic image features are open to various interpretations.

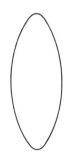

Fig. 29.9 An ambiguous image. The oval shape illustrated could be an elliptical object viewed from the side, or a circular object viewed obliquely. Extra information is needed to permit an unambiguous interpretation.

The pseudo-patterns that are sometimes detected in featureless regions of an image may produce a quite convincing appearance of a pathological lesion. On examining the lung fields on a normal chest radiograph, student radiographers are often convinced that they can see pathologically significant outlines where none exist.

It is thus vital that the observer is conscious of the dangers inherent in extra-polating two-dimensional image representations into three-dimensional solid structures, and of the tendency of the brain to create false visual patterns from totally unconnected visual information.

29.3.6   *Concentration*

Interpretation of diagnostic images requires concentration on the part of the observer. Physical discomfort due to poor ventilation, excessive temperature or humidity, distractions due to constant interruption or even anxieties caused by domestic or personal problems serve to upset concentration and may result in reduced efficiency and diagnostic accuracy. Pressures due to fatigue, poor health, overwork or shortage of time create similar results. It is too often the case that while high priority is given to the production of high-quality diagnostic images, relatively little thought is given to the provision of optimum conditions for the observer of the image. Thus, a proportion of the information in the image is wasted and the accuracy of diagnosis may be reduced.

29.4   Receiver operating characteristics (ROC)

It is possible to devise tests to evaluate the *overall* performance of an imaging system, including both the *objective* aspects of the system (e.g. its physical char-acteristics) and the *subjective* aspects of the system (e.g. the perceptual ability of the

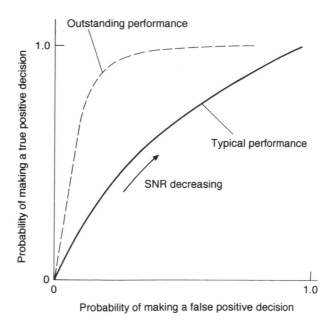

Fig. 29.10 Receiver operating characteristic (ROC) curve. The solid line represents the performance of a typical imaging system and observer, where the probability of making a correct judgement gradually reduces as the signal-to-noise ratio (SNR) reduces. The broken line illustrates the behaviour of an outstandingly good system, where the probability of making a correct judgement is higher and is maintained even when the SNR reduces.

observer). The tests are based on the detection in an image, of details (signals) which are only just above noise level; i.e. where the SNR is very low (Workman & Cowen, 1994). The results of such tests may be presented as a **receiver operating characteristic** (ROC).

In its simplest form, the ROC is obtained by forcing the observer to decide, for each of a series of images, whether or not a detail (signal) is present (see Chesters, 1982 and Gunn, 1994). There are four possible outcomes to each decision:

(1) **True positive** – if there *was* a signal, and it *was* detected.
(2) **True negative** – if there was *no* signal, and *none* was detected.
(3) **False negative** – if there *was* a signal, but it was *not* detected.
(4) **False positive** – if there was *no* signal, but one *appeared to be detected.*

The ROC curve (Fig. 29.10) shows the changing relationship between the likelihood of the observer making a true positive decision, and the likelihood of his making a false positive decision, as the signals get closer and closer to noise level.

ROC techniques have been applied in diagnostic imaging, and may help, for example, to determine which imaging system best suits a particular radiologist. ROCs also confirm that the perceptual performance of an observer may vary from moment to moment and is affected by external factors such as those described in section 29.3.6.

In this final chapter we have outlined some important influences on the way in which we perceive and interpret diagnostic images. The study of visual perception in diagnostic imaging is a fascinating and rapidly developing branch of science. There is much still to be discovered. We hope that the reader will continue to take an interest in the subject and actively participate in its further advancement.

References

Adrian-Harris D. (1979) Visual perception in radiography. *Radiography*, **XLV**, 237.

Aichinger H., Staudt F. & Kuhn H. (1992) Multiline grids for imaging in diagnostic radiology – a physical and clinical assessment. *Electromedica*, **60** (3/92), 74–81.

Ball J.L. & Moore A.D. (1986) *Essential Physics for Radiographers*. Blackwell Science Ltd, Oxford.

Berman L., de Lacey G., Twomey B., Welch T. & Eban R. (1985) Reducing errors in the accident and emergency department: a simple method using radiographers. *British Medical Journal*, **290**, 421–2.

Bowman S. (1990) *An investigation into abnormality identification in casualty radiographs – the 'red dot' system*. HDCR thesis, College of Radiographers.

Bramble J.M. & Templeton A.W. (1987) The importance of magnification radiology in the modern diagnostic imaging department. *Electromedica*, **55** (3/87), 91–4.

Breant C.M., Taira R.K. & Huang H.K. (1994) Interfacing aspects between the Picture Archiving Communications Systems, Radiology Information Systems, and Hospital Information Systems. *Journal of Digital Imaging*, **6** (2), 88.

Bushong S.C. (1988) *Magnetic Resonance Imaging – Physical and Biological Principles*. Mosby, St Louis.

Carter P.H. (ed.) (1994) *Chesneys' Equipment for Student Radiographers*. Blackwell Science Ltd, Oxford.

Chesney D.N. & Chesney M.O. (1981) *Radiographic Imaging*. Blackwell Scientific Publications, Oxford.

Chesters M.S. (1982) Perception and evaluation of images. In *Scientific Basis of Medical Imaging* (ed. P.N.T. Wells). Churchill Livingstone, Edinburgh.

Clark K.C. (1956) *Positioning in Radiography*. Heinemann, London.

Coleman N.J. & Cowen A.R. (1987) *A comparative assessment of video imaging films commercially available in the U.K.*, Report No. STD/87/20, Supplies Technology Division, NHS Procurement Directorate. HMSO, London.

Cowen A.R. & Coleman N.J. (1986) *A physical evaluation of the imaging performance of four different types of video imaging camera*, (FAXIL Assessment Report), STB/86/29. HMSO, London.

Cowen A.R., Coleman N.J., Workman A. & Maycock S.J. (1990) *The imaging sharpness of mammographic screen–film systems*, (Medical Devices Directorate Evaluation Report), STD/89/17. HMSO, London.

Eastman Kodak (undated) *Geometry of Image Formation*, Image Insight Workbook No. 2. Eastman Kodak Company, New York.

England N., Milward C. & Barratt P. (1990) *Physics in Perspective*. Hodder and Stoughton, London.

Evans D.H. (1988) Doppler ultrasound. In *Practical Ultrasound*, (ed. R.A. Lerski). IRL Press, Oxford.

Evans G. (1991) *An Evaluation of High Kilovoltage Chest Radiography*. HDCR thesis, College of Radiographers.

Evans J.A. (1988) Pulse-echo ultrasound. In *Practical Ultrasound*, (ed. R.A. Lerski). IRL Press, Oxford.

Forster E. (1985) *Equipment for Diagnostic Radiography*. MTP Press, Lancaster.

Fuji (1983) *Fundamentals of Sensitized Materials for Radiography*, (Fuji Film Technical Handbook). Fuji Photo Film Co Ltd, Tokyo.

Gregory R.L. (1976) *Eye and Brain – the Psychology of Seeing*. World University Library, London.

Gregory R.L. (1980) *The Intelligent Eye*. Weidenfeld and Nicolson, London.

Gunn C. (1994) *Roberts & Smith – Radiographic Imaging – A Practical Approach*. Churchill Livingstone, Edinburgh.

Harris J. (1969) Stereoradiography – some physiological, historical and practical considerations. In *Technical Papers on Radiography*. 3M, London.

Hay G.A. (1982) Traditional X-ray imaging. In *Scientific Basis of Medical Imaging*, (ed. P.N.T. Wells). Churchill Livingstone, Edinburgh.

HBN6 (1985) *Radiodiagnostic Department*. Health Building Note 6, DHSS & Welsh Office. HMSO, London.

Holwill M.E. & Silvester N.R. (1973) *Introduction to Biological Physics*. Wiley, London.

Horder A. (ed.) (1958) *The Ilford Manual of Photography*. Ilford Ltd, Ilford.

HPA (1977) *The Physics of Radiodiagnosis*. Hospital Physicists' Association, London.

HSE (1988) *COSHH Assessments*. Health and Safety Executive Document. HMSO, London.

HSE (1991) *Occupational Exposure Limits*, Health and Safety Executive Document, EH40/91. HMSO, London.

HSE (1992) *Glutaraldehyde and you* (information leaflet). Health and Safety Executive, London.

Hubel D.H. & Wiesel T.N. (1968) Receptive fields and functional architecture of monkey striate cortex. *Journal of Physiology*, **195**, 215–43.

Hufton A.P. & Russell J.G.B. (1986) The use of carbon fibre material in table tops, cassette fronts and grid covers: magnitude of possible dose reduction. *British Journal of Radiology*, **59** (698), 157–63.

Imhof K. (1989) The three-dimensional display of CT images: methods and capabilities. *Electromedica*, **57** (4/89), 154–9.

Jackson F.I. (1964) The air-gap technique: and an improvement by anteroposterior positioning for chest roentgenography. *American Journal of Radiology*, September, 688–91.

Jenkins D. (1980) *Radiographic Photography and Imaging Processes*. MTP Press, Lancaster.

Jenkins F.A. & White H.E. (1957) *Fundamentals of Optics*. McGraw-Hill, New York.

John D.H.O. (1967) *Radiographic Processing in Medicine and Industry*. Focal Press, London.

Kodak (1968) *Fundamentals of Radiographic Photography*. Kodak Ltd, London.

Kodak (1980) X-ray recording materials. In *Fundamentals of Radiographic Photography*, Vol. II. Kodak Ltd, Hemel Hempstead.

Kodak (1981) Image quality control. In *Fundamentals of Radiographic Photography*, Vol. I. Kodak Ltd, Hemel Hempstead.

Kodak (1982) Radiographic quality. In *Fundamentals of Radiographic Photography*, Vol. III. Kodak Ltd, Hemel Hempstead.

Kodak (1993) *Glutaraldehyde and you...*, Kodak Health Sciences Division information leaflet. Kodak Ltd, Hemel Hempstead.

Kreel L. (1981) *Clark's Positioning in Radiography*, Vol. 2. Heinemann Medical Books, London.

Lamb J.F., Ingram C.G., Johnston I.A. & Pitman R.M. (1986) *Essentials of Physiology*. Blackwell Scientific Publications, Oxford.

Liardet M. (1994) Seeing is believing. *Personal Computer World*, December, 586–91.

Longmore T.A. (1955) *Medical Photography – Radiographic and Clinical*. Focal Press, London.

M & B (1976) *Students' Manual to the Processing of Radiographic Films*. May & Baker Technical Services (Photographic), Dagenham.

MacAdam D.L. (1942) Visual sensitivities to color differences in daylight. *Journal of Optical Society of America*, **32**, 247–74.

Manton D.J., Roebuck E.J. & Fordham G.L. (1988) *Building and Extending a Radiology Department*. Royal Society of Medicine Services, London.

MDD (1994) *The testing of X-ray image intensifier–television systems*. (Medical Devices

Directorate Evaluation Report), MDD/94/07. HMSO, London.

NRPB (1988) *Guidance Notes for the Protection of Persons against Ionising Radiations arising from Medical and Dental Use.* HMSO, London.

Photosol (undated) *Fumes from X-ray chemistry*, (technical leaflet). Photosol Ltd.

Pizzutiello R.J. & Cullinan J.E. (eds) (1993) *Introduction to Medical Radiographic Imaging.* Eastman Kodak Company, New York.

Plummer D.T. (1989) *Biochemistry – the Chemistry of Life.* McGraw-Hill, London.

Roberts D.P. & Smith N.L. (1988) *Radiographic Imaging – A Practical Approach.* Churchill Livingstone, Edinburgh.

Rossman K. (1969) Point spread function, line spread function and modulation function. Tools for the study of imaging systems. *Radiology*, **93**, 257.

Sharp P.F. (1989) The gamma camera. In *Practical Nuclear Medicine* (eds P.F. Sharp, H.G. Gemmel & F.W. Smith). IRL Press, Oxford.

Siemens (1986) *Megalix 125/30/82C(G)*, (technical data leaflet). Siemens Medical Engineering Group, Erlangen.

Society of Radiographers (1991) *Preventing the Darkroom Disease – Health Effects of Toxic Fumes produced in X-ray Film Processing.* Society of Radiographers, London.

STD (1987) *Assessment of a Siemens Siregraph D remote control fluoroscopy/radiography package.* Report no. STD/87/33, Supplies Technology Division, NHS Procurement Directorate. HMSO, London.

Stockley S.M. (1986) *A Manual of Radiographic Equipment.* Churchill Livingstone, Edinburgh.

Strickland N.H. (1994) Practical problems when implementing a hospital-wide PACS. *Imaging*, **6**, 121.

Sykes J.B. (ed.) (1987) *The Concise Oxford Dictionary of Current English.* Oxford University Press, Oxford.

Todd K. (1951) More accurate use of the modified Sweet's eye localiser. *Radiography*, **XXIII** (267), 72–3.

Todd-Prokropek A. (1994) Communicating and archiving digital images in medicine. *Imaging*, **6**, 113.

Wackenheim A. (1987) Image perception and image processing. *Electromedica*, **55** (4/87), 116–21.

Wilks R. (1987) *Principles of Radiological Physics.* Churchill Livingstone, Edinburgh.

Williams P.L., Warwick R., Dyson M. & Bannister L.H. (eds) (1989) *Gray's Anatomy.* Churchill Livingstone, Edinburgh.

Workman A. & Cowen A.R. (1992) *A physical evaluation of computed radiography*, (Medical Devices Directorate Report), MDD/92/36. HMSO, London.

Workman A. & Cowen A.R. (1994) *Tutorial on the image quality characteristics of radiographic screen–film systems and their measurement*, (Medical Devices Directorate Evaluation Report), MDD/94/34. HMSO, London.

Xerox (1974/75) *Technical Applications Bulletin*, Nos 1–3. Xerox Corporation, Pasadena.

Index